CREATING SMART HEALTHCARE WITH BLOCKCHAIN AND ADVANCED DIGITAL TECHNOLOGY

CREATING SMART HEALTHCARE WITH BLOCKCHAIN AND ADVANCED DIGITAL TECHNOLOGY

Rishabha Malviya, PhD
Sonali Sundram, MPharm
Editors

APPLE ACADEMIC PRESS

First edition published 2025

Apple Academic Press Inc.
1265 Goldenrod Circle, NE,
Palm Bay, FL 32905 USA

760 Laurentian Drive, Unit 19,
Burlington, ON L7N 0A4, CANADA

CRC Press
2385 NW Executive Center Drive,
Suite 320, Boca Raton FL 33431

4 Park Square, Milton Park,
Abingdon, Oxon, OX14 4RN UK

Library and Archives Canada Cataloguing in Publication

CIP data on file with Canada Library and Archives

Library of Congress Cataloging-in-Publication Data

CIP data on file with US Library of Congress

ISBN: 978-1-77491-590-5 (hbk)
ISBN: 978-1-77491-591-2 (pbk)
ISBN: 978-1-00345-396-3 (ebk)

Dedication

Dear Healthcare Professionals,
We are dedicating this book to you. Our love for the profession shall live forever.
This book is also dedicated to the friendship of the editors.
We worked together and edited a fruitful book.

About the Editors

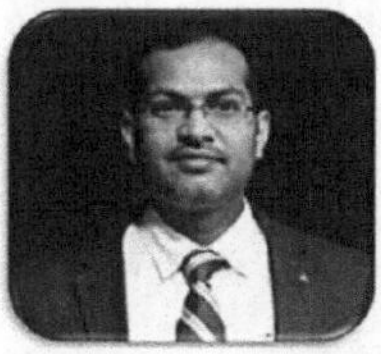

Rishabha Malviya, PhD
Associate Professor, Department of Pharmacy, School of Medical and Allied Sciences, Galgotias University, Greater Noida, Uttar Pradesh, India

Rishabha Malviya, PhD, completed a BPharm from Uttar Pradesh Technical University and an MPharm (Pharmaceutics) from Gautam Buddha Technical University, Lucknow, Uttar Pradesh, India. His PhD (Pharmacy) work was in novel formulation development techniques. He has 13 years of research experience and has been working as an Associate Professor in the Department of Pharmacy, School of Medical and Allied Sciences at Galgotias University for the past 11 years. His areas of interest include formulation optimization, nano formulation, targeted drug delivery, localized drug delivery, and characterization of natural polymers as pharmaceutical excipients. He has authored more than 150 research/review papers for national/international journals of repute. He has 51 patents (12 granted, 38 published, 1 filed) and publications in reputed national and international journals with more than 300 cumulative impact factors. He has also received an Outstanding Reviewer Award from Elsevier. He has authored and/or edited 70 books (Wiley, Springer Nature, De Gruyter, CRC Press/Taylor and Francis, River Publisher, Apple Academic Press, Nova Science Publishers, and OMICS International) and authored 125 book chapters. His name has been included in the world's top 2% scientist list for the years 2020, 2021, and 2022 by Elsevier BV and Stanford University. He is a reviewer/editor/editorial board member of more than 50 national and international journals of repute.

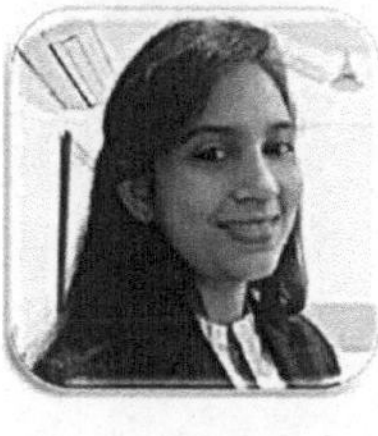

Sonali Sundram, MPharm
Assistant Professor, School of Medical and Allied Sciences, Galgotias University, Greater Noida, Uttar Pradesh, India

Sonali Sundram, MPharm, has worked as a research scientist on a project for ICMR at King George's Medical University, Lucknow. After that, she joined BBDNIIT, and currently, she is working at Galgotias University, Greater Noida. She completed her BPharm and MPharm (Pharmacology) degrees at AKTU, Lucknow, India. Her PhD (Pharmacy) work is in the area of neurodegeneration and nanoformulation. Her areas of interest include neurodegeneration, clinical research, and artificial intelligence. She has authored and/or edited more than 30 books (Wiley, CRC Press/Taylor and Francis, River Publisher, IOP Publishing, Apple Academic Press, etc.). She has attended as well as organized more than 15 national and international seminars/conferences/workshops. She holds more than eight national and international patents to her credit.

Contents

Contributors .... *xi*

Abbreviations .... *xv*

Foreword .... *xxi*

Preface .... *xxiii*

1. **Potential of Blockchain Technology for the Healthcare Domain** **1**
   Shailendra Singh Bhadauria, Aditi Chaudhary, and Sirisha Pingali

2. **Blockchain: A New Model for Health Information Exchanges** **41**
   Sushma Yadav, Avinash Tripathi, Shibu Das, Manish Yadav, and Shivkanya Fuloria

3. **Potential of Blockchain Technology in Tracking Disease and Pandemics** **53**
   Sunita Panchawat, Neeraj Sharma, Pradeep Kumar Jaiswal, and Deepika Bairagee

4. **Opportunities and Challenges of Blockchain Technology in Disease Outbreak Tracking** **91**
   Gera Jemimah, B. Maheshwari, G. S. N. Koteswara Rao, N. Raghavendra Naveen, Shams Aaghaz, A. V. S. S. S. Gupta, and Surya Kovvasu

5. **Blockchain Role in Medical Supply Chain Management** **115**
   Shashimala Tiwari

6. **Impact of Blockchain on Drug Traceability** **145**
   Mandeep Singh, Ruhul Amin Choudhury, and Vasudeva Kilaru

7. **Patient Selection and Treatment Strategies Using Computational Machine Analysis** **163**
   Anjali Gupta, Neha Sharma, and Pavan Kumar Arya Padarthi

8. **Artificial Intelligence in Healthcare to Improve the Quality of Life of the Elderly** **181**
   Gayatri Prajapati and Khwairakpam Sharmila

9. **Affordable Healthcare: The Promise of Blockchain** **213**
   Abhitav Tiwari, Mallika Tamminana, Shalini Perada, B. Srividya, Shivlal Yadav, Ankita Moharana, and Dhanalekshmi U. Meenakshi

10. **Smart Contracts: Medical Insurance Contracts for Patients** **241**
    Kamlesh Kumar Raghuvanshi, Subodh Kumar, Sushil Kumar, and Sunil Kumar

11. Remote Patient Monitoring with Blockchain: Powerful and Flexible Patient Observation Systems 279

Shweta Kumari, Vikash Kumar, Jyotirmaya Sahoo, Manjeet Kumar, Kamal Dua, and Sudhanshu Mishra

12. Secure Data Transmission Based on Deep Q-Learning Architecture with an Internet of Things Module in Healthcare Application 311

B. Sathiyaprasad and B. Satheesh Kumar

13. A Heterogeneous Graph-Based E-Health Solution in Cloud Computing with Semi-Supervision During Pandemic Periods 331

Antony Xavier Branson, Sai Shanmuga Raja, Sendilvelan Subramania, Larissa R. Sassykova, Francis Jency, Geetha Soman, Kanya Nataraj, and Mohandoss Sundaram

14. Autonomous Robots: A Disruptive Technology in the Health Sector.....365

Bikash Ranjan Jena, G. S. N. Koteswara Rao, Naga Jogayya Kothakota, Roja Rani Budha, L. Srinivas, J. Rajkumar, and Surya Kovvasu

15. Challenges to Digital Transformation in the Healthcare Industry.........399

Prachi Pachuary, Yashraj Sharma, Sharda Shambhakar, Sudhanshu Mishra, and Palak Gupta

Index...421

Contributors

Shams Aaghaz
Department of Pharmacy, School of Medical and Allied Sciences, Galgotias University, Greater Noida, Uttar Pradesh, India

Deepika Bairagee
Department of Pharmaceutical Sciences, Mohan Lal Sukhadia University, Udaipur, Rajasthan, India

Shailendra Singh Bhadauria
Faculty of Pharmaceutical Sciences, RAMA University, Mandhana, Kanpur, Uttar Pradesh, India

Antony Xavier Branson
Department of Computer Science and Engineering, Dr. M.G.R. Educational and Research Institute, Chennai, Tamil Nadu, India

Roja Rani Budha
Department of Pharmacology, Institute of Pharmaceutical Technology, Sri Padmavati Mahila Visvavidyalayam, Tirupati, Andhra Pradesh, India

Aditi Chaudhary
Faculty of Pharmaceutical Sciences, RAMA University, Mandhana, Kanpur, Uttar Pradesh, India

Ruhul Amin Choudhury
Department of Student Research and Project, Lovely Professional University, Jalandhar, Punjab, India

Shibu Das
Department of Pharmaceutical Chemistry, School of Pharmaceutical Sciences, Maharishi University of Information Technology, Lucknow, Uttar Pradesh, India

Kamal Dua
Faculty of Health, Australian Research Center in Complementary and Integrative Medicine, University of Technology, Sydney, Ultimo, NSW, Australia

Shivkanya Fuloria
Faculty of Pharmacy, AIMST University, Kedah, Malaysia

A. V. S. S. S. Gupta
Joginpally B.R. Pharmacy College, Yenkapally, Moinabad, Hyderabad, Telangana, India

Anjali Gupta
Parexel International Pvt. Ltd., Chandigarh, India

Palak Gupta
Department of Chemistry, University of Florida, Florida, United States

Pradeep Kumar Jaiswal
Department of Biochemistry and Biophysics, Texas A&M University, College Station, Texas, USA

Gera Jemimah
Joginpally B.R. Pharmacy College, Yenkapally, Moinabad, Hyderabad, Telangana, India

Bikash Ranjan Jena
School of Pharmacy and Life Sciences, Centurion University of Technology and Management, Jatni, Odisha, India

Francis Jency
Department of Computer Science and Engineering, Kumaraguru College of Technology, Coimbatore, Tamil Nadu, India

Vasudeva Kilaru
Department of Student Research and Project, Lovely Professional University, Jalandhar, Punjab, India

Naga Jogayya Kothakota
School of Pharmacy and Life Sciences, Centurion University of Technology and Management, Jatni, Odisha, India

Surya Kovvasu
Ambiopharm Inc., Beech Island, North Augusta, South Carolina, USA

B. Satheesh Kumar
Department of Computer Science and Engineering, Galgotia University, Yamuna Expressway, Greater Noida, Uttar Pradesh, India

Manjeet Kumar
School of Pharmacy, Arka Jain University, Jharkhand, India

Subodh Kumar
Department of Computer Science, Ramanujan College, University of Delhi, Delhi, India

Sunil Kumar
Department of Instrumentation, Shaheed Rajguru College of Applied Sciences for Women, University of Delhi, Delhi, India

Sushil Kumar
Department of Computer Science, Shyam Lal College(M), University of Delhi, North Campus, Delhi, India

Vikash Kumar
Narayan Institute of Pharmacy, Gopal Narayan Singh University, Jamuhar, Sasaram, Bihar, India

Shweta Kumari
T. John College of Pharmacy, Basavanapura, Bengaluru, Karnataka, India

B. Maheshwari
Joginpally B.R. Pharmacy College, Yenkapally, Moinabad, Hyderabad, Telangana, India

Dhanalekshmi U. Meenakshi
College of Pharmacy, National University of Science and Technology, Muscat, Oman

Sudhanshu Mishra
Department of Pharmaceutical Science and Technology, Madan Mohan Malaviya University of Technology, Gorakhpur, Uttar Pradesh, India; Department of Pharmacy, Banasthali Vidyapith, Vanasthali, Rajasthan, India

Ankita Moharana
Department of Pharmacy, Arka Jain University, Tata, Jamshedpur, Jharkhand, India

Kanya Nataraj
Department of Information Technology, Dr. M.G.R. Educational and Research Institute, Chennai, Tamil Nadu, India

N. Raghavendra Naveen
Sri Adichunchanagiri College of Pharmacy, Adichunchanagiri University, B.G. Nagar, Karnataka, India

Prachi Pachuary
Department of Management Studies, Kanya Gurukula, Haridwar, Uttarakhand, India

Pavan Kumar Arya Padarthi
University of Hertfordshire, Luton, United Kingdom

Sunita Panchawat
Department of Pharmaceutical Sciences, Mohan Lal Sukhadia University, Udaipur, Rajasthan, India

Shalini Perada
RITEE College of Pharmacy, Raipur, Chhattisgarh, India

Sirisha Pingali
Analyst, Lonza Biologics, Slough, United Kingdom

Gayatri Prajapati
Department of Human Development and Family Studies, School of Home Science, Babasaheb Bhimrao Ambedkar University, Lucknow, Uttar Pradesh, India

Kamlesh Kumar Raghuvanshi
Department of Computer Science, Ramanujan College, University of Delhi, Delhi, India

Sai Shanmuga Raja
Department of Computer Science and Engineering, Dr. M.G.R. Educational and Research Institute, Chennai, Tamil Nadu, India

J. Rajkumar
Department of Pharmaceutics, Vaageswari College of Pharmacy, Karimnagar, Telangana, India

G. S. N. Koteswara Rao
Department of Pharmacy, School of Medical and Allied Sciences, Galgotias University, Greater Noida, Uttar Pradesh, India

Jyotirmaya Sahoo
Sachchidanand Sinha College, Aurangabad Bihar, Under Magadh University, Bodh Gaya, Bihar, India

Larissa R. Sassykova
Faculty of Chemistry and Chemical Technology, Al-Farabi Kazakh National University, Almaty, Kazakhstan

B. Sathiyaprasad
Department of Computer Science and Engineering, Sathyabama Institute of Science and Technology, Rajiv Gandhi Salai, Chennai, Tamil Nadu, India

Sharda Shambhakar
Department of Pharmacy, Banasthali Vidyapith, Vanasthali, Rajasthan, India

Neeraj Sharma
Faculty of Pharmacy, Bhagwant University, Ajmer, Rajasthan, India

Neha Sharma
Department of Pharmacy, School of Medical and Allied Sciences, Galgotias University, Greater Noida, Uttar Pradesh, India

Yashraj Sharma
Department of Management Studies, Kanya Gurukula, Haridwar, Uttarakhand, India

Khwairakpam Sharmila
Department of Human Development and Family Studies, School of Home Science, Babasaheb Bhimrao Ambedkar University, Lucknow, Uttar Pradesh, India

Mandeep Singh
Department of Student Research and Project, Lovely Professional University, Jalandhar, Punjab, India

Geetha Soman
Department of Computer Science and Engineering, Dr. M.G.R. Educational and Research Institute, Chennai, Tamil Nadu, India

L. Srinivas
Department Pharmaceutics, Gitam Institute of Pharmacy, Gitam University, Visakhapatnam, Andhra Pradesh, India

B. Srividya
RITEE College of Pharmacy, Raipur, Chhattisgarh, India

Sendilvelan Subramania
Department of Mechanical Engineering, Dr. M.G.R. Educational and Research Institute, Chennai, Tamil Nadu, India

Mohandoss Sundaram
Department of Computer Science and Engineering, Dr. M.G.R. Educational and Research Institute, Chennai, Tamil Nadu, India

Mallika Tamminana
Bharat School of Pharmacy, Hyderabad, Telangana, India

Abhitav Tiwari
Guru Ghasidas Vishwavidalaya, Bilaspur, Chhattisgarh, India

Shashimala Tiwari
Specialist-FRU, India Health Action Trust, Uttar Pradesh Technical Support Unit, Lucknow, Uttar Pradesh, India

Avinash Tripathi
Department of Pharmaceutical Sciences, Sam Higginbottom University of Agriculture, Technology, and Sciences (SHUATS), Naini, Prayagraj, Uttar Pradesh, India

Manish Yadav
Sainik Pharmacy College, Mai Devkali, Hanumanganj, Prayagraj, Uttar Pradesh, India

Shivlal Yadav
Birla Institute of Technology, Mesra, Ranchi, Jharkhand, India; Department of Pharmacy, Central University of Rajasthan Ajmer, Rajasthan, India

Sushma Yadav
Sainik Pharmacy College, Mai Devkali, Hanumanganj, Prayagraj, Uttar Pradesh, India

Abbreviations

3D	three-dimensional
AA	attribute authority
ABE	attribute-based encryption
ACA	Affordable Care Act
ADSs	anomaly identification
AGVs	automated guided vehicles
AI	artificial intelligence
AMP	antimicrobial peptide
AMR	autonomous mobile robot
AO	administrative officer
API	active pharmaceutical ingredient
API	application programming interface
APTT	activated partial thromboplastin time
ARM	Association Rule Mining
ARs	autonomous robots
AUC	area under curve
BCT	blockchain technology
BLE	Bluetooth low-energy
BPMN	business process modeling notation
BuS	bottom-up summarization
CAD	coronary artery disease
CART	classification and regression tree
CDC	Centers for Disease Control and Prevention
CDM	clinical data management
CDSS	clinical decision support system
CIMD	computational intelligence medical data
CMS	Centers for Medicare and Medicaid Services
CNN	convolutional neural network
COPD	chronic obstructive pulmonary disease
COVID-19	coronavirus disease of 2019
CP-ABE	ciphertext-policy attribute-based encryption

CPABPP	ciphertext-policy attribute-based privacy preservation
CSID	Chinese skin image database
CT	computed tomography
DAGs	directed acyclic graphs
DAO	Decentralized Autonomous Organization
DApp	decentralized application
DDB	decentralized database
DDoS	distributed denial of service
DFS	distributed file system
DHT	digital health trend
DL	deep learning
DLT	distributed ledger technology
DNNs	deep neural networks
DO	dissolved oxygen
DOT	Department of Telecommunication
DPoS	delegated proof of stake
DQ-NNPP	Q-learning based Neural Network with Privacy Preservation technique
DSCSA	Drug Supply Chain Security Act
EBM	evidence-based medicine
ECG	electrocardiogram
EEA	Enterprise Ethereum Alliance
EEG	electroencephalogram
E-health	electronic-health
EHR	electronic health record
EMG	electromyogram
EMR	electronic medical record
EOA	externally owned account
EOG	electrooculography
EPC	electronic product codes
EPRS	European Parliamentary Research Service
EU	European Union
EVD	Ebola virus disease
FDA	Food and Drug Administration
F-DEMATEL	fuzzy-decision-making trial and evaluation laboratory
FHIR	fast healthcare interoperability resources
GAO	Government Accountability Office

GDSN	global data synchronization network
GIS	geographic information system
GP	genomes project
GSR	galvanic skin reaction
GUI	graphical user interface
HCI	human-computer interaction
HDFS	Hadoop distributed file system
HIE	health information exchange
HIPAA	Health Insurance Portability and Accountability Act
HIT	heparin-induced thrombocytopenia
HITECH	Health Information Technology for Economic and Clinical Health
HL7's	health level 7
HMV	hidden Markov model
HRI	human-robot interaction
HT-Scale	height scale
IBM	international business machines
ICT	information and communication technology
ICU	intensive care unit
IIS	internet information services
IoMT	internet of medical things
IoT	internet of things
IPFS	interplanetary file system
IS	information security
IT	information technology
JDBC	Java database connectivity
LAN	local area network
LiDAR	light detection and ranging
MAE	mean absolute error
MALDI	matrix-assisted laser desorption ionization
MB	megabyte
MDP	modern digital products
MDR	medical data release
MDS	medical data sharing
MEG	magnetoencephalogram
MERS	Middle East Respiratory syndrome
MITA	Medicaid information technology architecture
ML	machine learning

MLPQ	minimum-level priority queue
MMG	mechanomyogram
MoHAP	Ministry of Health and Prevention
MPI	master patient identifier
MRI	magnetic resonance imaging
MTF	mobile telepresence functionality
NCOA	National Council on Aging
NFC	near-field communication
NHS	National Health Service
NIST	National Institute of Standards and Technology
OCR	office for civil rights
ODBC	open database connectivity
OECD	Organization for Economic Cooperation and Development
OLAP	online analytical processing
P2P	peer-to-peer
PACS	picture archive and computer systems
PBFT	practical byzantine fault tolerance
PCI	percutaneous coronary intervention
PCR	polymerase chain reaction
PCTs	pragmatic clinical trials
PHI	personal health information
PHR	personal health record
PM	patient monitoring
PoA	proof-of-authority
PoB	proof-of-burn
PoD	proof-of-deposit
PoET	proof-of-elapsed time
PoI	proof-of-importance
PoS	proof-of-stake
PoW	proof-of-work
PPDP	privacy-preserving disease prediction
PPE	personnel protective equipment
PPS	pulse per second
Ppy	polypyrrole
PRE	proxy re-encryption
PSD	personal domains
PUD	public domains

RBI	Reserve Bank of India
RFID	radio-frequency identification
RHM	remote health monitoring
ROC	receiver operating characteristics
SAB-UAS	secure and anonymous biometric based-user authentication scheme
SARS	severe acute respiratory syndrome
SAR	socially assistive robots
SCM	supply chain management
SHALE	smart home assisted living for the elderly
SHG	semi-supervised heterogeneous graph
SNR	signal-to-noise ratio
SOFA	sequential organ failure assessment scores
SSI	self-sovereign identification
TA	trusted authority
TPAs	third-party administrators
TPR	true positive rate
TPS	transaction per second
TRU	traceable resource unit
UAVs	unmanned aerial vehicles
UNESCO	United Nations Educational, Scientific, and Cultural Organization
US CDC	United States Center for Disease Control and Prevention
US FDA	United States Food and Drug Administration
USA	United States of America
UV	ultraviolet
VBC	Vietnam Blockchain Corporation
VIRI	Virios Therapeutics, Inc.
VNA	vendor-neutral archives
VPU	vision processing unit
WBAN	wireless body-area network
WHO	World Health Organization
WHOSTNF	National Science Foundations and the White House Office of Science and Technology
WSN	wireless sensor networks

Foreword

We are in the era of the 4th Industrial Revolution, which is characterized by robotics, artificial intelligence (AI), data analytics, and data mining. Blockchain is one of the most important pioneering components of these revolutions. While the application of these techniques is widely available for money transfer, logistics, media, security, environment, etc., health is one of such sectors that has plenty of it, and probably only 20% has been explored. Coupled with healthcare, pharmaceutical sciences is the area that has limitless opportunities. This maiden attempt by Dr. Rishabha Malviya and Prof. Sonali Sundram to bring a multi-authored book, *Creating Smart Healthcare with Blockchain and Advanced Digital Technology,* is commendable.

Researchers and practitioners who are new to the field will benefit a lot from being able to quickly find information and access information on the potential and influence on the healthcare system rapidly. Additionally, this book will not only provide knowledge but also provide directions for researchers on a variety of topics, including medical supply chain management, various patient treatment modalities, accessible healthcare, medical insurance, patient monitoring, secure data transfer, and robotics in the healthcare system.

I compliment and congratulate the authors for their efforts, and I am sure the book will find a place for all stakeholders of medical and pharmaceutical sciences.

—**Prof. Ramesh K. Goyal**
Vice Chancellor,
Delhi Pharmaceutical Sciences and Research University,
Delhi, India

Preface

Society is going through big changes at the moment. Over the past few years, research on emerging technologies in Industry 4.0 has grown by leaps and bounds in both industry and academia. It's interesting that technologies like blockchain, deep learning (DL), and the Internet of Things (IoT) have been growing at an exponential rate. The Fourth Industrial Revolution had a wide range of effects and was made up of a mix of technologies from the physical, digital, and biological worlds.

Since the healthcare industry is one of the most affected areas by technological advancement, digitalization is having a profound impact on every aspect of how healthcare is delivered, from interactions between patients and caregivers to interactions between governments and stakeholders.

The healthcare industry's history is a sequence of technological innovations to improve patient outcomes and access to services. Blockchain, a recent healthcare breakthrough, is redefining the information architecture that underpins all healthcare services. Blockchain can make health information systems more safe, efficient, accessible, and dependable.

These advances in science and technology are expected to lead to new ways of diagnosing and treating diseases, such as precision medicine and medical cures. Medical and technological breakthroughs and improvements will make health and healthcare much more connected, precise, and open to everyone, leading to much better outcomes for people.

We have observed that very few books are available on the market that describe applications of blockchain technology in the pharmaceutical sector. So, keeping this in mind, we have edited a book that describes the basic concept of blockchain in relation to the pharmaceutical sector to advancement in blockchain technology in the healthcare sector.

This book explores how blockchain technology will transform healthcare in the upcoming decades.

This book offers a basic concept of blockchain, identifies its elements, and its application in healthcare. Along with this, this book provides a concise, novel, and broad representation of the application and challenges of digital technology used in healthcare.

The book covers the role of blockchain in patient selection and treatment strategies, in tracking disease and pandemics, in supply chain management, and in the health insurance sector.

—***Editors***

CHAPTER 1

Potential of Blockchain Technology for the Healthcare Domain

SHAILENDRA SINGH BHADAURIA,[1] ADITI CHAUDHARY,[1] and SIRISHA PINGALI[2]

[1]*Faculty of Pharmaceutical Sciences, RAMA University, Mandhana, Kanpur, Uttar Pradesh, India*

[2]*Lonza Biologics, Slough, United Kingdom*

ABSTRACT

The purpose of this chapter is to explore the blockchain in health for medical data release (MDR), medical data storage, medical data storage and key components of blockchain technology (BCT), application of blockchain in healthcare, working principle of blockchain in healthcare, benefits and drawbacks for healthcare application of blockchain, challenges and solutions of blockchain in healthcare. The acceleration of advanced digital healthcare has begun with artificial intelligence (AI) and is projected to accelerate further as the sector moves towards BCT. Blockchain is a decentralized, encrypted distributed ledger system. Initially designed for cryptocurrency and most usually referred to, there are an increasing number of applications outside of finance, many of which are crucial for medical imaging, aside from potential implementation challenges like public-private key access, distributed book size constraints, speed and complexity, and safety flaws. Examples of potential blockchain applications in medical imaging include image ownership of a patient, tracking medical devices, research, teleradiology, and AI. BCT opens up new avenues for complexity reduction, trust-free collaboration, and safe, unchangeable data. In this chapter, we provide a detailed evaluation of blockchain in healthcare, including its benefits and drawbacks, application,

Creating Smart Healthcare with Blockchain and Advanced Digital Technology.
Rishabha Malviya and Sonali Sundram (Eds.)

and operating principle. We quickly explore the issues and their solutions in light of numerous technologies that will assist researchers in the future. Blockchain has emerged in the last decade and added a lot of interest in the healthcare sector; future perspectives need for improved patient care, easier and more reliable research, and on-demand medical data access are driving digital health trends (DHTs).

1.1 INTRODUCTION

Healthcare companies listed on major stock exchanges perform vital functions for the healthcare sector as a whole. Doctors, nurses, hospitals, and other medical professionals from the private, public, and non-profit sectors all play a role in this broad field of medicine [1]. Donations from patients are the only source of revenue for many types of facilities, including those that provide housing, education, dental care, in-home healthcare, emergency care, in-patient care, outpatient care, and diagnostic and ambulatory testing. In addition to hospitals and doctors, this category also includes insurance firms and pharmaceutical and medical equipment corporations [2]. The application of blockchain technology in healthcare would have far-reaching positive effects [3]. But, picking the right Blockchain technology for the job is crucial to a smooth rollout. At the moment, public, proprietary, and consortium Blockchains are the three most common types. The level of security afforded to sensitive data in Blockchains, in terms of permissions, access, and so on, can vary widely [4]. There is a lack of consensus about what a Blockchain is and isn't at the moment, especially when it comes to different Blockchain implementations and uses [5]. Information of this nature is specially protected and confidential in the healthcare sector.

Everyone is familiar with and has some grasp of how public Blockchains like Bitcoin, Ethereum, etc., work [6]. Any person can freely explore these ecosystems. As an incentive for increased participation, the network itself offers perks to users. The healthcare industry, however, is not one where a decentralized Blockchain would be useful [7, 8]. It is common knowledge that there is a space problem with the blocks used by Bitcoin and Ethereum. Bitcoin's block size is just over 1 MB (megabyte), far too small for the kind of transactions and data storage required by medical research facilities. The second part of the question, "What were the results?" is also fairly standard fare [9]. In the Bitcoin network, about eight transactions per second are the maximum possible throughput. Bitcoin's consensus process requires miners to wait around 10 minutes before adding a new block to the blockchain [10]. This latency is, therefore, intolerable. Massive trade block processing with negligible latency is a common challenge for large medical institutions [11]. Delays of any kind could be disastrous. Because of its computationally intensive nature, bitcoin's proof-of-work (PoW) algorithm for reaching consensus in the blockchain requires a large number of processors to solve complex puzzles [12]. Consequently, it is not feasible for these organizations to invest so much money in consensus algorithms. An additional disadvantage is that public blockchains are open to everyone to see [13]. Clinical institutes may be hesitant to share data with anyone outside of their organization due to the sensitive nature of the data they handle, which could make medical organizations wary of participating in an open network. For this reason, it's possible that public blockchains won't function properly [14]. However, Blockchain technology comes in many flavors; the private Blockchain is particularly well-suited to healthcare institutions like hospitals [15].

To join the private blockchain network, new participants will need administrative approval. Hence, "permitted blockchain" is another name for private chains [16]. They are more than welcome to become a part of our private group.

This makes it possible to restrict some people's ability to contribute to the consensus process points of entry for potential new participants:

- People who are already a part of the ecosystem;
- An authoritative figure set the rules;
- Cooperation amongst many entities.

Companies that have joined the blockchain community can aid in maintaining the network's infrastructure. Licensed Blockchain system software is available in the form of the Hyperledger Fabric from the Linux Foundation [17, 18]. Those requirements were taken into account during its development. Private chains are a useful tool for conducting business because they provide anonymity, speed, and security.

In addition, the number of IoT products with medical applications has increased. These include internet-connected medical devices that can provide real-time patient monitoring [19]. The new Apple Watch includes electrocardiogram (ECG) functionality, which was developed in-house by Apple. For instance, Apple builds in-built heart rate monitors for a variety of their wearable and portable electronics [20].

With the advent of smart contracts, blockchains can now be used to record and then retrieve data at the user's request [21]. Nevertheless, advance contracts require expert assistance with management and upkeep, and they can be time-consuming to set up. Many studies detail the first steps toward introducing IoT into healthcare systems [22]. These conceptual designs are based on private Blockchains, which offer additional permission-based security. Smart contracts, which would be designed, implemented, and managed independently for each IoT device, are one possible solution [23].

1.2 THE INTERNET OF THINGS (IOT) IN THE HEALTHCARE INDUSTRY

The Internet of Things (IoT) in the healthcare industry may have access to a public Blockchain with a specialized smart contract and a common data format. Since this information pertains to a patient's health, both the smart contract and the data format must be secure [24]. With Blockchain technology, businesses would have to perform less paperwork, and more smart contracts could be put into place.

Researchers from many different fields have recommended using Blockchain for medical purposes [25]. To prevent counterfeiting, fraud, theft, and temperature switching, the blockchain network in this system is guided by stochastic simulation [26]. Even then, the recommended remedy enhances the supply chain in every conceivable way: efficiency, transparency, security, and dependability [27]. In order to draft and specify the smart contracts that make up the system, we used proof-of-authority (PoA) technology. Suggested information management and tracking systems would include monitoring drug shipments [28]. Both radio frequency identification and electronic product code information service are utilized to ensure the security of the pharmaceutical supply chain (EPCIS) [29].

The theoretical framework for this study was based on collective action theory and transaction cost theory. They set up a set of rules for how everyone involved in the distribution of medicines should act [30]. Drug manufacturers and advocacy groups face a serious problem with the illegal distribution of their products. Many international health organizations are working to address this issue, but pharmaceutical sales of these drugs continue to rise [31].

Advise a blockchain-based system for managing and tracking the distribution of medicines, in which all involved parties can monitor and verify the delivery of each batch. The proposed system was built on the back of a case study [32]. But it's crucial to ask if blockchain technology is the future of healthcare [33]. Fashions come and go. The blockchain is the cure for any broken system. New businesses may find many uses for the blockchain as a tool for solving problems [34]. The following are two examples of questions we might ask: Is this a private blockchain, or is it accessible to the general public? Second, how important is it to have a blockchain, if at all? If the first question can be answered by a private blockchain, then this isn't exactly ground-breaking. In order to respond to the second question, it is useful to think back to the original motivation for creating blockchain technology to safeguard against the dangers of centralization [35]. But the stakes have to be high before those dangers become noticeable. As an example, the pharmacy line can be managed centrally to avoid the need for distributed ledger technology (DLT) [36].

While blockchain's decentralization features are impressive, the technology itself is slow, inefficient, and requires a lot of energy and time to run [37]. Bitcoin transactions take about 10 minutes to be confirmed by the network. The line at the coffee shop is significantly longer than normal, which is problematic. If there is a concern about centralization, and only if, then Blockchain technology is the solution [38]. If there is no pressing need to decentralize some aspect of a system's operations, then there is probably no point in implementing blockchain technology [39].

Next, we'll go over some concrete uses for Blockchain technology, with an eye toward cutting-edge study and the possible future course of the healthcare sector, where it stands to have far-reaching positive effects [40].

1.3 POTENTIAL APPLICATION OF BLOCKCHAIN

This section depicts various healthcare-related use cases for Blockchain technology, highlighting the benefits realized by implementing this technology [41]. Benefits include decentralization, improved data security and privacy, health data ownership, greater availability, resilience, openness, trust, and verifiability of data [42].

1.3.1 INTEGRATION OF HEALTHCARE SERVICES

One of the most pressing medical concerns of the present day is the widespread dispersion of patients' medical histories across various databases maintained by different organizations [43]. Including blockchain-based medical records and transactions is one way to address this issue. Launching a smart contract to build a digital health ecosystem wherein only authorized medical professionals have access to a patient's medical records is one example of how this can be accomplished [44]. Figure 1.1 illustrates the various roles of blockchain in healthcare.

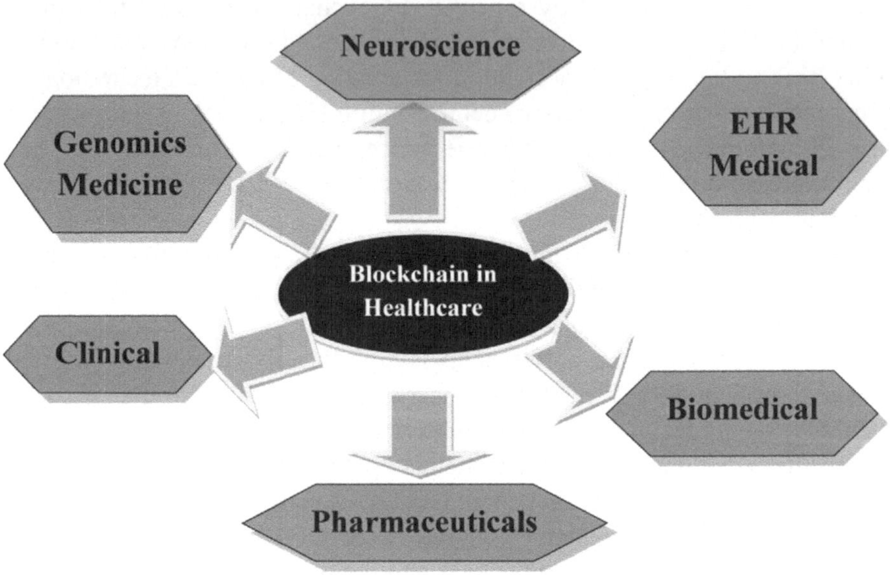

FIGURE 1.1 Roles of blockchain in healthcare.

The actions of doctors, such as taking notes, inserting scans, and conducting tests, are recorded as transactions. When a prescription is filled, the pharmacy logs the transaction in a distributed ledger called a "blockchain." By signing this form, the patient grants the insurer limited access to review medical records and receive payment for services [45]. Smart contracts are one way that patients show their appreciation to their doctors. It will be possible for doctors to offer advice or a second opinion on patient cases after reviewing them from a distance [46]. By tracking their health and wellness, health insurance policyholders can earn discounts or tokens from their providers. In addition, patients are allowed time-limited access to their medical records so that hospitals and other medical research facilities can perform their tests [47]. Patients may be issued tokens for use on the blockchain to store health data collected by wearable fitness equipment and perform financial transactions. Intelligent applications that analyze health data and prescribe lifestyle adjustments like diet and exercise will be possible to develop thanks to this blockchain-based healthcare ecosystem [48].

1.3.2 COUNTERFEIT DRUGS

Substitute medications made to look like the real thing are a contemporary issue. They are responsible for the deaths of between 1,20,000 and 1,000,000 people annually. Inefficient drug supply chains also result in higher prices [49]. Pharmaceutical companies must report extensive data because of regulatory constraints. In this regard, blockchain technology may contribute to the development of a remedy for these issues [50]. Better supply chain management (SCM) and the elimination of counterfeit medicines could be achieved through the integration of blockchain technology, AI, and cutting-edge data analytics. The manufacturing facility, distribution center, and logistics firm will all be rolled into one with the medical center or pharmacy [51]. The Blockchain allows for the tracking of individual drug packages. Customers can benefit greatly from this app because it allows them to verify the authenticity of the medicine they are purchasing [52]. The pharmaceutical supply chain is sealed off from counterfeit drugs. The use of AI and data analytics in logistics improves their effectiveness [53]. The effective distribution of pharmaceuticals will also contribute to the avoidance of price distortions. Automation of regulatory reporting and the facilitation of automatic payments along the supply chain will be permitted [54].

1.3.3 RELIEF EFFORTS IN THE WAKE OF A CATASTROPHIC EVENT

Blockchain technology allows us to rethink and demonstrate the efficacy of teamwork in disaster relief. Information from disparate sources, like emails or social media, can make it difficult to swiftly and effectively coordinate disaster relief efforts. When everyone involved can see the same information at the same time, coordination is easier, and productivity rises [55]. Blockchain technology makes it possible to link disparate autonomous systems via a decentralized network without requiring an overarching data infrastructure overseen by a single entity [56]. Imagine an island hit by an earthquake, where the UN has just launched a global humanitarian operation. Spread out across the island, A, B, and C groups each have their supply base from which they operate. Supplies water, B offers medical care, and C flies' people around in helicopters. Since the Blockchain is an immutable ledger, it is simple to ascertain which areas have a greater demand for resources [57]. So, let's say the B camp has to ferry over a large number of doctors and nurses to the other side of the island. Interface F is where the user enters their request, which is then distributed to all participants in the mission using Blockchain. The rest of the group will be alerted to the request and given the option to respond to the unique offer instantly [58]. Here, camp A might quickly send in the choppers. Smart contracts, simple open algorithms embedded in the Blockchain, will be agreed upon by all parties to ensure that the rules established by all are followed. If a request is a good fit for a given offer, the assistance is given without any additional steps being needed. One of the most essential characteristics is the potential of direct cooperation in a business process across businesses [59]. All Blockchain applications share a few commonalities. Blockchain technology ensures that each participant is truly independent and that they have full control over their data. Everyone contributes to the system and shares in its costs, but everyone benefits from the system's efficiency. This is simply one of many examples [60].

1.3.4 PHARMACY CHAIN SUPPLY

Among the most stringent requirements in the pharmaceutical sector are those for product stability and security. Blockchain technology, for instance, can be used to keep tabs on the supply chain in a way that is both secure and transparent. The potential for delays and mistakes made by humans to be greatly diminished is clear. It can be used at any point in the supply chain to monitor factors like cost, labor input, and environmental impact [61]. They can also be used to combat the counterfeit drug industry, which results in yearly losses of $200 billion, by tracking the origin of products. Many businesses, including chronicled, blockpharma, and modum, are already focusing on enhancing supply chain logistics using blockchain technology. Particularly, Modum satisfies European Union (EU) criteria, calling for proof that drugs have not been exposed to factors, such as temperature, that could affect their purity. Modum's answer was to create a sensor that logs data on the Blockchain about the conditions under which real goods are being transported [62].

1.3.5 GENOMIC MARKET

A new market for the secure exchange of genetic data between individuals is feasible through the use of blockchain networks [63]. The potential for individual genome sequencing has the potential to become a multibillion-dollar data industry [64]. And how can we best ensure that information travels securely from its origin to its final destination without any middlemen intervening? Without a doubt, the Blockchain is the solution. Genomic data can be more securely stored, acquired, and managed with blockchain, and the difficulties associated with handling genomic big data can also be overcome with this technology [65].

1.3.6 MEDICAL STAFF CREDENTIALING

It can be time-consuming and inconvenient to apply for a medical license the old-fashioned way, through channels such as the telephone, fax machine, and postal mail. Blockchains are well suited for credentials due to their verifiability and adaptability to incremental changes [66]. All participants in the chain can trust the information stored in the blockchain because of its immutability and the stringent controls in place. Each participant in the data has complete access to the ledger [67].

The credential "smart contract," which would use Blockchain's software as a live database of credentials, is another potential use case. It is expected that the credential data is dynamic, with contributions from users updating a centralized database [68]. In this way, whenever a request came in for credentialing information extending from the time of college graduation to the most current credentialing-relevant incidents, it wouldn't be necessary to scan many data sources. Instead, it would be readily available at any time, with the administrator having the option of manually or automatically displaying the practitioner's records [69]. Time and money would be saved by adopting this method because this is a routine process for which any delay results in increased expenses.

1.3.7 SAFEGUARDING THE INTERNET OF THINGS (IOT) FOR CONSTANT TRACKING

Using remote monitoring technology to ensure accountability for patients' health across all sensors and perceiving critical signals for patients are two of the most significant advances in digital health. In addition to providing curative care, doctors can now proactively screen for potential health issues and prevent others [70]. However, privacy and data accuracy are at stake in the IoT health sector, making security a top priority. A networked system may rely on [71] in times of crisis, such as when alerting a person's care provider about a heart attack or fall in an elderly person. It is also critical that your service has excellent defenses against attacks like distributed denial of service (DDoS). When personal information is stored on the Blockchain as a unique hash function, only authorized parties are granted access to the information [72]. This is because any change to the source data will result in a new hash function, and decoding the hash function into the source data requires a user to have a unique set of cryptographic keys.

There is very little chance that anyone will be able to access or make use of patient data if it is added as a hash function to the blockchain directory. Blockchain's decentralized architecture makes it possible for IoT devices to communicate directly with one another, bypassing the requirement for a centralized server. As a result, DDoS and man-in-the-middle attacks become more challenging to carry out while employing this method of communication [73].

It is not yet obvious if Blockchain is the proper technology to deploy [74], despite Blockchain's potential to improve IoT security in the healthcare sector. When considering how to secure remote monitoring devices, blockchain presents an exciting alternative for digital health organizations to investigate, but only as part of a much more comprehensive end-to-end security approach [75].

1.4 THE COMBINATION OF AI WITH BLOCKCHAIN TECHNOLOGY

The combination of blockchain and AI has the potential to revolutionize healthcare delivery. Healthcare will become more widely available and inexpensive as a result of cost savings in the healthcare business. AI relies on encrypted data, which can be stored and transferred on a blockchain. Blockchain technology will make it feasible to deduce the reasoning behind automated judgments [76].

Blockchain technology will help the healthcare industry reduce manual processes like data entry and reconciliation. In a predictive healthcare setting, AI can help us steer our efforts toward optimal service intensity. Information will be delivered in a way that makes sense for patients, professionals, and caregivers [77].

Consider the COVID-19 (coronavirus disease of 2019) case as a case study example. Using blockchain technology, hospitals and other healthcare facilities can conduct operations without worrying about the spread of the COVID-19 pandemic [78]. Therapeutic recommendations for future outbreaks (like coronavirus) can be established with the help of data from blockchains and AI systems, which can quickly identify the diagnosis and therapy for patients with COVID-19 [79]. Blockchain allows for the secure and private exchange of data between institutions such as hospitals, clinics, primary care doctors, and pediatricians. Data analysis is performed with the help of AI tools [80].

Take the COVID-19 case as an illustration. Blockchain technology underpins the COVID-19-secure clinical practice. By combining Blockchain technology with AI and COVID-19 to better prepare for future pandemics, the 19 people may be diagnosed and treated more quickly (similar to coronavirus). A blockchain-based solution enables the safe and confidential exchange of patient information amongst healthcare providers such as hospitals, primary care physicians, and pediatricians. Data analysis tools developed with AI are used. This conceptual framework can be used in the fields of risk management, pharmaceutical innovation, and therapeutic development [81, 82].

1.4.1 ADOPTION OF BLOCKCHAIN TECHNOLOGY

Blockchain technology is in its infancy; despite having been developed in 2008, It was created to serve as a public record of all Bitcoin transactions. Since 2008, there has been a dearth of high-quality output, and the underlying technology of Bitcoin has received little attention. Research gaps slow the spread of Blockchain technology. Business-wide implementation of this technology is hindered by the absence of "any legal structure to permit or support smart contracts" [82].

Deloitte discovered that 29% of respondents indicated a lack of awareness of Blockchain technology as one of the primary challenges to using this technology as part of their Global Blockchain Survey (Deloitte's 2019 global Blockchain Survey) conducted at the beginning of the year. On the other hand, bitcoin itself has been the subject of research rather than the blockchain itself. Around 22% of respondents in Deloitte's Global Blockchain Survey [83] feel there is not enough evidence of Blockchain's genuine usefulness.

1.4.2 THE COST OF MASS ADOPTION

To date, no products have emerged that are particularly well-suited for use with Blockchain. There is a significant time and money investment involved in developing new software, with estimates ranging from $10,000 for simple programs to $8,00,000 or more for highly specialized applications [84] when Blockchain is to be utilized for a specific purpose.

1.4.3 *DISPARITY BETWEEN THE DEMAND FOR AND SUPPLY OF BLOCKCHAIN SPECIALISTS*

There are two ways in which the shortage of expertise is hindering adoption. The number of employees in the innovation sector is insufficient to satisfy current needs. Second, the high price tag of retaining the best Blockchain talent is a direct result of their relative scarcity in the market. More people should become educated about Blockchain technology as interest in it increases [85].

1.4.4 *PEOPLE ARE RELUCTANT TO CHANGE*

This may hinder blockchain's mainstream acceptance, even though technology might drastically alter industries like contracts and financial markets. There are several examples of this throughout history. TCP/IP is used as an example of sluggish adoption by the Harvard Business Review. In 1972, when researchers were able to communicate via email, TCP/IP was widely adopted. In the 1980s, only a small number of companies were using TCP/IP; it wasn't until the mid-1990s that the protocol became widely used. If it took TCP/IP over two decades to reach people, it's unrealistic to think that everyone will use Blockchain in the next decade [86].

1.4.5 *REGULATION, LAW, AND POLITICS*

While there is much enthusiasm for blockchain technology, some hesitance in adopting it has been prompted by concerns about how it will be governed and what policies will be put in place to govern it [87]. Around 30% of people said that government oversight and regulation were the biggest challenges to further blockchain development. Some industries may be cautious about blockchain because of its association with the volatile cryptocurrency Bitcoin or simply because of the novelty of the technology. Fears that the blockchain is too dependent on a centralized server may also prevent it from being used to manage difficult issues like DSCSA (Drug Supply Chain Security Act) compliance [88]. Since blockchain relies on trust in data repositories rather than a trusted broker to validate transactions, it discourages healthcare organizations from storing and transferring sensitive data [89].

1.4.6 HEALTHCARE PAYMENTS

The healthcare industry loses thousands of dollars annually due to alleged mistakes and arguments caused by the inefficient and outdated healthcare payment process. Because of the simplicity of the agreements between the shareholders, there is no need for the sharing or exchange of information. If everyone in a company network could instantly tap into the same reliable information hub, it would be fantastic [89]. To put it simply, a blockchain is a distributed ledger that can be used to record and verify financial transactions and the ownership of assets without the intervention of a central authority. The end-to-end tracking of assets is made possible by the shared directory, which allows everyone to keep tabs on and analyze the status of those assets in near real-time.

There is currently a major issue with the pre-authorization process that is required by some insurance companies before they agree to pay for a given treatment. There are a number of factors that can make it difficult to ascertain whether or not an insurance policy will cover a certain expense for a member, including the involvement of multiple parties. The complexity, the number of manual stages, and the possible lack of adequate communication and technology may all stem from the payer-provider interaction. With Blockchain, all parties involved in a patient's care can access a single shared ledger, including information on the patient's entitlements and smart contracts that automate the pre-authorization process [91]. This allows for instantaneous benefit determination as data collection and dissemination are automated. Benefits of using Blockchain for pre-authorization include better patient treatment, precise payment to the provider, reduced administrative costs, and elimination of duplicate record-keeping [92, 93]. Claims submitted for patients who have since lost insurance or switched providers provide a further significant difficulty today. As ideal as it would be for doctors to verify patients' insurance coverage before seeing them, this is not often the case. Since validation is typically laborious and time-consuming, it is often skipped in the hopes that the patient would volunteer the information beforehand. When a patient seeks medical attention from a doctor or other medical professional, that visit initiates the claims process. Patients' health insurance companies are billed. Following adjudication of the claim, the insurer will communicate its decision to all parties. If the patient does not have insurance and the claim is denied because of coverage questions, the healthcare provider will be in the unpleasant position of trying to collect payment from the patient. If the patient's insurance information has changed, the doctor must resubmit the claim with the new information. This causes additional costs and often causes significant delays in overall therapy. Providers and people around the world face the same problem of how to enhance treatment without increasing costs. The aging of the population has increased the number of individuals with chronic ailments, and the increased need for services to help these individuals cope with their illnesses has been fueled by technological advancements and the growing autonomy of patients [94]. With this goal in mind, healthcare DT primarily utilizes the IoT, artificial intelligence (AI), machine learning (ML), and analytics. Improved diagnosis, treatment, and prevention are the ultimate goals of educating patients to make their own therapeutic decisions. Instead of viewing conversations on an "as-needed" basis, a physician might observe "real" exchanges as they occur [94]. Financial gains can be achieved through the application of organizational intelligence in the healthcare industry by making better use of available resources and services. Transaction transmission techniques, aging systems, a proliferation of data sources, and a lack of widespread adoption of data standards all contribute to a climate of fear in the healthcare business, where all parties involved are concerned for their security and privacy [95]. When it comes to patient care, this healthcare provider puts patient satisfaction and financial security first. The "digital maturity" of an organization is a measure of how well its information technology (IT) can meet the needs of a growing business.

1.5 THE KEY AIMS AND OBJECTIVES OF HEALTHCARE'S DIGITAL TRANSFORMATION

- Developing a real-time peer-to-peer (P2P) network to create a decentralized HC ecosystem.
- For the sake of maintaining the secrecy and security of user information.
- To a great extent, blockchain technology may improve medical treatment.
- Soon, we will have more effective diagnostic tools, therapeutic options, and prevention measures.

- Knowing that you have a healthcare provider that is both skilled and caring can make all the difference in the world.
- Value-based care is advantageous for both patients and doctors [96].

1.5.1 WHAT IS A BLOCKCHAIN SYSTEM?

There are essentially three pillars that make up the healthcare system:

- Primary care physicians and hospitals, examples include those who work in the medical field, such as doctors, nurses, technicians, and hospital administrators.
- Professions and operations related to an emerging need [97].
- Clientele in the healthcare industry, patients in particular.

This chapter looks at how constituent service providers can improve the health of their clients by using remote services that rely on technology [98]. Each year, more instances of medical industry security and privacy breaches become public knowledge. The medical records of 37 million people were compromised in more than 300 breaches between 2010 and 2017 [99]. As healthcare becomes increasingly digitized, concerns have arisen about patients' rights to control their data and how it is stored and used [100]. It has been suggested that blockchain might be used to solve some of healthcare's most serious issues [101], including the secure transfer of patient health records and the strict adherence to data privacy regulations.

1.5.2 HOW DOES BLOCKCHAIN HEALTHCARE SYSTEM WORK?

In a blockchain, the database is managed by the framework of verified nodes. The nodes themselves store blocks of information that cannot be altered and may be strongly shared across participants in the network. Data can be stored and recorded through the application of cryptographic signatures and the adoption of consensus procedures [102]. When applying the BCT to the healthcare industry, where there is a great deal of data to be distributed and exchanged, data preservation becomes an important consideration. There have been several iterations of blockchain development, and the technology has found usage in many different contexts. The focus is shifting from Bitcoin to other digital assets that may be stored and exchanged using blockchain technology in many industries, including real estate and finance [103]. In its third iteration, blockchain found various non-financial uses [104]. In addition, AI has propelled blockchain technology's current fourth stage of development, which is characterized by the emergence of features like data immutability [105]. Since Blockchain can permit trustless, distributed transactions, it has found applications in many different contexts. With potential uses in fields like automated claim authentication and public health management [106], blockchain technology appears to be a perfect fit for the healthcare sector. This technology allows patients to keep their data and make their own decisions about who can access it, which could ease problems with data ownership and sharing. The right authority can now employ consensus methods to instantly integrate, update, distribute, and retrieve recorded data [107]. It's advantageous to use this technology in healthcare since it does away with the requirement for third parties to store patient information [108]. More importantly, blockchain has the potential to strengthen accountability in data management procedures owing to human error, greatly lowering the risk of data misuse [109]. Given the optimistic overtones of the blockchain's impacts on social and business development, there appears to be a disagreement about the fundamental and derived benefits of the blockchain. Even if the benefits of blockchain technology are widely believed to be overblown, a recent study indicated that businesses are likely to adopt a cautiously pragmatic stance [110]. It might be argued that the widespread adoption of blockchain has led to the technology not living up to expectations [111], particularly in terms of regulatory obstacles to specific challenges. Lack of understanding of the technical features of blockchain and its benefits for data processing on the part of patients or doctors is a major obstacle to its widespread adoption. While this technology shows promise, it may be some time before it can be employed in all phases of organizational change [112] due to security and governance problems as well as organizational and societal impediments. This could be exacerbated by the existing fog around the role of blockchain technology in the administration of justice and governmental regulations. Current research efforts are directed at finding ways to get over these obstacles so that the blockchain can spread more quickly [113].

1.5.3 RESEARCH OBJECTIVES OF BLOCKCHAIN IN THE HEALTHCARE SYSTEM

- Studying how blockchain technology might be applied to the healthcare industry and making the resulting data set freely available to researchers worldwide.

- Strategic applications of blockchain technology have been made in the healthcare sector.
- Blockchain technology may be used to identify healthcare issues and restrictions.
- Applying a characterization framework to describe and differentiate existing healthcare blockchain systems is recommended.

1.5.4 CHALLENGES AND LIMITATIONS OF IMPLEMENTING BLOCKCHAIN TECHNOLOGY IN HEALTHCARE

Despite its complexity and limitations as a multidisciplinary idea, blockchain may find applications in many different areas. Researchers in this field are trying to figure out how to neutralize or at least mitigate the effects of these factors. Several challenges arise when applying blockchain technology to the healthcare industry (i.e., technical hurdles) [114].

1.5.4.1 THROUGHPUT

Increasing the number of checks performed is necessary as the volume of transactions and the number of nodes in the network both increase. For high-throughput healthcare systems, speeding up the diagnostic process may have unintended consequences. The proposed approach may also underperform if datasets are not labeled, as it is based on finding anomalies. A number of factors, such as the system's requirements for continuous updates, the size of the keyword set, the network setup, and the amount of disc space required by a blockchain type like Ethereum software, might impact a framework's scalability and performance. Similarly, Tanwar, Parekh, & Evans [115] suggest that larger performance-related expenses may be paid by introducing specialized characteristics into existing systems, such as forming global smart agreements. In addition, a small number of studies have related problems with the performance of a proposed system to how nodes within that system are managed.

1.5.4.2 LATENCY

The time it takes for a block to be validated is thus potentially short enough to allow an attack to succeed. Since healthcare networks are complex, it's important to employ them as soon as possible during analysis to prevent compromising the results [116].

1.5.4.3 SECURITY

It's possible that having 51% of the votes might decrease the efficiency of the entire network. If the healthcare system were to fail, healthcare organizations would also be negatively impacted, making this a critical issue that has to be addressed.

1.5.4.4 RESOURCE CONSUMPTION

Using this method could waste a lot of resources because of the energy needed for mining. However, the implementation of blockchain could lead to high computing and energy costs due to the necessity for numerous devices to keep track of patients, which in turn increases the already high cost of patient monitoring (PM). It is challenging for businesses to manage these expenses [117]. In a medical blockchain, important roles are issue, preservation, and medical data sharing (MDS).

1.5.4.5 MEDICAL DATA RELEASE (MDR)

When a person visits a medical facility like a hospital, they become part of a system that keeps track of their medical history and any further tests they undergo. Entering the issuer's private key and generating a digest and hash of medical data allows the doctor to upload the data to the blockchain. Medical data codes are encrypted with symmetric keys, while real data is encrypted with public keys. All of us are arriving at the hospital at the same time to see the patient [118].

1.5.4.6 MEDICAL DATA STORAGE (MDS)

After the medical facility has received the information, the patient verifies their signature. Using the original medical data's private decryption key, we can read the signature and decrypt the encrypted medical data, and then we can build a new encryption key for cloud storage and a cloud signature.

1.5.4.7 MEDICAL DATA SHARING (MDS)

Users can grant access to a third-party institution, such as a hospital, for limited access to their health records and remove that access at any moment through the access control system. The medical blockchain will store the decryption keys, permissions to use them, and expiration dates for third-party agencies. In recent years, blockchain technology has received considerable attention as a potential means of protecting sensitive patient information, facilitating the transmission of biomedical and electronic health records (EHR), simulating cognitive processes, and more. The blockchain infrastructure relies heavily on a decentralized P2P network. Distributed consensus algorithms combine methods, encryption, and mathematics to get over the limitations of conventional methods of synchronizing distributed databases. Blockchain technology is characterized by open-source software, immutability, anonymity, decentralization, and transparency [119].

1.6 KEY COMPONENTS OF BLOCKCHAIN TECHNOLOGY

1.6.1 DECENTRALIZED

There is no restriction on who can use the database because it uses a completely open-access control model. Numerous systems exist that can access, monitor, store, or update data.

1.6.2 TRANSPARENT

It may be simple for potential users to update the data that is gathered and stored on a blockchain. As a counterpoint, the impossibility of tampering with or stealing data, thanks to the blockchain's inherent transparency, is an attractive prospect.

1.6.3 IMMUTABLE

The consensus of more than 51% of the network's nodes is required to make changes to a record after it has been saved.

1.6.4 AUTONOMY

A record cannot be changed after it has been saved unless more than 51% of the network's nodes agree to make the change.

1.6.5 OPEN SOURCE

Due to blockchain technology, all users on a network will have access to publicly available source code. As a bonus, this infinite flexibility opens the door to a wide range of potential future applications, including making it simpler for everyone to study papers in the open.

1.6.6 ANONYMITY

This technology is more secure and reliable because its origin and destination cannot be determined. Each new transaction in this network must be validated by a participating node. Blockchain transactions become increasingly immutable as they are verified by every node in the network [120].

1.7 APPLICATION OF BLOCKCHAIN IN HEALTHCARE

Instead, the banking and cryptocurrency sectors have been the primary adopters of blockchain technology. This technological potential is best illustrated by the fact that blockchain can be used to stabilize and secure data sets that enable users to communicate with specialized genetics, medicine, monitoring, and neuroscience transactions [121].

1.7.1 ELECTRONIC HEALTH RECORDS (EHRS)

There is no need for any kind of manual intervention when integrating EHR software into a central blockchain directory, beginning at the time of data production and continuing through the time of data recovery.

1.7.2 CLINICAL RESEARCH

Blockchain technology has created a decentralized, secure environment for all possible exchanges of data in clinical research. This paves the way for trustworthy information sharing amongst various academic institutions.

1.7.3 MEDICAL FRAUD DETECTION

Blockchain can be used to spot fraudulent activity and make a transaction that is both transparent and secure because it does not allow transactions to be duplicated or altered [122].

1.7.4 NEUROSCIENCE RESEARCH

The potential applications of Blockchain are numerous, and they range from cognitive enhancement to reproduction to perhaps replication of the brain itself. It seems clear that blockchain technology is the future of brain storage platforms.

1.7.5 PHARMACEUTICAL INDUSTRY AND RESEARCH

When it comes to the pharmaceutical industry, blockchain has the potential to provide total traceability by keeping tabs on the whole supply chain. By documenting the product's history from production to sale, counterfeiters and thieves of pharmaceuticals are foiled [123].

1.7.6 WORKING PRINCIPLES IN HEALTHCARE

Blockchain technology has many potential uses in the healthcare industry, including the management and processing of data. Its unrivaled safety and capacity for sharing medical data and resources are mostly attributable to its section flexibility and capacity to do so. Blockchain is at the heart of many cutting-edge medical advances being made today [124]. You can classify new healthcare solutions built on the blockchain into four broad categories:

- Data sources blockchain platforms;
- Healthcare apps;
- Stakeholder participation; and
- New possibilities are arising as a result of developments in electronic medical records (EMR), cloud data protection and privacy rules, health information management, and easy access to and interchange of patient data.

Companies that rely heavily on data, such as those in the healthcare industry, have a responsibility to ensure, store, exchange, and manage the seamless incorporation of their data. These critical problems are amenable to reliable and efficient solutions using blockchain technology. There has been a significant uptick in interest in blockchain technology from people and businesses of all sizes. There are a number of characteristics that make this a reality, including anonymity, decentralization, appropriateness, and perseverance [125].

High-performance teams are necessary for developing a healthcare system that is more patient-centered, integrated, and fruitful. The healthcare industry is crucial to medical billing. This means that without a reliable price structure, quality service cannot be guaranteed. A patient's therapy can officially begin during the check-out phase once they've been admitted to the hospital [126, 127].

1.8 BENEFITS AND DRAWBACKS FOR HEALTHCARE APPLICATIONS OF BLOCKCHAIN

In this section, we examined the benefits and drawbacks of utilizing blockchain technology in the healthcare industry, and we have included Tables 1.1 and 1.2 to illustrate these points. Give an account of both the upsides and the potential drawbacks of using blockchain technology in healthcare [128].

Table 1.1 demonstrates the advantages of blockchain in healthcare. While Table 1.2 shows the disadvantages of blockchain in healthcare.

TABLE 1.1 Advantages of Blockchain in Healthcare

Advantages	Description
Data security and privacy have been upgraded.	Blockchain technology makes it impossible to edit, delete, or tamper with data once it has been saved, making it an ideal medium for storing sensitive medical information. Medical records stored on a blockchain are typically encrypted, timestamped, and chronologically linked. Patient's identities and personal information can be safeguarded when medical records are stored on a blockchain network using cryptographic keys.
Health data ownership	Patients should have access to and ownership of their data. A patient's health information must be protected from unauthorized access and use, and this activity must be detected. In the future, advanced cryptographic protocols and Blockchain-based smart contracts may be able to fulfill these requirements.
Availability/ robustness	Due to the records being stored on multiple nodes, a blockchain can withstand attacks on its data integrity, data deficiency, and accessibility.
Transparency and trust.	The decentralized nature of blockchain makes it ideal for usage in the healthcare industry. It may be helpful to give healthcare workers easier access to these apps.
Data verifiability	The authenticity and veracity of the records stored on a blockchain can be confirmed even if the user does not have access to the underlying plaintext. This tool could be useful for evaluating documents related to supply chain management and insurance claims.
Decentralization	Many different groups and individuals have a vested interest in healthcare; hence, its management must be decentralized. Blockchain has the potential to serve as a decentralized backbone for data management, making it possible for all parties involved to have equal access to and authority over the same medical records.

TABLE 1.2 Disadvantages of Blockchain in Healthcare

Drawbacks	Description
Data Ownership	Where do you see medical records going in the future? Who will have permission to view the materials? Nothing of such has been established as of the time of this writing.
Cost	Without an up-front understanding of the resources required for healthcare blockchain technology, it will be difficult to get widespread adoption.
Rules and regulations	Blockchain technology opens up many possibilities in the medical area. The HIPAA Act and other current privacy regulations may conflict with developing healthcare blockchain initiatives.
Uncertainty	There are now just a small number of initiatives using undefined but promising blockchain technology. Not having an urgent need for such a solid blockchain paradigm is a significant barrier.

1.9 CONCEPTION AND IMPLEMENTATION OF ETHEREUM-BASED SYSTEMS

The final product of development inside this framework is a distributed application (DApp) that communicates with a private blockchain network and a distributed file system (DFS). The smart contract infrastructure for the medical blockchain was developed on Ethereum. The network is open source and rapidly growing, with a sizable public DApp library and a substantial user base. In the platform's current consensus algorithm to create distributed systems, two of the most promising consensus methods are delegated proof-of-stake (DPoS) and practical byzantine fault tolerance (PBFT) [129]. When DFS data is compared to ledger entries, the DApp can spot discrepancies, unauthorized data additions, and missing entities. There are auditable checkpoints at every stage. These solidity-based smart contracts rely on functions, events, state variables, and modifiers. Transactions have been made using smart contracts on the Remix and Kovan test networks. Building a smart contract requires three stages: coding in the Solidity programming language, compilation, and public announcement. The real-time compiler Solidity is used to generate the bytecode. The Ethereum Wallet allows smart contract installations to be made public on the Ethereum blockchain when this smart contract is deployed on the blockchain; it transforms machine-level byte code, with each byte representing an operation. One of the miners has recognized it. Therefore, block-1 can now be validated. EVM-2 queries the web-based data, merges it into transaction (TX), and then deploys it to the blockchain as soon as a user submits a request through the online interface. Within Block 2, adjustments were made to TX's existing condition. To see how TX affects the contract states it has recorded, Node 3 must synchronize to Block-2 or above [130].

Ethereum smart contracts are used to construct digital representations of current medical records that are distributed across the network's nodes; this allows for improved healthcare delivery based on the blockchain. Metadata, permissions, and data integrity are all constructed into the contracts we create. Cryptographically signed instructions for the administration of these assets are transmitted via blockchain transactions in our system. Data alterations are enforced by legitimate transactions and are performed through the contract's state-transition functionalities. If the rules governing a given medical record can be represented computationally, they can be incorporated into the structure of these regulations [131]. The policy may need two distinct consent transactions to be sent from patients and healthcare providers before allowing access to a third party, for instance. Blockchain smart contracts are the foundation of a system we developed specifically for healthcare's intricate workflows. Medical workflows can be streamlined with the help of smart contracts, which can also be used to control who has access to certain pieces of patient information.

A smart contract on blockchain technology can manage rights and access data. Different parties participate in this scheme. This enhances the doctor-patient dialog. Smart contracts allow data permission. It traces ID actions from origin to surrender. Smart contracts have well-described functions and processes. Smart contracts reduce the need for one organization to oversee and approve operations, saving administrative costs [132].

Data transactions are sealed by private keys (patient or doctor). The system's blocks represent the ownership and access levels of members' data. Smart contracts on the blockchain automate and log transitions between states (for instance, a new system record being created or a shift in viewing privileges). Using Ethereum smart contracts, we keep track of who has access to a patient's medical record and how to retrieve it (information pointers). A cryptographic hash is added to the blockchain to guarantee the authenticity of all transactions. Records can be shared between patients and doctors. In either situation, the recipient is alerted so they can double-check the accuracy of the updated data before giving their final verdict. This helps to maintain the interest of the record keepers. This system emphasizes accessibility by centralizing the patient-provider connections of its users. We employ public-key cryptography to verify identities and domain name system lookups to associate a given name or Social Security number with an individual's Ethereum address [133]. After the blockchain verifies permissions, an off-chain synchronization mechanism handles the exchange of information between the patient and the provider's database. P2P network PEDIGREE 9x by 2020. Smart contracts on the blockchain automate and log transitions between states. We implement a cryptographic hash into the blockchain to guarantee the authenticity of all transactions. Documentation between patients and doctors can be shared. Medical processes have been established using blockchain smart contracts. Care for patients in need of routine medical treatment, diagnosis, or surgery. When it comes to healthcare, smart contracts help patients, doctors, and institutions minimize delays in a medical database retrieval, analysis, and management system [134].

1.9.1 INFORMATION SHARING REGARDING LAB TESTS AND RESULTS

The primary goal is to facilitate communication between the various parties involved in a patient's care by using blockchain smart contracts to enable the sharing of therapeutic information among laboratories, physicians, emergency rooms, and other partners. Here's a scenario: a patient needs blood work and makes a trip to the lab. Patients are notified through the Ethereum blockchain when their processed test results are ready; patients have the option of allowing the laboratory to encode information and place it on the Ethereum blockchain, and laboratories then save the processed results in patients' medical records. Patients provide their permission to have their information stored on a distributed ledger. An unresponsive patient would not prevent emergency room professionals from accessing their medical records on the Ethereum blockchain and providing individualized care in the event of a medical emergency. Patients can save time and effort by not having to physically bring lab results or organize faxing data to many providers because they are already kept digitally on the healthcare blockchain [135]. Furthermore, he makes sure that his doctors have all the data they need to give him the best care possible. By eliminating the need to print and mail or fax individual test results to suppliers, laboratories can save money on regulatory fees. Patients and medical facilities can also get payments from insurance companies through the healthcare blockchain.

1.9.2 IMPROVEMENTS IN PATIENT-PROVIDER INTERACTION THROUGH IMPROVED COMMUNICATION

Through the use of smart contracts, this request is immediately transmitted to the primary care physician. A physician's response to a patient's request for a referral to a specialist should reflect careful thought about the situation. All data about a patient's treatment history must be recorded in the EHR. Importantly, smart contracts on the Ethereum blockchain define the particular rules for who can access a patient's record and to what extent in a local database. Here, the patient has again formally requested a certain course of medical care; therefore, the agreement's stringent framework dictates that this application is forwarded to the appropriate expert [136]. When a primary care physician determines that a patient might benefit from seeing a specialist, they will make the recommendation, and the patient will be transferred to that specialist's care. The EHR should contain all data relevant to the patient's treatment history. Remember that smart contracts on the Ethereum blockchain regulate the access privileges for patient records stored in a nearby database. Here, medical professionals won't have to delay attending to patients while they await an answer from the insurance company. All of this will be managed automatically by smart contracts, reducing the number of appeals brought about by the incorrect reading of manually generated prior authorization forms, saving time, and minimizing human error associated with reviewing and responding to prior authorization requests. Medical insurance providers can now make their coverage guidelines available to the public in the form of blockchain smart contracts. Providers can use the blockchain to submit requests for specialist visits, treatments, and prescriptions [137]. The payer's medical insurance smart contract could potentially make authorization choices automatically using the request data and the patient's medical history stored on the Ethereum blockchain. After that, the medical care provider receives a timely response to the authorization request. The patient and any approved third parties (laboratory, pharmacy, specialist, etc.) would have immediate access to information confirming that the therapy is covered by insurance.

1.9.3 INFORMATION FLOW

The primary goal is to streamline the time it takes to get paid by the healthcare system. As a result, doctors can continue caring for patients without having to wait for insurance companies to reply. As a result of the execution of automated smart contracts, the entire procedure will be monitored. Reduce the number of appeals that are initiated due to misinterpretation of manually written prior authorization forms and, ultimately, eliminate the need for human assessment of prior authorization requests. The health insurance company publishes its plans on the blockchain in the form of smart contracts. To get approval for a specialist visit, treatment, or prescription, a provider can use the blockchain to make the request [117]. Using the request details and the patient's medical history stored on the Ethereum blockchain, the smart contract for the payer's medical insurance may make authorization decisions automatically. When the authorization is complete, the information will be promptly sent back to the medical center. Not only could the patient but also any delegated laboratories, pharmacies, specialists, or other stakeholders could check the status of their insurance authorization in real-time. Payers now spend a large amount of time manually examining and responding to requests, which might be avoided with an automated prior authorization process. It will allow doctors to continue caring for patients without having to wait for a response from insurance companies. In addition, consumers won't have to wonder if their health plan will pay for the care their doctor prescribes. When patients and doctors have access to up-to-the-minute information on prior authorization, they can more effectively collaborate on a treatment strategy that takes into account both the individual's needs and the insurance policy's provisions [139].

1.9.4 SMART CONTRACTS ON ETHEREUM FOR HUMAN CLINICAL TRIALS

Compared to the current approach, which often requires substantial expenditures to purchase patient contact information from independent data providers and to execute comprehensive pull-marketing campaigns, this method offers a simpler and more cost-effective alternative for the pharmaceutical and medical device industries to recruit participants for clinical trials. Making it feasible to execute smart contracts for clinical trials on the Ethereum network is the primary goal, with the expectation that this will encourage more individuals to participate in medical research and ultimately result in better care for those who do. Protocol registration, common research data, screening, and enrollment records will all be managed via this method's use of smart contracts [140].

The pharmaceutical company queries the Ethereum blockchain for participant details. After patients have been selected, the organization gives them a message with a link to a mobile app where they may view their whole medical history, including the outcomes of any lab tests they may have participated in. With the patient's approval, a pharmaceutical company's bill paid through a smart contract would be split between the patient and the labs that provided the accurate test results. Drug and medical device companies can save a lot of money on marketing and data collection if they focus their efforts on the most likely consumers. While patients would be compensated for their time and effort in participating in trials, they would also have the opportunity to try out promising new therapies. Participating laboratories would have a fresh avenue for making money off their findings [141].

1.9.5 HEALTHCARE REIMBURSEMENT DATA FLOW

Getting compensated by the healthcare system faster is the key focus. Therefore, doctors can continue treating patients without waiting for responses from insurance companies. The entire process will be tracked as a result of the execution of automated smart contracts. Several payment methods have been used for healthcare reimbursement, with differing degrees of efficiency. Regardless of the arrangement in which these mechanisms are employed, the resulting systems must pay according to the volume, complexity, and caliber of care provided. In addition to increasing the precision and effectiveness of reimbursement processes, extending the use of the electronic medical record (EMR) to track patient behavior, provider practices, and organizational operations may also raise the standard of healthcare.

1.10 CHALLENGES AND SOLUTIONS OF BLOCKCHAIN IN HEALTHCARE

This new technology offers a wide variety of applications across a wide range of industries.

1.10.1 PRIVACY AND SECURITY OF DATA

In the event of an unexpected medical crisis, the patient must appoint one or more representatives who have access to the patient's records and health information without the consent of the third party. Patient data privacy and security are now in jeopardy because the agent can grant access to a group of people. Incorporating high-security technologies into data may restrict users' access to certain conversations. The security of blockchain networks may be compromised by a 51% assault. More than half of the blockchain is being used by miners in this attack. To prevent subsequent transactions from being processed without their consent, miners are given the power to govern the network. According to Coin Desk's reporting, this latest attack increases the risk that private, inaccurate information about a patient is stored in the patient's medical record [143].

1.10.2 MANAGING STORAGE CAPACITY

With blockchain, transaction data of a restricted kind can be kept and processed without the need for massive amounts of storage, which is an issue related to the efficient usage of available storage space. The scope of the healthcare sector-wide storage problems became increasingly apparent. Huge volumes of data are processed daily in the healthcare sector. All nodes in the blockchain network have access to medical images, including X-rays and MRI scans. It is possible to get your hands on any of them. Moreover, the databases used in this software are transactional; thus, they require high throughput. The transactional performance of record searches and reads diminishes dramatically as the database size increases. As a result, it's important to look for a blockchain solution that can handle high volumes of users and survive disruptions.

1.10.3 INTEROPERABILITY ISSUES

Another issue with blockchains is interoperability or the ability for different blockchains to communicate with each other reliably and properly across different channels of communication. Because of this problem, information sharing is impaired [138, 144].

1.10.4 STANDARDIZATION CHALLENGES

Although blockchain technology has the potential to improve healthcare, it is still in its infancy in this field. In addition, there will be numerous options for tried-and-true international benchmarks. These already existing standards may be used to guide the types, sizes, and forms of data used in blockchain-based applications. The information we share should be protected, too, by adhering to these guidelines.

1.11 CONCLUSION

Blockchain technology will improve data privacy, confidentiality, and interoperability in the healthcare industry of the future, where the patient will occupy center stage. HIE (health information exchange) allows for these records to be shared in a way that is more streamlined, decentralized, and safe than ever before. The benefits, disadvantages, and future applications of the digital revolution in healthcare are investigated with the use of blockchain technology. Although blockchain is still a young technology, its applications in the medical field have expanded quickly in recent years. Technology based on distributed ledgers, or blockchains, may simplify processes while simultaneously facilitating trustless collaboration and the safekeeping of immutable data. For example, in a blockchain-based system, encryption can be used to verify a patient's identity and strengthen the reliability of stored information. Distributed ledger technology (DLT) allows authorized users to add transaction records to a shared ledger but not delete or modify existing ones. All transactions are encrypted, and the blockchain ensures that the network is tested before use. This study examines the usage of blockchain technology in healthcare, the challenges it faces, and how it could be utilized to build a robust system for storing and exchanging medical records.

ACKNOWLEDGMENT

The authors are highly thankful to the Department of Pharmacy, Faculty of Pharmaceutical Sciences Rama University, for providing library facilities for the literature survey.

FUNDING

This research did not receive any type-specific grant from funding agencies in the public, commercial, or not-for-profit sector.

CONFLICT OF INTEREST

The authors have no conflicts of interest to declare.

KEYWORDS

- **artificial intelligence**
- **blockchain**
- **digital health trends**
- **electronic health**
- **healthcare**
- **Internet of things**
- **neuroscience**

REFERENCES

1. Malik, H., Farooq, M. S., Khelifi, A., Abid, A., Qureshi, J. N., & Hussain, M. (2020). A comparison of transfer learning performance versus health experts in disease diagnosis from medical imaging. *IEEE Access, 8*, 139367–139386.
2. Scheerhagen, M., Van, S. H. F., Birnie, E., Franx, A., & Bonsel, G. J., (2015). Measuring client experiences in maternity care under change: Development of a questionnaire based on the WHO responsiveness model. *PloS One, 10*(2), e0117031.
3. Liao, L., Chen, M., Rodrigues, J. J., Lai, X., & Vuong, S., (2012). A novel web-enabled healthcare solution on HealthVault system. *Journal of Medical Systems, 36*(3), 1095–1105.
4. Devadass, L., Sekaran, S. S., & Thinakaran, R., (2017). Cloud computing in healthcare. *International Journal of Students' Research in Technology & Management, 5*(1), 25–31.
5. Talesh, S. A. (2018). Data breach, privacy, and cyber insurance: How insurance companies act as "compliance managers" for businesses. *Law & Social Inquiry, 43*(2), 417–440.
6. McCoy, T. H., & Perlis, R. H., (2018). Temporal trends and characteristics of reportable health data breaches, 2010–2017. *JAMA, 320*(12), 1282–1284.
7. Meinert, E., Alturkistani, A., Foley, K., Osama, T., Car, J., Majeed, F., Van, V. H., et al. (2019). *Implementation of Blockchains in Healthcare: Protocol for a Systematic Review. JMIR Res Protoc. 8*(2), e10994.
8. Rupasinghe, T., Burstein, F., Rudolph, C., & Strange, S., (2019). Towards a blockchain-based fall prediction model for aged care. In: *Proceedings of the Australasian Computer Science Week Multiconference* (pp. 1–10).
9. Angraal, S., Krumholz, H. M., & Schulz, W. L., (2017). Blockchain technology: Applications in health care. *Circulation: Cardiovascular Quality and Outcomes, 10*(9), e003800.
10. Hölbl, M., Kompara, M., Kamišalić, A., & Nemec, Z. L., (2018). A systematic review of the use of blockchain in healthcare. *Symmetry, 10*(10), 470.

11. Agbo, C. C., Mahmoud, Q. H., & Eklund, J. M., (2019). Blockchain technology in healthcare: A systematic review. In: *Healthcare* (Vol. 7, No. 2, p. 56). MDPI.
12. O'Donoghue, O., Vazirani, A. A., Brindley, D., & Meinert, E. (2019). Design choices and trade-offs in health care blockchain implementations: Systematic review. *Journal of Medical Internet Research, 21*(5), e12426.
13. Abou, J. J., & Saade, R. G., (2019). Blockchain applications–usage in different domains. *IEEE Access, 7*, 45360–45381.
14. Hasselgren, A., Kralevska, K., Gligoroski, D., Pedersen, S. A., & Faxvaag, A., (2020). Blockchain in healthcare and health sciences—A scoping review. *International Journal of Medical Informatics, 134*, 104040.
15. Risius, M., & Spohrer, K., (2017). A blockchain research framework. *Business & Information Systems Engineering, 59*(6), 385–409.
16. Ozdagoglu, G., Damar, M., & Ozdagoglu, A., (2020). The state of the art in blockchain research (2013–2018): Scientometrics of the related papers in Web of Science and Scopus. *Digital Business Strategies in Blockchain Ecosystems*, 569–599.
17. Kitchenham, B., Brereton, O. P., Budgen, D., Turner, M., Bailey, J., & Linkman, S., (2009). Systematic literature reviews in software engineering–a systematic literature review. *Information and Software Technology, 51*(1), 7–15.
18. Aznoli, F., & Navimipour, N. J., (2017). Cloud services recommendation: Review the recent advances and suggest future research directions. *Journal of Network and Computer Applications, 77*, 73–86.
19. Gopalakrishnan, S., & Ganeshkumar, P., (2013). Systematic reviews and meta-analysis: Understanding the best evidence in primary healthcare. *Journal of Family Medicine and Primary Care, 2*(1), 9.
20. Mendling, J., Weber, I., Aalst, W. V., Brocke, J. V., Cabanillas, C., Daniel, F., Debois, S., et al., (2018). Blockchains for business process management challenges and opportunities. *ACM Transactions on Management Information Systems (TMIS), 9*(1), 1–6.
21. Kuo, T. T., Gabriel, R. A., & Ohno-Machado, L., (2019). Fair compute loads enabled by blockchain: Sharing models by alternating client and server roles. *Journal of the American Medical Informatics Association, 26*(5), 392–403.
22. Swan, M., (2015). *Blockchain: Blueprint for a New Economy.* "O'Reilly Media, Inc.
23. Efanov, D., & Roschin, P., (2018). The all-pervasiveness of the blockchain technology. *Procedia Computer Science, 123*, 116–421.
24. Miau, S., & Yang, J. M., (2018). Bibliometrics-based evaluation of the blockchain research trend: 2008–March 2017. *Technology Analysis & Strategic Management, 30*(9), 1029–1045.
25. Yli-Huumo, J., Ko, D., Choi, S., Park, S., & Smolander, K., (2016). Where is current research on blockchain technology?—A systematic review. *PloS One, 11*(10), e0163477.
26. Angelis, J., & Da Silva, E. R., (2019). Blockchain adoption: A value driver perspective. *Business Horizons., 62*(3), 307–314.
27. Adanur, B., Bakir-Güngör, B., & Soran, A., (2020). Blockchain-based fog computing applications in healthcare. In: *2020 28th Signal Processing and Communications Applications Conference (SIU)* (pp. 1–4). IEEE.
28. Zhang, P., White, J., Schmidt, D. C., Lenz, G., & Rosenbloom, S. T., (2018). FHIRChain: Applying blockchain to securely and scalably share clinical data. *Computational and Structural Biotechnology Journal, 16*, 267–278.

29. Mettler, M., (2016). Blockchain technology in healthcare: The revolution starts here. In: *2016 IEEE 18th International Conference on e-Health Networking, Applications, and Services (Healthcom)* (pp. 1–3). IEEE.
30. Kuo, T. T., Kim, H. E., & Ohno-Machado, L., (2017). Blockchain distributed ledger technologies for biomedical and health care applications. *Journal of the American Medical Informatics Association, 24*(6), 1211–1220.
31. Soltanisehat, L., Alizadeh, R., Hao, H., & Choo, K. K., (2020). Technical, temporal, and spatial research challenges and opportunities in blockchain-based healthcare: A systematic literature review. *IEEE Transactions on Engineering Management.*
32. Cios, K. J., & Moore, G. W., (2002). Uniqueness of medical data mining. *Artificial Intelligence in Medicine, 26*(1, 2), 1–24.
33. Ji, Y., Zhang, J., Ma, J., Yang, C., & Yao, X., (2018). BMPLS: Blockchain-based multi-level privacy-preserving location sharing scheme for telecare medical information systems. *Journal of Medical Systems, 42*(8), 1–3.
34. Ito, K., Tago, K., & Jin, Q., (2018). i-Blockchain: A blockchain-empowered individual-centric framework for privacy-preserved use of personal health data. In: *2018 9th International Conference on Information Technology in Medicine and Education (ITME)* (pp. 829–833). IEEE.
35. Taherdoost, H. (2023). The Role of Blockchain in Medical Data Sharing. *Cryptography 7*, 36.
36. Precht, H., & Marx, G. J., (2021). Usage of multiple independent blockchains for enhancing privacy using the example of the bill of lading. In: *International Congress on Blockchain and Applications* (pp. 300–309). Springer, Cham.
37. Afrooz, S., & Navimipour, N. J., (2017). Memory designing using quantum-dot cellular automata: Systematic literature review, classification, and current trends. *Journal of Circuits, Systems, and Computers, 26*(12), 1730004.
38. Ahmad, M. O., Dennehy, D., Conboy, K., & Oivo, M. (2018). Kanban in software engineering: A systematic mapping study. *Journal of Systems and Software, 137*, 96–113.
39. Mehta, N., & Pandit, A., (2018). Concurrence of big data analytics and healthcare: A systematic review. *International Journal of Medical Informatics, 114*, 57–65.
40. Zhang, R., Simon, G., & Yu, F., (2017). Advancing Alzheimer's research: A review of big data promises. *International Journal of Medical Informatics, 106*, 48–56.
41. Behera, R. K., Bala, P. K., & Dhir, A., (2019). The emerging role of cognitive computing in healthcare: A systematic literature review. *International Journal of Medical Informatics, 129*, 154–166.
42. Page, M. J., McKenzie, J. E., Bossuyt, P. M., Boutron, I., Hoffmann, T. C., Mulrow, C. D., Shamseer, L., et al., (2021). The PRISMA 2020 statement: An updated guideline for reporting systematic reviews. *Systematic Reviews, 10*(1), 372.
43. Yaqoob, I., Salah, K., Jayaraman, R., & Al-Hammadi, Y., (2021). Blockchain for healthcare data management: Opportunities, challenges, and future recommendations. *Neural Computing and Applications*, 1–6.
44. Du, X., Chen, B., Ma, M., & Zhang, Y. (2021). Research on the application of blockchain in smart healthcare: Constructing a hierarchical framework. *Journal of Healthcare Engineering.*
45. Badr, S., Gomaa, I., & Abd-Elrahman, E., (2018). Multi-tier blockchain framework for IoT-EHRs systems. *Procedia Computer Science, 141*, 159–166.

46. Casado-Vara, R., & Corchado, J., (2019). Distributed e-health wide-world accounting ledger via blockchain. *Journal of Intelligent & Fuzzy Systems, 36*(3), 2381–2386.
47. Dagher, G. G., Mohler, J., Milojkovic, M., & Marella, P. B., (2018). Ancile: Privacy-preserving framework for access control and interoperability of electronic health records using blockchain technology. *Sustainable Cities and Society, 39*, 283–297.
48. Dhagarra, D., Goswami, M., Sarma, P. R., & Choudhury, A. (2019). Big data and blockchain supported conceptual model for enhanced healthcare coverage: The Indian context. *Business Process Management Journal.*
49. Dwivedi, A. D., Srivastava, G., Dhar, S., & Singh, R., (2019). A decentralized privacy-preserving healthcare blockchain for IoT. *Sensors, 19*(2), 326.
50. Fan, K., Wang, S., Ren, Y., Yang, K., Yan, Z., Li, H., & Yang, Y., (2018). Blockchain-based secure time protection scheme in IoT. *IEEE Internet of Things Journal, 6*(3), 4671–4679.
51. Firdaus, A., Anuar, N. B., Razak, M. F., Hashem, I. A., Bachok, S., & Sangaiah, A. K., (2018). Root exploit detection and features optimization: Mobile device and blockchain-based medical data management. *Journal of Medical Systems, 42*(6), 1–23.
52. Griggs, K. N., Ossipova, O., Kohlios, C. P., Baccarini, A. N., Howson, E. A., & Hayajneh, T., (2018). Healthcare blockchain system using smart contracts for secure automated remote patient monitoring. *Journal of Medical Systems, 42*(7), 1–7.
53. Guo, R., Shi, H., Zhao, Q., & Zheng, D. (2018). Secure attribute-based signature scheme with multiple authorities for blockchain in electronic health records systems. *IEEE Access, 6*, 11676–11686.
54. Hussein, A. F., ArunKumar, N., Ramirez-Gonzalez, G., Abdulhay, E., Tavares, J. M., & De Albuquerque, V. H., (2018). A medical records management and security blockchain-based system supported by a genetic algorithm and discrete wavelet transform. *Cognitive Systems Research, 52*, 1–11.
55. Hyla, T., & Pejaś, J., (2019). eHealth integrity model based on permissioned blockchain. *Future Internet, 11*(3), 76.
56. Islam, N., Faheem, Y., Din, I. U., Talha, M., Guizani, M., & Khalil, M. (2019). A blockchain-based fog computing framework for activity recognition as an application to e-healthcare services. *Future Generation Computer Systems, 100*, 569–578.
57. Jamil, F., Hang, L., Kim, K., & Kim, D., (2019). A novel medical blockchain model for drug supply chain integrity management in a smart hospital. *Electronics, 8*(5), 505.
58. Kaur, H., Alam, M. A., Jameel, R., Mourya, A. K., & Chang, V., (2018). A proposed solution and future direction for blockchain-based heterogeneous Medicare data in cloud environment. *Journal of Medical Systems, 42*(8), 1–1.
59. Lee, S. H., & Yang, C. S., (2018). Fingernail analysis management system using microscopy sensor and blockchain technology. *International Journal of Distributed Sensor Networks, 14*(3), 1550147718767044.
60. Lee, S. J., Cho, G. Y., Ikeno, F., & Lee, T. R., (2018). BAQALC: Blockchain applied lossless efficient transmission of DNA sequencing data for next-generation medical informatics. *Applied Sciences, 8*(9), 1471.
61. Li, H., Zhu, L., Shen, M., Gao, F., Tao, X., & Liu, S., (2018). Blockchain-based data preservation system for medical data. *Journal of Medical Systems, 42*(8), 1–3.
62. Li, X., Huang, X., Li, C., Yu, R., & Shu, L., (2019). EdgeCare: Leveraging edge computing for collaborative data management in mobile healthcare systems. *IEEE Access, 7*, 22011–22025.

63. Mamoshina, P., Ojomoko, L., Yanovich, Y., Ostrovski, A., Botezatu, A., Prikhodko, P., Izumchenko, E., et al., (2018). Converging blockchain and next-generation artificial intelligence technologies to decentralize and accelerate biomedical research and healthcare. *Oncotarget, 9*(5), 5665.
64. Steinfeld, B., Scott, J., Vilander, G., Marx, L., Quirk, M., Lindberg, J., & Koerner, K., (2015). The role of lean process improvement in implementation of evidence-based practices in behavioral health care. *The Journal of Behavioral Health Services & Research, 42*(4), 504–518.
65. Nguyen, D. C., Pathirana, P. N., Ding, M., & Seneviratne, A. (2019). Blockchain for secure EHRs sharing of mobile cloud-based e-health systems. *IEEE Access, 7*, 66792–66806.
66. Al Omar, A., Bhuiyan, M. Z., Basu, A., Kiyomoto, S., & Rahman, M. S., (2019). Privacy-friendly platform for healthcare data in the cloud based on a blockchain environment. *Future Generation Computer Systems, 95*, 511–521.
67. Rahmadika, S., & Rhee, K. H., (2019). Toward privacy-preserving shared storage in untrusted blockchain P2P networks. *Wireless Communications and Mobile Computing., 2019.*
68. Shen, B., Guo, J., & Yang, Y., (2019). MedChain: Efficient healthcare data sharing via blockchain. *Applied Sciences, 9*(6), 1207.
69. Tian, H., He, J., & Ding, Y. (2019). Medical data management on blockchain with privacy. *Journal of Medical Systems, 43*(2), 1–6.
70. Uddin, M. A., Stranieri, A., Gondal, I., & Balasubramanian, V., (2018). Continuous patient monitoring with a patient-centric agent: A block architecture. *IEEE Access, 6*, 32700–32726.
71. Crosby, M., Pattanayak, P., Verma, S., & Kalyanaraman, V., (2016). Blockchain technology: Beyond Bitcoin. *Applied Innovation, 2*(6–10), 71.
72. Wong, D. R., Bhattacharya, S., & Butte, A. J. (2019). Prototype of running clinical trials in an untrustworthy environment using blockchain. *Nature Communications, 10*(1), 1–8.
73. Yang, J., Onik, M. M., Lee, N. Y., Ahmed, M., & Kim, C. S., (2019). Proof-of-familiarity: A privacy-preserved blockchain scheme for collaborative medical decision-making. *Applied Sciences, 9*(7), 1370.
74. Zhang, A., & Lin, X., (2018). Towards secure and privacy-preserving data sharing in e-health systems via consortium blockchain. *Journal of Medical Systems, 42*(8), 1–8.
75. Zheng, X., Sun, S., Mukkamala, R. R., Vatrapu, R., & Ordieres-Meré, J., (2019). Accelerating health data sharing: A solution based on the internet of things and distributed ledger technologies. *Journal of Medical Internet Research, 21*(6), e13583.
76. Tandon, A., Dhir, A., Islam, A. N., & Mäntymäki, M., (2020). Blockchain in healthcare: A systematic literature review, synthesizing framework, and future research agenda. *Computers in Industry, 122*, 103290.
77. Chukwu, E., & Garg, L., (2020). A systematic review of blockchain in healthcare: Frameworks, prototypes, and implementations. *IEEE Access, 8*, 21196–21214.
78. Celesti, A., Ruggeri, A., Fazio, M., Galletta, A., Villari, M., & Romano, A., (2020). Blockchain-based healthcare workflow for tele-medical laboratory in federated hospital IoT clouds. *Sensors, 20*(9), 2590.

79. Fusco, A., Dicuonzo, G., Dell'Atti, V., & Tatullo, M., (2020). Blockchain in healthcare: Insights on COVID-19. *International Journal of Environmental Research and Public Health, 17*(19), 7167.
80. Agbo, C. C., & Mahmoud, Q. H., (2020). Blockchain in healthcare: Opportunities, challenges, and possible solutions. *International Journal of Healthcare Information Systems and Informatics (IJHISI), 15*(3), 82–97.
81. Mazlan, A. A., Daud, S. M., Sam, S. M., Abas, H., Rasid, S. Z., & Yusof, M. F., (2020). Scalability challenges in healthcare blockchain system—A systematic review. *IEEE Access, 8*, 23663–23673.
82. Khatoon, A., (2020). A blockchain-based smart contract system for healthcare management. *Electronics, 9*(1), 94.
83. Dubovitskaya, A., Xu, Z., Ryu, S., Schumacher, M., & Wang, F., (2017). Secure and trustable electronic medical records sharing using blockchain. In: *AMIA Annual Symposium Proceedings* (Vol. 2017, p. 650). American Medical Informatics Association.
84. Azaria, A., Ekblaw, A., Vieira, T., & Lippman, A., (2016). MedRec: Using blockchain for medical data access and permission management. In: *2016 2nd International Conference on Open and Big Data (OBD)* (pp. 25–30). IEEE.
85. Alwen, J., Blocki, J., & Harsha, B. (2017). Practical graphs for optimal side-channel resistant memory-hard functions. In: *Proceedings of the 2017 ACM SIGSAC Conference on Computer and Communications Security* (pp. 1001–1017).
86. Lei, A., Cruickshank, H., Cao, Y., Asuquo, P., Ogah, C. P., & Sun, Z. (2017). Blockchain-based dynamic key management for heterogeneous intelligent transportation systems. *IEEE Internet of Things Journal, 4*(6), 1832–1843.
87. Huang, J., He, D., Obaidat, M. S., Vijayakumar, P., Luo, M., & Choo, K. K., (2021). The application of the blockchain technology in voting systems: A review. *ACM Computing Surveys (CSUR), 54*(3), 1–28.
88. Zhou, T., Shen, J., He, D., Vijayakumar, P., & Kumar, N. (2020). Human-in-the-loop-aided privacy-preserving scheme for smart healthcare. *IEEE Transactions on Emerging Topics in Computational Intelligence.*
89. Qian, Y., Shen, J., Vijayakumar, P., & Sharma, P. K. (2021). Profile matching for IoMT: A verifiable private set intersection scheme. *IEEE Journal of Biomedical and Health Informatics, 25*(10), 3794–3803.
90. Lin, C., He, D., Kumar, N., Huang, X., Vijayakumar, P., & Choo, K. K. (2019). HomeChain: A blockchain-based secure mutual authentication system for smart homes. *IEEE Internet of Things Journal, 7*(2), 818–829.
91. Saeed, H., Malik, H., Bashir, U., Ahmad, A., Riaz, S., Ilyas, M., Bukhari, W. A., & Khan, M. I., (2022). Blockchain technology in healthcare: A systematic review. *Plos One, 17*(4), e0266462.
92. De Aguiar, E. J., Faiçal, B. S., Krishnamachari, B., & Ueyama, J., (2020). A survey of blockchain-based strategies for healthcare. *ACM Computing Surveys (CSUR), 53*(2), 1–27.
93. Ganesan, R., Devi, T., Kumar, S. R., & Gayathri, N., (2022). Securing healthcare information using blockchain technology: A deep insight. In: *Blockchain Security in Cloud Computing* (pp. 253–263). Springer, Cham.
94. Xu, M., Chen, X., & Kou, G., (2019). A systematic review of blockchain. *Financ. Innov., 5*, 27.

95. Hoy, M. B., (2017). An introduction to the blockchain and its implications for libraries and medicine. *Medical Reference Services Quarterly, 36*(3), 273–279.
96. Gilboy, M. B., Heinerichs, S., & Pazzaglia, G., (2015). Enhancing student engagement using the flipped classroom. *Journal of Nutrition Education and Behavior, 47*(1), 109–114.
97. Zheng, Z., Xie, S., Dai, H. N., Chen, X., & Wang, H., (2018). Blockchain challenges and opportunities: A survey. *International Journal of Web and Grid Services, 14*(4), 352–375.
98. Gutiérrez, O., Romero, G., Pérez, L., Salazar, A., Charris, M., & Wightman, P., (2020). HealthyBlock: Blockchain-based IT architecture for electronic medical records resilient to connectivity failures. *International Journal of Environmental Research and Public Health, 17*(19), 7132.
99. Roehrs, A., Da Costa, C. A., & Da Rosa, R. R., (2017). OmniPHR: A distributed architecture model to integrate personal health records. *Journal of Biomedical Informatics, 71*, 70–81.
100. Tosh, D. K., Shetty, S., Liang, X., Kamhoua, C. A., Kwiat, K. A., & Njilla, L., (2017). Security implications of blockchain cloud with analysis of block withholding attack. In: *2017 17th IEEE/ACM International Symposium on Cluster, Cloud and Grid Computing (CCGRID)* (pp. 458–467). IEEE.
101. Wood, G., (2014). Ethereum: A secure, decentralized generalized transaction ledger. *Ethereum Project Yellow Paper, 151*(2014), 1–32.
102. Wahsheh, H. A., & Al-Zahrani, M. S., (2021). Secure and usable QR codes for healthcare systems: The case of COVID-19 pandemic. In: *2021 12th International Conference on Information and Communication Systems (ICICS)* (pp. 324–329). IEEE.
103. Tikhomirov, S., (2017). Ethereum: State of knowledge and research perspectives. In: *International Symposium on Foundations and Practice of Security* (pp. 206–221). Springer, Cham.
104. O'Dwyer, K. J., & Malone, D.. (2014). *Bitcoin Mining and its Energy Footprint.*, 280–285.
105. McFarlane, C., Beer, M., Brown, J., & Prendergast, N. (2017). *Patientory: A Healthcare Peer-to-Peer EMR Storage Network v1*. Entrust Inc.: Addison, TX, USA.
106. Li, Z., Wang, W. M., Liu, G., Liu, L., He, J., & Huang, G. Q., (2018). Toward open manufacturing: A cross-enterprises knowledge and services exchange framework based on blockchain and edge computing. *Industrial Management & Data Systems.*
107. Xia, Q. I., Sifah, E. B., Asamoah, K. O., Gao, J., Du, X., & Guizani, M., (2017). MeDShare: Trustless medical data sharing among cloud service providers via blockchain. *IEEE Access, 5*, 14757–14767.
108. Noh, S. W., Sur, C., Park, Y. H., Shin, S. U., & Rhee, K. H., (2017). Blockchain-based user-centric records management system. *Int. J. Control Autom., 10*(11), 133–144.
109. Sterne, J. A., Savović, J., Page, M. J., Elbers, R. G., Blencowe, N. S., Boutron, I., Cates, C. J., et al., (2019). Rob 2: A revised tool for assessing risk of bias in randomized trials. *BMJ*, 366.
110. Higgins, J. P., Sterne, J. A., Savovic, J., Page, M. J., Hróbjartsson, A., Boutron, I., Reeves, B., & Eldridge, S., (2016). A revised tool for assessing risk of bias in randomized trials. *Cochrane Database of Systematic Reviews, 10*(Suppl 1), 29–31.

111. McGhin, T., Choo, K. K., Liu, C. Z., & He, D. (2019). Blockchain in healthcare applications: Research challenges and opportunities. *Journal of Network and Computer Applications, 135*, 62–75.
112. Gopal, G., Suter-Crazzolara, C., Toldo, L., & Eberhardt, W., (2019). Digital transformation in healthcare–architectures of present and future information technologies. *Clinical Chemistry and Laboratory Medicine (CCLM), 57*(3), 328–335.
113. Siyal, A. A., Junejo, A. Z., Zawish, M., Ahmed, K., Khalil, A., & Soursou, G., (2019). Applications of blockchain technology in medicine and healthcare: Challenges and future perspectives. *Cryptography, 3*(1), 3.
114. Dimitrov, D. V., (2019). Blockchain applications for healthcare data management. *Healthcare Informatics Research, 25*(1), 51–56.
115. Tanwar, S., Parekh, K., & Evans, R., (2020). Blockchain-based electronic healthcare record system for healthcare 4.0 applications. *Journal of Information Security and Applications, 50*, 102407.
116. Pandey, P., & Litoriya, R., (2020). Implementing healthcare services on a large scale: Challenges and remedies based on blockchain technology. *Health Policy and Technology, 9*(1), 69–78.
117. Khan, F. A., Asif, M., Ahmad, A., Alharbi, M., & Aljuaid, H., (2020). Blockchain technology, improvement suggestions, security challenges on smart grid and its application in healthcare for sustainable development. *Sustainable Cities and Society, 55*, 102018.
118. Laskowski, M., (2017). A blockchain-enabled participatory decision support framework. In: *International Conference on Social Computing, Behavioral-Cultural Modeling and Prediction and Behavior Representation in Modeling and Simulation* (pp. 329–334). Springer, Cham.
119. Hirtan, L., Krawiec, P., Dobre, C., & Batalla, J. M., (2019). Blockchain-based approach for e-health data access management with privacy protection. In: *2019 IEEE 24th International Workshop on Computer Aided Modeling and Design of Communication Links and Networks (CAMAD)* (pp. 1–7). IEEE.
120. Al Omar, A., Bhuiyan, M. Z., Basu, A., Kiyomoto, S., & Rahman, M. S., (2019). Privacy-friendly platform for healthcare data in the cloud based on a blockchain environment. *Future Generation Computer Systems, 95*, 511–521.
121. Devibala, A., (2019). A survey on security issues in IoT for blockchain healthcare. In: *2019 IEEE International Conference on Electrical, Computer and Communication Technologies (ICECCT)* (pp. 1–7). IEEE.
122. Brunese, L., Mercaldo, F., Reginelli, A., & Santone, A., (2019). A blockchain-based proposal for protecting healthcare systems through formal methods. *Procedia Computer Science, 159*, 1787–1794.
123. Tuan, M. N., Thanh, N. N., & Le Tuan, L., (2019). Applying a mindfulness-based reliability strategy to the Internet of Things in healthcare–a business model in the Vietnamese market. Technological *Forecasting and Social Change, 140*, 54–68.
124. Tripathi, G., Ahad, M. A., & Paiva, S., (2020). S2HS-A blockchain-based approach for smart healthcare system. In: *Healthcare* (Vol. 8, No. 1, p. 100391). Elsevier.
125. Ray, P. P., Dash, D., & De, D. (2019). Edge computing for internet of things: A survey, e-healthcare case study, and future direction. *Journal of Network and Computer Applications, 140*, 1–22.

126. McGhin, T., Choo, K. K., Liu, C. Z., & He, D. (2019). Blockchain in healthcare applications: Research challenges and opportunities. *Journal of Network and Computer Applications, 135*, 62–75.
127. Sharma, A., Malviya, R., & Sundram, S. (2022). *Role of Deep Learning, Blockchain and Internet of Things in Patient Care* (pp. 48–50). Scrivener Publishing.
128. Stephanie, L., & Sharma, R. S. (2020). Digital health eco-systems: An epochal review of practice-oriented research. *International Journal of Information Management, 53*, 102032.
129. Koshechkin, K. A., Klimenko, G. S., Ryabkov, I. V., & Kozhin, P. B., (2018). Scope for the application of blockchain in the public healthcare of the Russian Federation. *Procedia Computer Science, 126*, 1323–1328.
130. Mertz, L., (2018). (Block) chain reaction: A blockchain revolution sweeps into health care, offering the possibility for a much-needed data solution. *IEEE Pulse, 9*(3), 4–7.
131. Liu, W., Zhu, S. S., Mundie, T., & Krieger, U., (2017). Advanced blockchain architecture for e-health systems. In: *2017 IEEE 19th International Conference on e-Health Networking, Applications, and Services (Healthcom)* (pp. 1–6). IEEE.
132. Hussain, S., & Lee, S., (2015). Semantic transformation model for clinical documents in big data to support healthcare analytics. In: *2015 Tenth International Conference on Digital Information Management (ICDIM)* (pp. 99–102). IEEE.
133. Chen, Y., Ding, S., Xu, Z., Zheng, H., & Yang, S., (2019). Blockchain-based medical records secure storage and medical service framework. *Journal of Medical Systems, 43*(1), 1–9.
134. Zubaydi, H. D., Chong, Y. W., Ko, K., Hanshi, S. M., & Karuppayah, S., (2019). A review of the role of blockchain technology in the healthcare domain. *Electronics, 8*(6), 679.
135. Restuccia, F., D'Oro, S., & Melodia, T., (2018). Securing the internet of things in the age of machine learning and software-defined networking. *IEEE Internet of Things Journal, 5*(6), 4829–4842.
136. Jiang, S., Cao, J., Wu, H., Yang, Y., Ma, M., & He, J., (2018). Blochie: A blockchain-based platform for healthcare information exchange. In: *2018 IEEE International Conference on Smart Computing (SmartComp)* (pp. 49–56). IEEE.
137. Dimitrov, D. V., (2019). Blockchain applications for healthcare data management. *Healthcare Informatics Research, 25*(1), 51–56.
138. Park, Y-H,, Kim, Y., & Shim, J. (2021). Blockchain-Based Privacy-Preserving System for Genomic Data Management Using Local Differential Privacy. *Electronics. 10*(23), 3019.
139. Onik, M. M., Aich, S., Yang, J., Kim, C. S., & Kim, H. C., (2019). Blockchain in healthcare: Challenges and solutions. In: *Big Data Analytics for Intelligent Healthcare Management* (pp. 197–226). Academic Press.
140. Srivastava, S., Singh, S. V., Singh, R. B., & Shukla, H. K., (2021). Digital transformation of healthcare: A blockchain study. *International Journal of Innovative Science, Engineering & Technology, 8*(5).
141. Prisco, G., (2016). *The Blockchain for Healthcare: Gem Launches Gem Health Network with Philips Blockchain lab.* Bitcoin Magazine.
142. Britton, J. R. (2015). Healthcare Reimbursement and Quality Improvement: Integration Using the Electronic Medical Record Comment on "Fee-for-Service Payment--an Evil

Practice That Must Be Stamped Out?". *Int J Health Policy Manag. 2015 May 8;4*(8), 549–551.

143. Healthcombix, (2016). Retrieved from: https://www.crunchbase.com/organization/healthcombix (accessed on 4 December 2023).

34. *Blockchain in Healthcare, Patient Benefits and More – Blockchain Unleashed*, (2018). IBM Blockchain Blog. Retrieved from: https://www.ibm.com/blogs/blockchain/2017/10/blockchain-in-healthcare-patient-benefitsandmore/ (accessed on 4 December 2023).

144. Jones, G., (2017). *Universal Health Coin (UHC)*. Retrieved from: https://www.everand.com/book/524248311/Universal-Health-Coin-The-Story-of-a-Public-Benefit-Corporation-Creating-a-Cash-Based-Health-Cost-Sharing-System-That-Utilizes-Blockchain-Technology (accessed on 4 December 2023).

CHAPTER 2

Blockchain: A New Model for Health Information Exchanges

SUSHMA YADAV,[1] AVINASH TRIPATHI,[2] SHIBU DAS,[3] MANISH YADAV,[1] and SHIVKANYA FULORIA[4]

[1]Sainik Pharmacy College, Mai Devkali, Hanumanganj, Prayagraj, Uttar Pradesh, India

[2]Department of Pharmaceutical Sciences, Sam Higginbottom University of Agriculture, Technology, and Sciences (SHUATS), Naini, Prayagraj, Uttar Pradesh, India

[3]Department of Pharmaceutical Chemistry, School of Pharmaceutical Sciences, Maharishi University of Information Technology, Lucknow, Uttar Pradesh, India

[4]Faculty of Pharmacy, AIMST University, Kedah, Malaysia

ABSTRACT

The technology that has changed our lives the most in the last 10 years is Blockchain. The financial and banking sectors are fully aware of the potential applications of blockchain technology. However, being a decentralized and distributed tool, Blockchain may be used as a strong tool for a large variety of daily purposes. Instead of centralized, concealed, exclusive, and changeable alternatives, Blockchain supports comprehensive, networked, open, unchangeable, and secure architectural approaches. Security policy, patient security, data management, sharing of information, data immutability, trust, and openness are all difficulties that contemporary healthcare systems face. Blockchain is being used more and more in the healthcare sector, which

Creating Smart Healthcare with Blockchain and Advanced Digital Technology.
Rishabha Malviya and Sonali Sundram (Eds.)

has a significant influence on the system. Indeed, the sharing and storing of health data on a web powered by Blockchain can resolve a number of issues with medical data. Interoperability is essential for a competent and efficient medical care arrangement because it enables software applications and technological platforms to enable secure and easy data sharing and make use of data exchanged between healthiness organizations and app vendors. Consequently, a lack of interconnection results in fragmented and segregated data, delayed communications, and the heterogeneous workflow tools that plague healthcare today. The following services make up a full view of a blockchain-based healthcare system: a digital health card, doctor services, mentoring insurance, and health document notary services. Blockchain allows access to longitudinally, complete, and tamper-aware medical records that are stored in dispersed systems in a secure and pseudo-anonymous way. The obstacles associated with the use of Blockchain in the healthcare sector include governance, a lack of historical precedent, privacy, sustainability, scalability, participant acceptance, and operational costs. Describes the challenges and prospects of implementing blockchain-based in the healthcare industry. It also provides a list of key manufacturers and health-related blockchain technologies. Clinical studies of telecare hospital information systems and E-health (electronic-health) were also examined and evaluated in terms of data security. This study examined conceivable future challenges such as sustainability and storage space, blockchain size, global compatibility, and uniformity. This research examined potential future obstacles such as regularity, global compliance, sustainability, and storage capacity.

2.1 INTRODUCTION

Blockchain may be a rising inventory of the business or block that is maintained by a shared or distributed database. By establishing trust, accountability, and transparency, blockchain knowledge, also known as the chain of hope, can facilitate transaction processing technologies and marketing process optimization operations [1]. A ledger system called Blockchain is assumed to assist with data management and storage in time-stamped blocks across all computing networks and connect with the utilization of encryption [2]. In 2008, the cryptocurrency Bitcoin launched blockchain technology, which has inherited properties like decentralization, transparency, and anonymity. With around 400 million transactions executed as of March 19, 2019, Bitcoin is a convincing use-case for how well blockchain technology functions [3]. Healthcare information systems have changed due to the financial use of blockchain technology. By transferring ownership of medical data to the patients themselves, blockchain technology can provide an answer that is beneficial to guard the documenting and sharing of health records while also guaranteeing the confidentiality of each patient's information [4]. We propose that blockchain technology features a wide selection of applications that can be utilized in public programs within the American healthcare system [5]. The fundamental good thing about Blockchain is that it offers answers for problems with accountability and disclosure between businesses and people that are in both parties' best interests (Figure 2.1). The employment of blockchain equipment within the healthcare business has exciting opportunities for securing stakeholder communications, delivering clinical reports quickly, and mixing different kinds of personal health information (PHI) on a safe infrastructure [6].

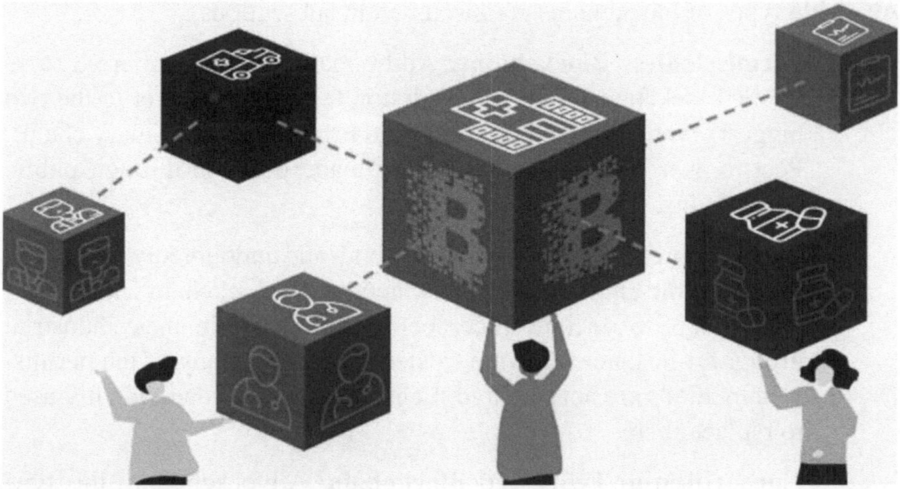

FIGURE 2.1 Blockchain technology.

2.2 BACKGROUND OF BLOCKCHAIN TECHNOLOGY

A distributed ledger that efficiently, inexpensively, and securely records transactions is how blockchain technology is described. Bitcoin's core technology, known as the Blockchain, was unveiled in 2008 by an anonymous developer going by the name Satoshi Nakamoto [7]. He created a system that functioned as a permissionless paradigm, allowing flexible joining and leaving of the node without the need for prior knowledge of consensus nodes.

From among the many possibilities available, Satoshi chose testimony-of-work as the consent method for managing the ledgers, which a few other coins now employ [8]. Since then, the business, financial, and healthcare sectors have all been using blockchain technology. Blockchain technology can safeguard patient data in the healthcare sector [9]. The majority of medical facilities are fully accessible to a central authority, which is currently in use and client-server-based. Due to a lack of privacy or security, fraudsters would be able to access patient data in this situation if a system malfunctions [10]. This technological strategy primarily immutably stores digital data in a decentralized manner to enable the secure movement of created data or metadata between networks and users. A blockchain is a listing of statistics that can be connected collectively to the usage of cryptography [11].

2.2.1 TYPES OF BLOCKCHAIN

Available types of blockchains are discussed in subsections.

1. **Permissionless Blockchains:** Additionally, they are referred to as public blockchains. Public permission fewer chains refer to the two biggest cryptocurrencies, Bitcoin and Ethereum (the primary chain). Peer-to-peer (P2P) connections are made possible through public blockchains, which include Bitcoin.
2. **Permissioned Blockchain:** The second, and undoubtedly most well-known, is the undisclosed Blockchain. It is a blockchain with known participants to operate under permissions. Within their industrial group, for instance, they are trusted; therefore, many of the permission methods are not required. Legal contracts are occasionally used to replace them.
3. **Consortium or Federated Blockchain:** A blockchain of this type eliminates the power that is given to one person. Therefore, rather than a single body, power is given in this instance to a number of people or people who form groups called federations or consortiums. Such as Quorum, Corda, and Hyperledger [12].

2.3 E-HEALTH METHOD

E-health is an innovative tool that has grown significantly in importance over time, ranging from PHR from several on-site sensors to assist in diagnosis to wireless monitoring to patient-recorded patient records, such as electronic health records (EHRs). The capacity of Blockchain to store medical data via decentralized storage on several branches of the blockchain platform is demonstrated by a complete analysis of earlier studies in the E-health system in terms of objectives, case studies, major discoveries, and security aspects (Figure 2.2) [13].

2.4 CURRENT SCENARIO OF BLOCKCHAIN TECHNOLOGY

Numerous researchers have previously explored how blockchain technology may improve healthcare data exchange and help with a range of other diagnosis applications [14]. Furthermore, an evaluation of the security, privacy, and effectiveness of patient care management systems was carried out [15]. These concerns about data safety and confidentiality can be addressed with blockchain technology. This is because, in this situation, Blockchain consists of a shared, encrypted database that serves as an everlasting, unchangeable public store of knowledge [16]. Using their public keys, patients can store their medical records on the Blockchain network, and transactions, including that information, can be stored using both the patients' distinctive IDs and community keys. Medical care organizations are able to utilize only smart contracts to admittance the patient's non-personal information when the two unique IDs match [17]. Additionally, the infrastructure for current data storage has been connected. The system can receive data input from a variety of sources, including hospital servers, doctor's offices, etc. The suggested approach successfully decentralizes medical records while maintaining security. Their framework utilized a POW-based consensus algorithm and a smart contract mechanism in order to verify a fresh block in their smart contracts system [18]. This Blockchain's secure consensus method was initially applied for the applications of Bitcoin and other cryptocurrencies. To solve a numerically difficult puzzle game, miners must find a hash of the block submitted to the transaction pool with a value less than the default. This is the basic premise of the PoW technique [19]. The miner who calculates this hash value initially verifies the transactions (or other entries) contained in the block and receives a reward. When used on a big blockchain, the PoW protocol has a significant energy consumption issue. This is demonstrated by the fact that the electricity now used for Bitcoin mining is comparable to the demands of a bigger one in the country [20].

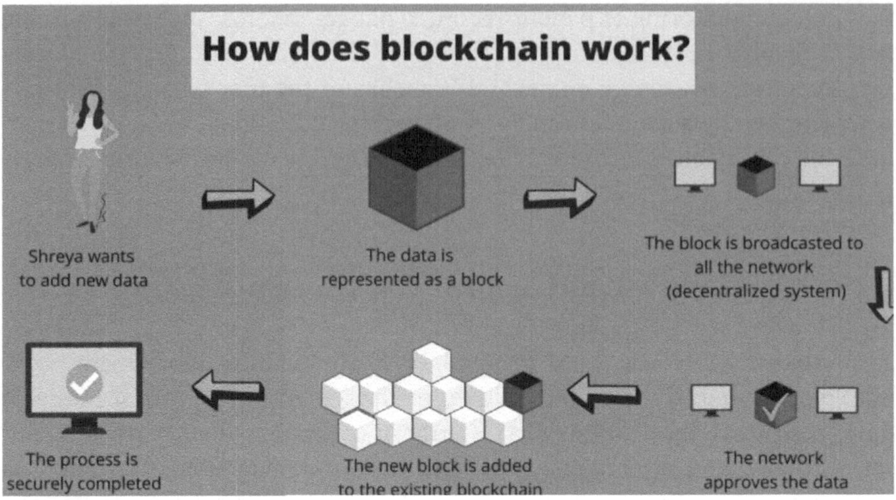

FIGURE 2.2 Blockchain process.

2.5 DATA SHARING

While delivering one of the greatest opportunities for healthcare improvement, data sharing also presents one of the biggest privacy concerns. Powles and Hodson address the need for transparency regarding the sharing of patient data with third parties by using the case study of the DeepMind relationship with the Royal Free London NHS Foundation Trust [21]. A major hindrance to effective healthcare is the absence of globally accepted patient identities and information-blocking policies. Interoperability is important as well, especially during an epidemic like the coronavirus pandemic [22]. In that instance, the appropriate hospitals and doctors from other countries should be aware of the medical details of the patients in order to offer better healthcare services. With the patient's agreement and responsibility over the data, the necessary parties in other countries might easily receive the patient's medical data using blockchain-based techniques [23]. The privacy and security of that data are seriously at stake now that this representative can grant access to a group of people to the same patient's records. The receivers will only have access to some or all of the data since high-security measures make it difficult to move the data from one block to another [24]. A blockchain-based data-sharing framework for cloud settings has been presented to handle the admittance management issue related to responsive information [25].

2.6 APPLICATION

Many industries and professions could be disrupted and revolutionized by blockchain technology. Although blockchain applications have moved to other industries, blockchain-based cryptocurrency applications are well-known and used. Numerous businesses recognize its value and begin researching its potential. Today, we are beginning to see certain blockchain use cases outside of finance and banking, including supply chain management (SCM), advertising verification, energy conservation, and healthcare [26]. Blockchain technology is used far more than just decentralized coins because of its distinctive properties. Blockchain systems can change a number of business procedures, including asset management, electronic voting, vehicle rentals, movie theaters, and many others [27, 28].

2.6.1 MEDICAL DATA MANAGEMENT

Major data sources for the healthcare industry include patient health records, complex billing, clinical trials, medical research, etc. BC aspires to enable access to a patient's complete medical history from all providers in one location for both the patient and their doctor. Blockchain can track patient health records securely, privately, and thoroughly. It increases the efficacy, disintermediation, and security of electronic medical records (EMRs). Additionally, it improves the interoperability, efficiency, and security of health information exchanges (HIEs) [24]. These facts become more important when the Centers for Medicare and Medicaid Services (CMS) begin to tie financial support to provider adoption and "meaningful use" attestation by providers. Given these approaching milestones and the varying degrees of implementation success, there are considerable questions regarding the future of the widespread adoption of EHR systems and the structure of the American healthcare system in the following 10 years [30].

2.6.2 FINANCIAL APPLICATIONS

The success of blockchain-based cryptocurrency platforms has paved the way for numerous possible applications in various financial sectors. Trusted intermediaries typically handle financial transactions between people and institutions. Blockchain can replace the services offered by these reliable middlemen, particularly the avoidance of duplicate financial transactions and the registration and confirmation of financial activity, according to its enabled design features and characteristics [31].

2.6.2.1 HEALTHCARE

Healthcare is one of those fields where a ton of data is produced. The management of scientific studies, dealing with health assurance claims, and archiving health accounts are a few examples of daily reporting on patient monitoring (PM). By decentralizing the aforementioned processes and making patients, physicians, and insurance providers the users and record managers, blockchain technology is being used in the healthcare industry [32].

2.6.2.2 ETHEREUM

Vitalik Buterin, a researcher and programmer in the field of cryptocurrencies, has developed a Next-Generation Smart Contract and Decentralized Application (DApp) Platform [5]. It makes use of a Blockchain-based distributed computing infrastructure and a Turing-complete scripting language to allow the processing of smart contracts on the Blockchain [33].

2.6.2.3 ENERGY

For the generation and delivery of energy, the energy industry is one of the most important industries in every nation. However, in the energy industry, controlling operations, including bills, trade selling, and well-groomed network and network management, is necessary for transparency regarding the marketing and selling of energy and representation for the chemical industry's piece of the equipment-machine electrical marketplace in order to give each network member actual data. Mengelkamp and other blockchain experts are the most decentralized tools intended for the micro-web power sector, according to this study's findings. The smart grid serves a crucial role in the energy sector; however, while data is being transmitted there, many risks could exist [34].

2.6.3 CHALLENGES FOR HEALTHCARE INTEROPERABILITY IN BLOCKCHAIN-BASED APPLICATIONS

The concept that data are easily changeable is one that many programs are built on. This presumption is true for the majority of centralized systems where data are handled by a dependable third party, such as Amazon Web

Services. A blockchain-based application with decentralized storage makes it difficult to alter data en masse, and its change record is logged as an unchangeable log, ensuring the record structure described in a blockchain (via smart contract) is made to enable development when necessary. Limiting change is thus a crucial issue when implementing blockchain technology in the design of health systems [35].

2.6.3.1 PUBLIC SAFETY

Addressing the problem of inadequate agency cooperation might make public safety delivery more efficient by offering a shared source of reality that each agency individually interacts with following predetermined conditions. For essential evidence to be accepted, establishing a chain of custody is frequently necessary. Blockchain technology may make it easier to trace the beginning of the chain of custody for such evidence [29].

2.7 CONCLUSION

Additionally, the study's timetable has been impacted by an increase in blockchain activity in the medical sector. The objective of this study is to ascertain the gap between Blockchain and those businesses by assessing the significant blockchain studies that have already been conducted in the health sector. Many researchers have studied how blockchain technology is used in the healthcare sector. In this study, studies on the Blockchain and healthcare underwent bibliometric analysis. This study significantly influences the growth of the healthcare sector. Researchers and practitioners have access to research opportunities in a variety of areas, including the process of exchanging health data, experimental trials, the pharma business, updates along with accessing large information, artificial intelligence (AI), 5G ultrasonic devices, safety measures, and confidentiality. The research covered the inspiration for academics and scholars as well as difficulties that could arise when analyzing Blockchain in the healthcare system.

CONFLICT OF INTEREST

The authors have no conflict of interest.

FUNDING

No funding.

KEYWORDS

- **blockchain**
- **e-health**
- **financial applications**
- **healthcare**
- **medical data management**
- **peer-to-peer insurance**
- **security**

REFERENCES

1. Sadiku, M. N., Eze, K. G., & Musa, S. M., (2018). Blockchain technology in healthcare. *Int. J. Adv. Sci. Res. Eng.*, *4*(5), 154–159.
2. Prokofieva, M., & Miah, S. J., (2019). Blockchain in healthcare. *Australasian Journal of Information Systems*, *23*.
3. Jadhav, V. D., & Moosafintavida, D. S., (2020). Blockchain in healthcare industry and its application and impact on COVID-19 digital technology transformation. *MuktShabd Journal*, *9*, 479.
4. Alla, S., Soltanisehat, L., Tatar, U., & Keskin, O., (2018). Blockchain technology in electronic healthcare systems. In: *IIE Annual Conference. Proceedings* (pp. 901–906). Institute of Industrial and Systems Engineers (IISE).
5. Randall, D., Goel, P., & Abujamra, R. (2017). Blockchain applications and use cases in health information technology. *Journal of Health & Medical Informatics*, *8*(3), 8–11.
6. Gökalp, E., Gökalp, M. O., Çoban, S., & Eren, P. E., (2018). Analyzing opportunities and challenges of integrated blockchain technologies in healthcare. *Eurosymposium on Systems Analysis and Design*, 174–183.
7. Alla, S., Soltanisehat, L., Tatar, U., & Keskin, O., (2018). Blockchain technology in electronic healthcare systems. In: *IIE Annual Conference; Proceedings* (pp. 901–906). Institute of Industrial and Systems Engineers (IISE).
8. Saha, A., Amin, R., Kunal, S., Vollala, S., & Dwivedi, S. K., (2019). Review on Blockchain technology-based medical healthcare system with privacy issues. *Security and Privacy*, *2*(5), e83.

9. Abu-Elezz, I., Hassan, A., Nazeemudeen, A., Househ, M., & Abd-Alrazaq, A., (2020). The benefits and threats of blockchain technology in healthcare: A scoping review. *International Journal of Medical Informatics*, *142*, 104246.
10. Tanwar, S., Parekh, K., & Evans, R., (2020). Blockchain-based electronic healthcare record system for healthcare 4.0 applications. *Journal of Information Security and Applications*, *50*, 102407.
11. Prokofieva, M., & Miah, S. J., (2019). Blockchain in healthcare. *Australasian Journal of Information Systems*, *23*.
12. Siyal, A. A., Junejo, A. Z., Zawish, M., Ahmed, K., Khalil, A., & Soursou, G., (2019). Applications of blockchain technology in medicine and healthcare: Challenges and future perspectives. *Cryptography*, *3*(1), 3.
13. Zubaydi, H. D., Chong, Y. W., Ko, K., Hanshi, S. M., & Karuppayah, S., (2019). A review of the role of blockchain technology in the healthcare domain. *Electronics*, *8*(6), 679.
14. Azogu, I., Norta, A., Papper, I., Longo, J., & Draheim, D., (2019). A framework for the adoption of blockchain technology in healthcare information management systems: A case study of Nigeria. In: *Proceedings of the 12th International Conference on Theory and Practice of Electronic Governance* (pp. 310–316).
15. Harshini, V. M., Danai, S., Usha, H. R., & Kounte, M. R., (2019). Health record management through blockchain technology. In: *2019 3rd International Conference on Trends in Electronics and Informatics (ICOEI)* (pp. 1411–1415). IEEE.
16. Saha, A., Amin, R., Kunal, S., Vollala, S., & Dwivedi, S. K., (2019). Review on "Blockchain technology-based medical healthcare system with privacy issues. *Security and Privacy*, *2*(5), e83.
17. Hussien, H. M., Yasin, S. M., Udzir, N. I., Ninggal, M. I. H., & Salman, S., (2021). Blockchain technology in the healthcare industry: Trends and opportunities. *Journal of Industrial Information Integration*, *22*, 100217.
18. Hasselgren, A., Kralevska, K., Gligoroski, D., Pedersen, S. A., & Faxvaag, A., (2020). Blockchain in healthcare and health sciences—A scoping review. *International Journal of Medical Informatics*, *134*, 104040.
19. Bell, L., Buchanan, W. J., Cameron, J., & Lo, O. (2018). *Applications of Blockchain within Healthcare. Blockchain* in Healthcare Today.
20. Attaran, M., (2022). Blockchain technology in healthcare: Challenges and opportunities. *International Journal of Healthcare Management*, *15*(1), 70–83.
21. Kumar, T., Ramani, V., Ahmad, I., Braeken, A., Harjula, E., & Ylianttila, M., (2018). Blockchain utilization in healthcare: Key requirements and challenges. In: *2018 IEEE 20th INTERNATIONAL Conference on e-Health Networking, Applications and Services (Healthcom)* (pp. 1–7). IEEE.
22. Siyal, A. A., Junejo, A. Z., Zawish, M., Ahmed, K., Khalil, A., & Soursou, G., (2019). Applications of blockchain technology in medicine and healthcare: Challenges and future perspectives. *Cryptography*, *3*(1), 3.
23. Zubaydi, H. D., Chong, Y. W., Ko, K., Hanshi, S. M., & Karuppayah, S., (2019). A review of the role of blockchain technology in the healthcare domain. *Electronics*, *8*(6), 679.
24. Baiod, W., Light, J., & Mahanti, A. (2020). Blockchain technology and its applications across multiple domains: A technology review. *Journal of International Technology and Information Management*, *29*(4), COV3-COV3.

25. Panda, S. K., Jena, A. K., Swain, S. K., & Satapathy, S. C., (2021). *Blockchain Technology: Applications and Challenges*. Springer International Publishing.
26. Sadiku, M. N., Eze, K. G., & Musa, S. M., (2018). Blockchain technology in healthcare. *Int. J. Adv. Sci. Res. Eng.*, *4*(5), 154–159.
27. Randall, D., Goel, P., & Abujamra, R. (2017). Blockchain applications and use cases in health information technology. *Journal of Health & Medical Informatics*, *8*(3), 8–11.
28. Sharma, A., Malviya, R., & Sundram, S., (2022). *Role of Deep Learning, Blockchain and Internet of Things in Patient Care* (pp. 50–51). Scrivener Publishing.
29. Esposito, C., De Santis, A., Tortora, G., Chang, H., & Choo, K. K. R., (2018). Blockchain: A panacea for healthcare cloud-based data security and privacy? *IEEE Cloud Computing*, *5*(1), 31–37.
30. Jena, A. K., & Dash, S. P., (2021). Blockchain technology: Introduction, applications, challenges. In: *Blockchain Technology: Applications and Challenges* (pp. 1–11). Springer, Cham.
31. Tasatanattakool, P., & Techapanupreeda, C., (2018). Blockchain: Challenges and applications. In: *2018 International Conference on Information Networking (ICOIN)* (pp. 473–475). IEEE.
32. Akram, S. V., Malik, P. K., Singh, R., Anita, G., & Tanwar, S., (2020). Adoption of blockchain technology in various realms: Opportunities and challenges. *Security and Privacy*, *3*(5), e109.
33. Navadkar, V. H., Nighot, A., & Wantmure, R., (2018). Overview of blockchain technology in government/public sectors. *International Research Journal of Engineering and Technology*, *5*(6), 2287–2292.
34. Edemekong, P. F., Annamaraju, P., & Haydel, M. J., (2018). Health insurance portability and accountability act.
35. Liang, X., Zhao, J., Shetty, S., Liu, J., & Li, D. (2017). Integrating Blockchain for data sharing and collaboration in mobile healthcare applications. In: *2017 IEEE 28th Annual International Symposium on Personal, Indoor, and Mobile Radio Communications (PIMRC)* (pp. 1–5). IEEE.

CHAPTER 3

Potential of Blockchain Technology in Tracking Disease and Pandemics

SUNITA PANCHAWAT,[1] NEERAJ SHARMA,[2]
PRADEEP KUMAR JAISWAL,[3] and DEEPIKA BAIRAGEE[1]

[1]*Department of Pharmaceutical Sciences, Mohan Lal Sukhadia University, Udaipur, Rajasthan, India*

[2]*Faculty of Pharmacy, Bhagwant University, Ajmer, Rajasthan, India*

[3]*Department of Biochemistry and Biophysics, Texas A&M University, College Station, Texas, USA*

ABSTRACT

Numerous issues have arisen as an outcome of the COVID-19 (coronavirus) pandemic over the globe. Building a framework for efficiently managing the COVID-19 outbreak requires the use of blockchain technology (BT). The most recent information on the Blockchain and how it might be used to address difficult problems brought on by the COVID-19 epidemic is collated and discussed using searches in PubMed, Scopus, and Google Scholar. In this study, we suggest a pandemic-fighting infrastructure based on blockchain technology. Furthermore, to tackle the COVID-19 pandemic problem, we identified and presented nine key blockchain applications. The World Health Organization (WHO) had to designate COVID-19 as a pandemic just one month after it began to spread quickly due to its extreme severity. The absence of a specific way to discover newly infected individuals and predict the risk of coronavirus contagion is the major issue most countries confront. Therefore, we require a technologically capable

Creating Smart Healthcare with Blockchain and Advanced Digital Technology.
Rishabha Malviya and Sonali Sundram (Eds.)

solution to address the COVID-19 problem. Decentralization, transparency, and immutability are just a few of the many attributes of blockchain technology that can help with pandemic management by spotting outbreaks early, accelerating medication distribution, and defending patient confidentiality during action.

3.1 INTRODUCTION

The medical sector is searching for new, cutting-edge technology to locate and stop the COVID-19 (coronavirus) pandemic during this period of global health crisis. Therefore, reliable and precise data are necessary to monitor and control the propagation of any infection. The current state of affairs, however, prevents the use of technology to offer accurate information regarding the spread or epidemic of a new coronavirus. Public hospitals and clinical laboratories are among the places where COVID-19 pandemic patients may be found; nevertheless, the information they provide may not be reliable since it is not monitored, properly stored, and possibly not documented in line with the specified regulations [1, 2].

Blockchain technology (BT), defined as a digital database with information that can be utilized and shared simultaneously within a vast, decentralized, and open net, can play a crucial role in resolving these kinds of issues by making it simple to track the coronavirus's spread, recognize high-risk patients, and be extremely knowledgeable to regulate the contamination in real-time. Diabetes patients have already benefited from the usage of telemedicine in the fight against the COVID-19 pandemic [1, 3]. Several technologies, such as Industry 4.0, biosensors, 3D scanning, and multi-agent systems [3, 4], can be used to identify infected patients.

A blockchain-based digital ledger that is widely dispersed, decentralized, and openly accessible. Blockchain technology is made up of three main parts: blocks, miners, and nodes. The chains are constructed from several blocks, and each block has a hash, a nonce, and data. The miners create fresh chains by engaging in a process called mining. The electronic components known as nodes keep a copy of the Blockchain and make sure that the net is running properly [6, 7]. Figure 3.1 shows how blockchain technology was utilized to treat the COVID-19 epidemic or to gather information on patients who were still actively unwell.

- Gathering the necessary information from the blockchain nodes that are participating and
- Generating raw data before converting it into a large amount of data.

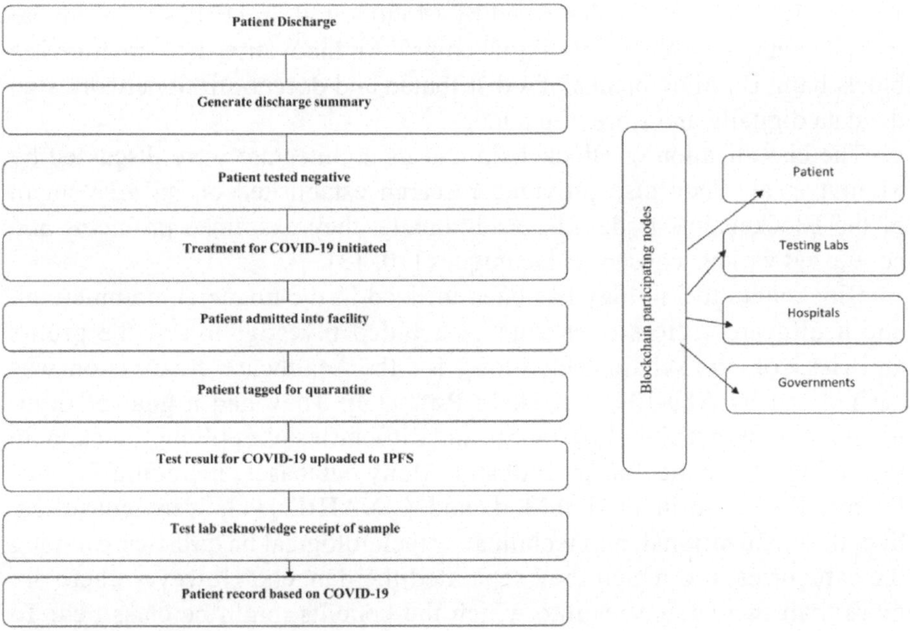

FIGURE 3.1 Blockchain technology's contribution to the COVID-19 epidemic [1].
Source: Adapted from Ref.[1]

These steps are used to build the digital document ledger that is accessible online. Blockchain technology guarantees the safety of the gathered data and aids in preserving its confidentiality. Different artificial intelligence (AI)-based technologies are used to examine blockchain-secured data. BT provides a variety of practical alternatives for the COVID-19 pandemic, including management of the medical supply chain, tracking of outbreaks, and tracking of contributions. Additionally, it is utilized to set up dependable, trustworthy, and quick data sharing among the stakeholders. Hospitals and populations confront a global lack of medical supplies to combat this epidemic [8, 9].

3.2 RESEARCH AND LITERATURE REVIEW

3.2.1 OVERVIEW OF BLOCKCHAIN TECHNOLOGY

Satoshi Nakamoto developed blockchain technology in Japan as a sort of cryptocurrency system, with the original version being known as Bitcoin [10,

12, 13]. Blockchain was described by Monrat et al. in [13] as "The fundamental technology of various digital coins." An innovative data structure is a blockchain. Building blocks of a distributed and decentralized network sign the data digitally and store it in a ledger.

The classification of Blockchain and its architecture were discussed by Monrat et al. They also provided research established on an assessment of the Blockchain's trade-offs. Additionally, they examined problems and contrasted various consensus techniques [10, 13].

Blockchain technology has been utilized in the financial, commercial, and healthcare sectors over time. A detailed investigation of the profits and risks of blockchain technology for the healthcare subdivision was carried out by Abu-Elezz et al. in Ref. [12]. They had a goal of organizing and researching the benefits and difficulties of applying blockchain technology to the healthcare industry. Many databases, including Science Direct, IEEE, Springer, PubMed, and CINAHIL [11], were consulted. Social, organizational, and technical or technological hazards were among the categories into which they separated the dangers. However, there are more than two categories into which the benefits might be classified. To validate Blockchain in healthcare, Fusco et al. provided a traceroute for a COVID-19-safe clinical practice [10, 14]. Liao created several social marketing success metrics to boost the potency of health promotion via the application of an optimization technique. He decided to make use of the F-DEMATEL (fuzzy-decision-making trial and evaluation laboratory) [10, 15]. Shen et al. [16], who suggested an effective data-sharing network named MedChain, highlighted the challenges of collecting medical exam information. The plan integrates structured P2P networks, digest chains, and blockchain technologies to solve problems with medical data gathering.

Healthcare-related processes may also be made easier with the use of blockchain capabilities like immutability, decentralization, transparency, and traceability [12]. Decentralization is the action of shifting power from a centralized organization to a dispersed network [10, 12, 17]. Data cannot ever be modified because of immutability and the consistency of blockchain entries. Contrarily, traceability is the process of locating data through time. On the other hand, transparency mentions the clarity of the data, i.e., the capacity of all network users to view the data included in a blockchain transaction [10, 12].

Blockchain is defined as "a chain of blocks associated by a link" in the dictionary. Block construction is a grouping of legitimate transactions.

Any node in the network can start the transaction, which is subsequently broadcast to every node. Then, by leveraging previous transactions, a validation procedure may be carried out by employing cryptographic techniques. The transactions will be included in the current Blockchain after these two primary procedures are finished. Each block comprises a variable number of transactions. The block size at the time Satoshi invented Bitcoin was around 1 MB. It increased to 8 MB in March of 2018. The greater block size required increases as more transactions are completed, yet faster processing is obtained [15].

The blockchain network's block connections are depicted in Figure 3.2. The reference, also known as the link between the blocks, is a hash in a binary context, and it is a part of the parent block, the preceding block. The primary block without a parent block is named the genesis block.

All participants in the public Blockchain who have the required authority may see every transaction as well. It follows that there are no control alternatives available to some operator or thing [10, 12]. On the other hand, anyone who needs to interact with the Blockchain in a private system must first get permission to do so. The transactions in this system are only accessible to participants who have been granted access.

While hybrid blockchains have flexible options, positive data can be reserved, secluded, or made open to the community. This is referred to as consortium in certain studies [10, 12].

A thorough evaluation and analysis of the most recent blockchain consensus techniques were published by Xiao et al. in Ref. [17]. They identified the consensus protocol as the crucial piece of technology supporting the reliability and efficiency of the Blockchain. To boost the speed of the blockchain network or satisfy specific application requirements, a variety of consensus strategies have been proposed, from small adjustments to the Nakamoto consensus protocol to inventive new consensus processes. For instance, in cutting-edge block proposal methods that need less computing power to mine, Blockchain researchers are interested in proofs of stake (PoS), proofs of authority (PoA), and proofs of elapsed time (PoET) [10, 17].

Blockchain technology was thoroughly examined by Zheng et al. in Ref. [18]. Before examining several common consensus approaches that are applied in various blockchains, they first offer an overview of the blockchain architecture. A brief discussion of technological challenges and recent advancements is also included.

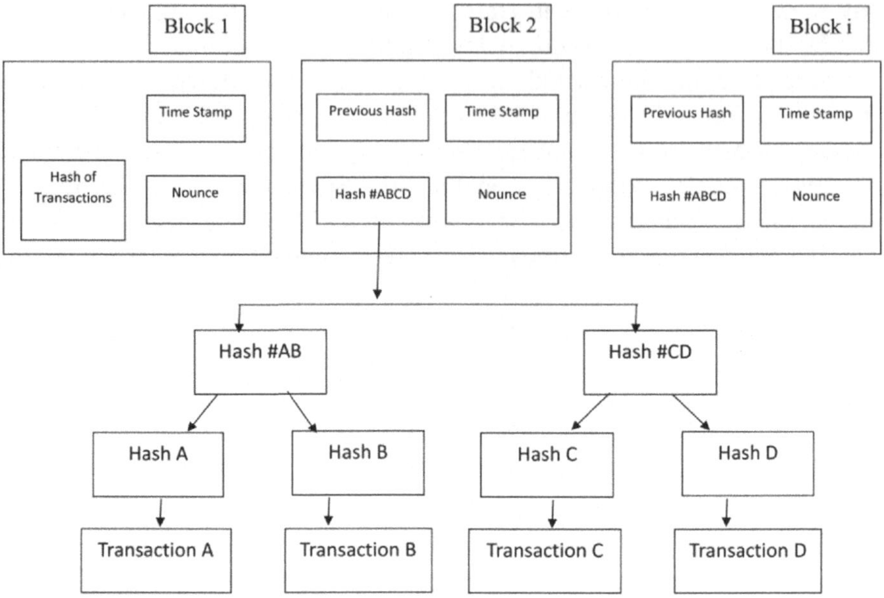

FIGURE 3.2 Block connectivity.

Source: Adapted from Ref. [10]

3.2.1.1 BLOCK STRUCTURE

The body and the header are the two basic parts of a block [14]. Parent block hash, block version, timestamp, nBits, Merkle tree root hash, and nonce are some of the metadata that make up the header [10, 16]. The body block is the basis for the transactions and transaction counter. The transactions section lists every transaction that has been recorded for the block, and the counter indicates how many additional transactions have been placed since [10].

Within its system, Blockchain employs several algorithms. It makes use of asymmetric cryptographic encryption to validate and authenticate the transaction. Additionally, it makes use of digital signatures to guarantee the environment's dependability. The person who started the transaction and the minors who are being verified both sign transactions using digital signatures. For these two techniques, a private key and public key pair are held by each node in the network [10]. Figure 3.3 depicts the block hierarchy.

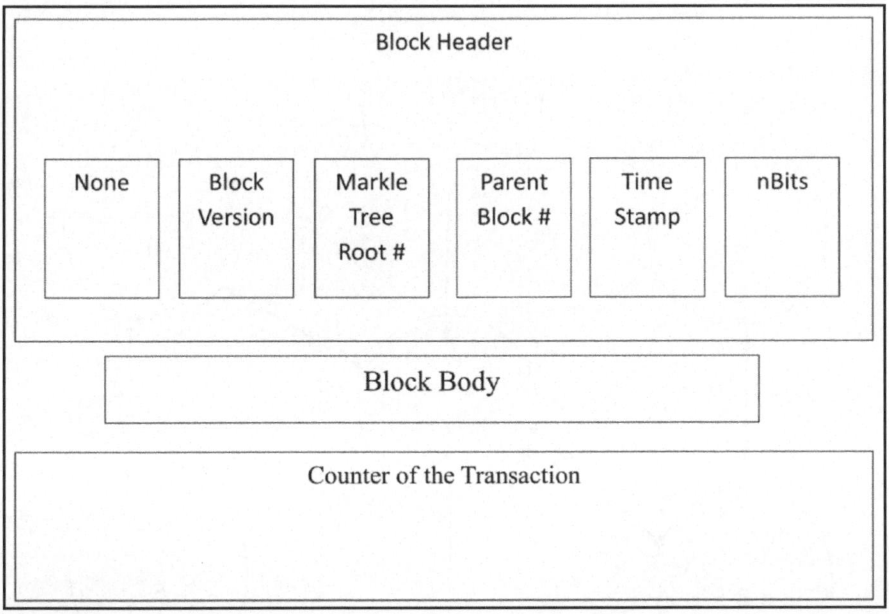

FIGURE 3.3 Block structure.

Source: Adapted from Ref. [10]

3.2.1.2 NODES NETWORK

Information added to other nodes of the blockchain system cannot be changed. In addition to decentralizing, this technique ensures dispersal. Consistency across nodes may be supported by preserving the local copy in the blockchain system and refreshing each timestamp. The single point of failure issue can be solved since there is no trust between nodes. The collective execution of transactions is the responsibility of each node [10, 17]. The node can also start mining, validate transactions, and carry out several tasks at once [10, 12]. A blockchain network's node connection is depicted in Figure 3.4 [10].

Let's say that a user initiates a transaction on the blockchain network, which leads to the formation of a new block to demonstrate how the nodes function. Once a block has been replicated, each node in the network receives a copy of it, but they do not add it to their copy of the Blockchain until they are certain there has not been any tampering [12, 13, 17]. Peer-to-peer (P2P) is a decentralized technology used by blockchain [10].

Public-private keys, digital signatures, and hashing are the three primary algorithms and operations used. As seen in Figure 3.2, the hash function joins

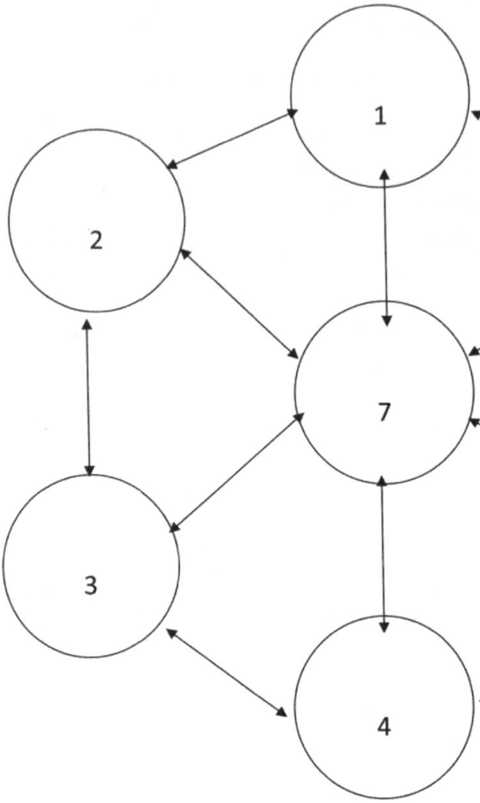

FIGURE 3.4 Blockchain nodes connectivity.
Source: Adapted from Ref. [10]

the blocks of the blockchain scheme to prevent tampering, and the digital signature is used to verify an individual's identity. In addition, it shields the system from non-repudiation. Additionally, according to researchers [20], the application determines whether a blockchain's design is authorized or permissionless [19].

Scalability is one of Blockchain's main problems [21]. The authors in Ref. [22] suggest using connector software and a blockchain system to raise the presentation and quality of the system. Public Blockchain was used to describe the smart contract as a computational model in Ref. [10]. The writers present a blockchain lesson and explain how it works in Ref. [23].

The trust chain can conduct transactions without centralized supervision, according to a somewhat modified formulation of the issue in Ref. [24]. These transactions may also be used to foster trust among strangers. The dealer and owner use the Internet information services (IIS) approach, according to researchers in Ref. [24], to certify a novel communicating undisputable autograph business [25].

3.2.1.3 SMART CONTRACTS

The technology of smart contracts is not new. According to American computer scientist Nick Szabo [27], who developed the digital currency "Bit Gold" in 1998 [26], smart contracts are computerized contract protocols that carry out the positions of an agreement. The application of smart contracts was postponed throughout the global shutdown to convert all paper-based contracts since the paper-based infrastructure is no longer effective and cannot manage such contracts. Governments and financial institutions must thus take action to maintain the operations of the enterprises [3].

A comprehensive answer and superior replacement for paper-based contracts is a blockchain with smart contracts. It does not require the real presence of the consumer because it is one of the fundamental components. Additionally, it eliminates third-party middlemen and attendant processing delays. For all parties involved, it is, therefore, a quicker, less expensive, and quicker resolution [3].

3.2.2 THE THREE PILLARS OF BLOCKCHAIN TECHNOLOGY

3.2.2.1 DECENTRALIZATION

In a decentralized blockchain system, info is dispersed diagonally in the network rather than being held by a single organization. Decentralization resolves trust concerns because it allows various parties to govern a network without requiring users to trust a single central authority. Due to its lesser likelihood of systemic failure, it inspires user trust.

3.2.2.2 TRANSPARENCY

The degree of responsibility that transparency adds is one that many firms need. In an open blockchain, all transactions can be tracked and searched. Although this feature can conflict with the privacy and security features of a blockchain, they can coexist. Blockchain can shield your data from unauthorized users while giving certain authorized individuals flexible access.

3.2.2.3 IMMUTABILITY

For many businesses, the immutability feature of Blockchain represents a game changer. Data placed onto the Blockchain cannot be changed once it is there. The cryptographic hash purpose is the cause of this Blockchain's characteristics. Through the use of a cryptographic technique, each block may be uniquely identified [28].

3.3 CHALLENGES OF BLOCKCHAIN TECHNOLOGY

Lack of interoperability and lack of scalability are the key issues with Blockchain. Due to the relatively low storage capacity of Blockchain, adding large amounts of contact data would have a significant negative impact on its effectiveness [29]. Utilizing off-chain storage mechanisms would significantly reduce the load of storing outside the Blockchain.

For several demographic groups, including the elderly and young individuals, technology provides both benefits and drawbacks. There are methods to include them, but it could alter how any system rolls out transactions. They can use any system thanks to a variety of cutting-edge technologies, including wireless IoT and wearable technology.

It is a proven truth that centralized systems perform better economically than decentralized ones. On the other hand, the decentralized blockchain system may protect privacy far better than a centralized system, which can significantly reduce the reluctance to implement the technology due to concerns about potential violations of hominoid honesties. This will encourage others to embrace our proposed strategy, which will be essential in the long run for saving a billion lives every day [28].

3.3.1 SMART CONTRACT SECURITY

Individual immunity passports, the verification of COVID-19 vaccination records, and the fulfillment of contractual obligations are all possible with smart agreements. Additionally, cryptocurrencies and assets like vaccinations or PPE (personnel protective equipment) may be followed using smart contracts [30].

Using smart contracts to manage the COVID-19 epidemic may present certain difficulties owing to the way blockchain technology is built; they have several benefits, such as cost-effectiveness and simplicity of correction. Public blockchain systems are among these difficulties; data and transactions are accessible to the general public, opening the system up to manipulation by malevolent users. Furthermore, the infrastructure on which smart contracts run is decentralized due to the possibility that malicious operators who use pseudonyms and regulator nodes for illegal purposes might expose smart contracts to several security threats. Criminals can, for instance, get phony vaccination certificates for individuals who haven't received the shot using smart contracts that leverage control nodes. Furthermore, the enlargement of clever agreements is hampered by the non-technical users of blockchain technology [30, 31].

These tools – FSolidM, KEVM, Security, MAIAN, and Mythril – according to Ref. [32], assist in finding vulnerabilities and protecting smart contracts from potential assaults. It is vital to establish safety procedures that are founded on particular aims to strengthen safety in keen agreements, even though approaches and tools are utilized to close gaps and address issues faced by users of smart contracts [30].

3.3.2 PEOPLE'S PRIVACY PRESERVATION

To counteract COVID-19, the use of Blockchain has been suggested as an essential component of digital contact tracking [30]. Blockchain technology has been used to create applications that track COVID-19 patients and follow up on their bags, enforcing the social isolation that is required by governments.

Although the COVID-19 tracking apps that employ blockchain technology have certain benefits, some problems must be taken into account.

One of these tests is protecting operator confidentiality and sensitive info, such as home addresses and phone numbers from the government [33]. Anyone may access user data thanks to open blockchain systems (like Bitcoin). As a result, misuse of people's privacy is possible.

Governments should thus enact legislation and provide additional resources to stop these abuses [39]. Other approaches to resolving these problems, such as the mixing strategy or maintaining anonymity while utilizing blockchain technology, were offered [34].

As an alternative, we may deploy private blockchain systems that operate in a measured situation (like Quorum) to secure operator information [30].

3.3.3 PROCESSING DATA RELATED TO COVID-19

The COVID-19 pandemic is the subject of a wealth of ever-evolving data. It's crucial to track geographic information, calculate the period, and update it often on the Blockchain for the data collected through digital contact tracing. As data velocity rises, data processing becomes more difficult [30].

That is, when utilized to handle data linked to COVID-19, public blockchain systems have a 20 transaction per second (TPS) throughput and privacy constraint, which causes issues [35]. Contrarily, private blockchain platforms may be speedy, secure, and able to process thousands of transactions per second, but they are not a dependable fix for Corona's data processing problems [30]. The current data pre-processing frameworks can be improved by adding an extra edge- or fog-based layer [36].

Additionally, data compression techniques and communication through external channels can lower the pace of transactions, which will help to solve the data processing issue [37].

3.3.4 CREATE AN INTEROPERABLE BLOCKCHAIN-BASED SYSTEM

We might benefit from interoperability characteristics that enable diverse blockchain-based systems to continually connect [10] when developing an interoperable blockchain-based system. Supporting the blockchain platform's interoperability can increase productivity and the supply chains for PPE and vaccines since it enables users to see and transfer data across several blockchain platforms independently (without the requirement for translation service) [30]. The variety of technologies that are used and the variations in software designs using blockchain platforms have made it difficult to develop an interoperable Blockchain-based COVID-19 outbreak management system [10].

The differences between the supported languages-suggested consensus techniques and data protection and transaction concerns in smart contracts have not been addressed by any solutions. As a result, additional study is required to resolve this problem [10].

3.3.5 LIMITED ADOPTION OF BLOCKCHAIN TECHNOLOGY

People's lifestyles and society have altered as a consequence of the COVID-19 outburst, requiring governments and other organizations to discover remedies and use cutting-edge technology to address the problems the epidemic has brought about. Blockchain technology was, therefore, applied to digital contact tracing. As previously indicated, digital contact tracing aids governments or authorities in limiting the spread of the coronavirus and enforcing social segregation among residents. The traceability and decentralization capabilities of blockchain technology, which boost confidence between governments and producers, can also make it easier to import PPE, vaccinations, and medical supplies [38]. Additionally, digitizing the vaccination certificate and adding a tracking function can help to limit the number of fake certificates [30, 39].

Although blockchain technology has benefits that can help battle the COVID-19 epidemic, its uptake has been delayed and uneven.

This is primarily caused by several things, such as the following: (i) a dearth of rules regulating blockchain technology and specific plans to manage risks; (ii) a lack of corporate encouragement and initiative to change their traditional business practices; (iii) a lack of sufficient blockchain technology expertise; (iv) the increased incidence of power consumption, which either affects the efficiency of mining projects for a framework blockchain and limits its ability to adapt; and (v) the lack of corporate support for changing they are traditional corporate practices.

To assist organizations and enterprises in better adapting to combat COVID-19, more research should be done to find norms and standards that may be applied to blockchain technology [10].

3.4 BLOCKCHAIN TECHNOLOGY APPLICATIONS TO COMBAT COVID-19

The COVID-19 situation can be significantly mitigated because of blockchain technology. It's one. One of the most advanced technologies is significant in this circumstance. This section lists the key blockchain applications that benefit the most impacted industries. With the least amount of harm, keep them operating. Figure 3.5 illustrates how such apps work, including locating contacts, exchanging data with healthcare partners, immunization and online education, supply chain management (SCM), smart contracts, vaccination certificates, electronic government, and secure certification.

3.4.1 CONTACT TRACING

Contact tracking is a crucial component to contain severe epidemic outbreaks. It aims to halt the spread of illness and has assisted in containing the COVID-19 epidemic in various areas [40]. Calculating any case's crossponding physical contact throughout the incubation phase is crucial. The

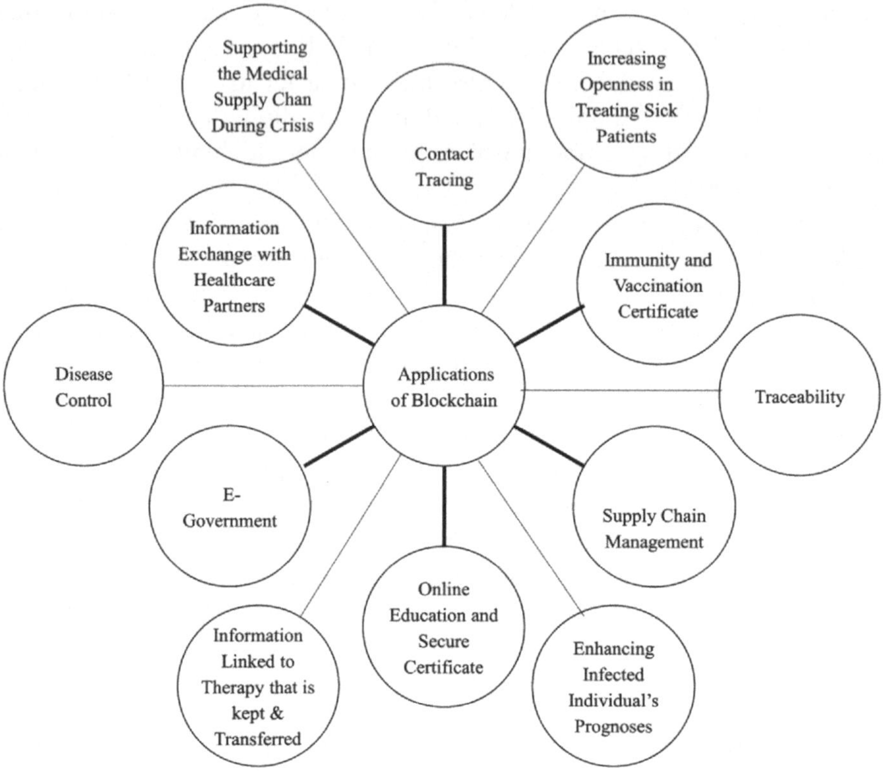

FIGURE 3.5 Blockchain technology used in the COVID-19 epidemic.

Source: Adapted from Ref. [10]

researchers in Ref. [10] found that SARS-CoV-2 (COVID-19) would take roughly 5.5 days to incubate before exhibiting symptoms and that not all infected individuals manifested symptoms. This might result in a decreased extent of COVID-19's dissemination [37].

Many authorities have introduced notable changes to mobile contact tracing applications in response to the unexpected COVID-19 epidemic to help with the challenging task of tracking down every contact of freshly identified sick individuals [1]. Contact tracing can be used to determine social interaction. By taking the initiative and providing the public with a study of the virus's scope, it seeks to stop the spread of COVID-19. Following the analysis are directions that can be used to diagnose, counsel, and quarantine people in situations of genuine risk. IoT and smartphones can improve the efficacy of this application. Although the contact-tracing program will breach users' privacy policies, the government and the healthcare industries embraced it [37].

If the Blockchain is utilized often, data collection will have a high degree of accuracy and dependability [37]. For the impacted locations, it provides real-time data. Blockchain, on the other hand, keeps an eye on and reports on virus-free or safe zones [1, 10]. GIS (geographic information system) and AI are two examples of additional technologies that blockchain technology works with to gather data [1].

Mass surveillance and P2P mobile applications are the two platforms that make use of contact tracing [10]. The Internet of Things (IoT) is a critical constituent of the mass surveillance system in smart cities and e-governments. In difference, the P2P-Mobile submission makes use of facilities to show the collected data to the surveillance system and the blockchain network and may show users the possibility of contracting COVID-19 [10].

3.4.1.1 ARCHITECTURE OVERVIEW

There are three main categories of users: Contact Tracer, patient, and administrator. Depending on their level of control over the system, each of these users has granular access to it. Every app user who has been granted access promises to abide by the privacy rules and protocols to protect Individual Data. These operators would cooperate with the GUI (graphical user interface) of the system's DApp (decentralized application) browser, which would demonstrate all of the recommended framework's functionality. Users would interact with other system modules based on their responsibilities. Blockchain technology is used to accomplish the suggested framework's functionality. The finest distributed platform for our proposed system is provided by a blockchain, which is founded on a P2P architecture where all nodes have equivalent rights. Separately, transactions on the blockchain are safe and tamper-proof, thanks to some consensus rules.

The cryptographic technique is suggested for trustworthy communication to increase security and privacy. Each user is given a unique address for the recommended structure, which aims to promote trust among operators in an announcement system [28].

3.4.1.2 CONTACT TRACING WORKFLOW

All confirmed cases must undergo contact tracing to stop fresh transmission chains. If a person has direct physical interaction with a proven circumstance for an additional 15 minutes, is within one meter of the confirmed case, or is physically caring for the confirmed case without wearing appropriate protective equipment, they are considered contacts. Finding contacts is the first stage in contact tracing. The best ways to identify someone are through extensive case investigations and interviews with the patient or, in certain cases, their caregiver. The contact tracing team must find contacts based on the environment and social customs. The contact tracing team would compile a list of individuals who are physically interacting with the confirmed patient while providing therapy. Each individual who has been identified as a contact should be informed and given instructions on how to self-quarantine, what symptoms to watch out for, whom to contact for testing and treatment if the disease gets worse, and any other questions or concerns the contact may have. Contacts who are participating in self-quarantine must self-report any indications or indications, including the absence of any. If contact is proven to be asymptomatic after a certain period, self-quarantine should end.

3.4.1.3 SMART CONTRACT

Basic procedures are carried out using smart contracts. They play a significant role in DApps. These agreements provide users with system access and let them carry out certain operations on the records. Contact Tracing Records is the contract that is a part of our suggested system. The functionality of our suggested contact tracking system is implemented in this contract. It establishes roles and grants access to those roles to carry out specific tasks. The prerequisites for each of the processes contained in the suggested system are defined. It also explains how to give access to different roles so they may carry out certain activities [28].

3.4.1.4 VULNERABILITY ANALYSIS

A critical component of every organization is the protection of important and valuable data. The code must be secure and devoid of vulnerabilities that might result in future losses [42]. The proposed system's whole functionality is defined by the smart contract; therefore, the code must be rigorously tested to ensure that it is complete and secure. This code inspection functionality is available in several security analysis tools. Oyente, a smooth agreement auto-auditing tool, analyzes smart contracts and alerts users to any possible fault attacks like the well-known DAO (Decentralized Autonomous Organization) attack [43]. This was produced in January 2016 by National University of

Singapore researchers. It provides analysis reports with a variety of features that attest to the reality of security issues.

3.4.1.5 TRANSACTION

This section describes the system's features and how they are included throughout system implementation:

1. **Assign Roles:** A trusted administrative organization that is tasked with establishing a user's duties within the system is in charge of this phase of the DApp. The Blockchain receives (Role Name, Roll Address) from the Assign Roles. Both of these act as a user's unique identifier on the system. The roles would be of two types since the system includes two distinct kinds of users, i.e., Assign Roles may allocate roles to Contact Tracer, or Assign Roles may also assign roles to patients. Assign Roles transmits (Role Name, Role Address) to the Blockchain in the role list for the Contact Tracer and Patient Tracer, which are two independent entities. Users must first authenticate themselves to access the system's various capabilities because of the symmetric key encryption employed to protect it.
2. **Add Patient Records:** The patient is now given the role to perform several DApp duties. The patient sends the document to be added to the Blockchain while requesting that records relevant to biodata be included.
3. **View Patient Records:** The patient accesses his medical records using the Role address, which was given to him. To carry out this function, the system would adhere to the following steps: following a user's login, the system now compares the patient's address with the record that is currently recorded in Blockchain. Once step 1's validation is complete, the user's system has access to the record R.
4. **Add Patient Symptoms and Test Record:** For the contact tracer to monitor and maintain track of the patient's health, the patient will record and submit his symptoms regularly. To carry out this action, the system would do as follows: The patient can contribute the test results and symptoms to an off-chain system called IPFS (InterPlanetary File System) after authentication. IPFS uses a dispersed hash bench to store the data. The information file saved using IPFS is given a hash. Transmits the hash data to the Blockchain.

5. **Get Message:** The contact tracer can send messages to the patient about safety precautions or emergency information in case something goes wrong. The system will automatically produce the message that appears initially on the screen from the contact tracer once the patient logs in.
6. **Add Contacts:** If the patient's test for the condition is positive, he can enter contact information. He will provide information on everyone he has been near for more than 15 minutes during the past three, four, or seven days, roughly within the range of one meter. To stop the transmission of this disease, the contact tracer must monitor contacts as soon as feasible.
7. **Send Message:** Contact Tracer would be able to provide the patient with timely information about their health, preventative actions, or emergency information after assessing the patient's symptoms. To carry out this task, the system would do the actions listed below: contact tracer gives the patient's address and the message he wishes to deliver. This communication would be promptly delivered to a specific patient and stored on the Blockchain [28].

3.4.1.6 USAGE SCENARIO FOR "ALGORITHM 1"

To address the privacy and data abuse issues that Contact Tracing faces, role-based access is introduced in the solution we've developed. This ensures that only parties who have been validated will have access to the Algorithm 1 service and that no unauthorized parties will be able to change the contact tracing data. As its name implies, Algorithm 1's initial function, Assign Roles, is used to assign characters to the appropriate accounts so they have granular admission to the system. In the course of their duties, the administrator should handle this operation for several accounts. The patient then completes the next action and adds the patient record, following validation. All of the information will be stored after everything is in order.

Both the contact tracer and the patient can use the Retrieve Data feature, but they must first authenticate themselves. Retrieving the specific data according to the patient ID requires a patient ID as input. After confirmation for totaling test archives to the system, the patient can also execute the function of adding test records. These test documents would be protected via IPFS, and the Blockchain would store the hash. The next function is Send message, which is carried out by the contact tracer and transmits messages or instructions to the patient. Patient ID must be supplied as an argument. The patient's ID for that specific patient would receive a notification. The last action in Algorithm 1 is Get message, which requires an enduring id as a quarrel. Once the patient's validation process has been accomplished, the screen will inquire whether there is any message associated with that patient's ID [28].

3.4.1.7 WORKFLOW OF THE PLANNED SYSTEM

In the future, dispersed blockchain-based contact tracking, users, and network administrators will be the two main user entities. There are two categories of users: Contact Tracer and Patient. The administrator's responsibility is to specify the duties of the new accounts. Each user would have a public account address and role name. The suggested blockchain network introduces a list of every user with certain duties.

Users interact with the system to request the services they need. The system would initially check the list of responsibilities assigned by the administrator before entertaining the request and providing the appropriate response. The blockchain network encrypts every communication to guarantee anonymity. The AES128 cryptographic technique is employed for encryption in the suggested approach. To save data given by users, IPFS, a distributed secure record-keeping system, is employed. After storing, it creates appropriate hashes. The blockchain network then stores these hashes. On the DApp browser, all additional operations are also possible.

3.4.1.8 APPLICATION OF THE SUGGESTED FRAMEWORK

1. **Access Granted:** Let's today comprehend the process a user, or patient, would go through to input his daily observations and medical data into the system. The beginning of procedure starts with the Administrator, a trusted employee of the hospital or healthcare organization. The administrator is in charge of distributing the Roles to different system users. This person would also need some technical knowledge and expertise to comprehend and operate the system. The administrator's role assignment, which includes the part name and account address of the operator to whom the role is being assigned, would thus be the initial step. Each user would require a

character name and account address to utilize the proposed system. Thus, the first step would be the administrator's role assignment, which would comprise the character name and account address of the user to whom the role is being given. Each user would require a role name and account address to be using the proposed system. Therefore, once the administrator assigns a role to this user, the role name and account address are saved in a roles list in case further validation is required.

A patient must request before doing any operations on the designated system once tasks have been allocated. After comparing the patient's role name and account address to those in the Roles List, the system provides the patient authorization to carry out these tasks. The system would save the data on the Blockchain when the patient completes the required activities and carries out transactions using that data. When a transaction is completed, the system receives a notification from the blockchain sheet, which the patient may observe on the DApp browser. As a result, the entire recommended system is now accessible.

2. **Access Denied:** Now that we've established the situation, let's examine what would happen if a user attempted to access system features without having been given a part by the manager or without utilizing the explanation address to which the parts have been allocated. When a user asks for access to the system's dashboard in this process, the system evaluates the Roles List to decide whether or not the user should be permitted to utilize the system's different functionalities. The system denies admission to the operator and indicates the operator is unsuccessful in authorizing if the user is not given a role to carry out these duties [28].

3.4.2 INFORMATION EXCHANGE WITH HEALTHCARE PARTNERS

Important data that must be communicated across healthcare partners include information about patients, treatments that were administered, preventative measures that were employed by physicians and other healthcare professionals, and so forth. These data are essential to COVID-19 research because they allow researchers to identify innovative treatment approaches that can lower the mortality toll. These data are supplied by hospitals and health organizations. Therefore, to safeguard the confidentiality of data, particularly patient information, international agencies and organizations utilize HIPAA (Health Insurance Portability and Accountability) rules [44]. However, there are challenges to expanding the data-sharing system.

The decentralization and transparency of blockchain technology can be utilized to enhance the healthcare system. Decentralization may be used to improve data security and privacy for patients, strengthen data control, and do away with paper-based medical records. This will make data exchange across hospitals and health organizations simpler and quicker. Additionally, the transparency feature may be utilized to stop data fraud and defend patient privacy against misuse or exploitation [44].

3.4.3 IMMUNITY AND VACCINATION CERTIFICATE

Tests to check if somebody has developed protection against a virus (such as COVID-19) after fully recovering from the disease include immunoserology, antibody testing, and immunizer.

The viruses or illnesses against which he or she has received a vaccination or immune protection are listed on the immunity (vaccination) certification. By enabling officials and authorities to make preparations and by facilitating cross-border transit for persons who possess this certification, the certificate aids in limiting and restricting the scope of COVID-19 [45]. Governments' primary duties in minimizing travel-related frauds, therefore, revolve around the certificate's deception security, strong discretion measures, and cost-effectiveness. Utilizing blockchain-based vaccine certification and immunity testing, a suitable and reliable data management method that is manageable, secure, and cost-effective has been developed [10].

Blockchain employs numerical signatures to protect together examinations and certificates and asymmetric encryption and decryption patterns [46]. Decentralization also boosts user confidence by preserving information authenticity and protection, which verifies the safety of such data in contradiction to malicious assaults or a solitary point of disappointment.

The aforementioned certificates may be verified in a trustworthy, cutting-edge way, and they protect the privacy of user information. For instance, many businesses can promote and implement policies that restrict who is permitted to return to work at reopened markets after the COVID-19 issue and only permit employees with a valid electronic vaccination license (immunity passport) to do so. Here, the implementation of Blockchain ensures that only "COVID-19 clear case" personnel may continue their employment. The crucial traceability and transparency components of blockchain technology make it feasible to establish the data provenance of the COVID-19 lab findings. Furthermore, evaluating the reliability of PCR (polymerase chain reaction) testing kits for the COVID-19 test may be highly beneficial for organizations. For the operators to register on the record, it produces an immunity passport.

3.4.4 SUPPLY CHAIN MANAGEMENT (SCM)

Factories have been unable to handle this shutdown because of the extra processes, such as fleshly interaction and community isolation, which has caused major harm to the supply chain internationally. As a result, the worldwide supply chain's imports and exports have been prohibited [44]. According to Ref. [47], "75% of enterprises have had significant or highly unfavorable consequences on their organizations," "94% of businesses are facing stock chain commotions from COVID-19," and "55% of corporations expect to lower their growth outlooks." Due to the increased demand, supply chains for the medical and pharmaceutical industries are scarce. The demand for local commodities in the supply chains has also significantly increased [44].

Blockchain is one of the greatest choices to take into account while managing the supply chain. Because of its property transparency, it can link all the stakeholders over a single decentralized universal network while safely exposing the data from the silos. A variety of blockchain networks in the SCM area were proposed, as indicated in Ref. [37]. As was said in the sections above, blockchain technology reduces operational risk, speeds up data handling, and reduces processing time across all areas and applications. The VeChain technology, which ensures the dependability and legitimacy of masks imported from China, is one example that was used in China. It verifies all linked jobs, resources, packages, and codes [10, 47].

3.4.5 ONLINE EDUCATION AND SECURE CERTIFICATION

Although numerous colleges and institutions have been locked throughout the globe as a result of the quarantine, this does not indicate that education is coming to an end or taking a break. Because of its irreplaceable nature, education is difficult to operate online.

The certification of students' credentials (degrees, transcripts, and other certifications), among other issues, is still a concern due to inadequate cross-platform coordination [44].

Platforms for online learning built on the Blockchain can help with these issues [44]. Authorized users can have access to decentralized blockchain-based storage while other users' data is kept protected [3]. When one of an institution's issuing authorities uploads a credential to a blockchain-based organization, it provides safe issuance and distribution of verified educational credentials, which is known as a blockchain [10]. The MOODLE platform, a worldwide blockchain-based network, provides the aforementioned benefits and is one of the greatest examples [44].

3.4.6 E-GOVERNMENT

Numerous operations and services within the governmental institution sector have been put on hold as a result of the coronavirus pandemic, lockdowns, and quarantines. This has caused several governments that do not largely rely on information and communications technology (ICT) to adopt the idea of electrical government, often known as e-government, and they have begun to digitize every element of their services. Public utilities (such as water, gas, electricity, and sanitary facilities), tax collection, wage payment, and other services are a few examples of these [10, 44].

By minimizing delays and service operating expenses, Blockchain boosts the efficiency of e-government services. Additionally, it provides access to shared databases and blockchain automation capability [44]. Any attempt at counterfeiting will be immediately discovered. Blockchain offers several improvements for data secrecy and consistency when it comes to security. Some of the advantages that blockchain technology offers to e-governments include data integrity and immutability [44].

A summary of the ways that blockchain technology is being utilized to fight the COVID-19 pandemic is given in Table 3.1, along with the types of Blockchain that may be used in each application and the transaction fees.

TABLE 3.1 Existing Applications for Blockchain [10]

Application	Expected Latency	Expected Scalability	Types of Blockchain	Transaction Cost
Smart contract	Within hours Within days	10–10,000 per system institute per day.	Consortium Private	0–0.01 No cost
Contract tracing	Within hours	360–1,440 transactions per phone per day.	Public	0–0.01 USD
Information exchange with healthcare partners	Within seconds Within hours	1,000–1,00,000 transactions per minute.	Private Consortium	No cost 0–0.01 USD
Immunity and vaccination certificate	Within hours	NAN	Consortium	No cost
Supply chain management	Within day Within minutes	100–10,000 per system per day.	Private Consortium	No cost 0–0.01 USD
Online education and secure certification	Within minutes Within minutes	100–10,000 per municipality per day.	Public Public	0–0.01 USD No cost
E-Government	Within days	100–10,000 per municipality per day.	Consortium	0–0.01 USD

3.4.7 DISEASE CONTROL

Disease surveillance has to be precise and successful to control infectious diseases and stop the pandemic [48]. Among the diseases that may be tracked and managed with blockchain technology are the Middle East respiratory syndrome (MERS), coronavirus, cholera in Africa, Nipah in Asia, and the Ebola virus. By incorporating it into the electronic devices used by locals, the blockchain network may be utilized to track the spread of COVID-19 contagions amongst people on a global scale. Blockchain technology is crucial in the COVID-19 pandemic to assist virus sufferers by documenting patients' illness symptoms incorruptibly.

3.4.8 TRACEABILITY

The capacity to track infected patients is referred to as traceability. The propagation of the coronavirus must be stopped. With the use of blockchain technology, it is now feasible to track the travels of infected individuals, offer real-time information on impacted areas, and document direct combat operations. Blockchain technology can be used to track individuals' movements in virus-free environments [49]. Chain blocks are used to keep track of safe zone data such as population, location, and coronavirus epidemic status. Regular tracking of supplies and items is necessary to provide transparency across the medical supply chain. For this tracing, the blockchain network's transaction recording and monitoring capabilities may be leveraged.

3.4.9 SUPPORTING THE MEDICAL SUPPLY CHAIN DURING THIS CRISIS

The healthcare industry is facing a major problem in this pandemic crisis: keeping a steady source of nutrients and medications. The trade supply chain and the supply chain for commodities have both benefited greatly from blockchain technology [50]. By securely connecting blocks and transactions it may guarantee the medical chain's dependability. Blockchain encryption is therefore utilized to safeguard the anonymity of supply chain data. Recently, IBM (international business machines) unveiled the "rapid supplier connect" initiative, a blockchain net that will provide the medical source chain during COVID-19.

3.4.10 INCREASING OPENNESS IN TREATING SICK PATIENTS

Transparency is a crucial aspect of blockchain technology. It is crucial to safeguard the private information and data of patients getting treatment. Since fake news is so common on social media sites, its unreliability promotes panic and despair. Blockchain technology may provide a feasible option to assure the correctness of data assessment because of its ability to analyze data and supply real-time data updates. It could make it easier to transition from interoperability driven by patients to interoperability driven by institutions [51].

3.4.11 ENHANCING INFECTED INDIVIDUALS' PROGNOSES

If a sick person receives treatment promptly, their chance of recovery can be increased. Effective quarantine case monitoring is made possible in hospitals and at home thanks to blockchain technology. Faster medicine delivery is made possible by this, and infected patients' recuperation will benefit greatly. Blockchain enables highly private patient symptoms, location, and past health condition records during the COVID-19 pandemic. Decentralized networks of end users, healthcare providers, and governments make up the data block [52].

3.4.12 INFORMATION LINKED TO THERAPY THAT IS KEPT AND TRANSFERRED

One of the most important and difficult jobs during this COVID-19 epidemic is to preserve and transmit the obtained data. In 2009 and 2017, data breaches resulted in the exposure of more than 176 million patient records. With the use of blockchain technology, a decentralized, see-through, and unalterable record of patient data may be kept. Thanks to blockchain technology, patients, doctors, and other healthcare professionals may safely and quickly transmit the same information [53].

3.4.13 BETTER HEALTHCARE PROTECTION

Platforms that focus on providing access to high-quality, affordable healthcare were enabled by blockchain technology [54]. It could offer an effective way to monitor the coronavirus epidemic and shield more patients from the pandemic. It enables real-time regular checking to track the whereabouts of infected individuals so they can receive the necessary care when they need it. Misdiagnosis would be less likely if hospitals and medical staff had access to a safe and accurate database of patient records.

3.4.14 EFFECTIVE HEALTHCARE MANAGEMENT DURING THE CRISIS

An effective healthcare management system is required to address the COVID-19 catastrophe both now and in the future. Frontline health responders require more than 89 million masks, 39 million gowns, 76 million gloves, and 2.9 million liters of hand sanitizer each month to defend themselves and others against COVID-19, according to the WHO. The supply of all of the aforementioned items is managed using blockchain technology [54]. It is also envisaged that improvements will be made to biomedical and healthcare ledgers, the upkeep of medical data, the processing of insurance claims, and the conduct of clinical and biomedical research during this COVID-19 crisis [55].

3.5 BLOCKCHAIN COVID-19 ONGOING RESEARCH

3.5.1 DESIGN OF A P2P MOBILE APPLICATION USING BLOCKCHAIN

As a solution to the major issues related to COVID-19, it is suggested to analyze the outcomes of developing a blockchain-based, decentralized P2P, real-time dispensation mobile request arrangement for assisting everyone in classifying the spots of infection inside a crowded group of people. Users will be able to automatically determine the possibility of a COVID-19 viral outbreak using the most recent version of the highly recommended P2P mobile application, which will also help the authorities locate patients who are secretly afflicted. The system is largely composed of four subsystems: a mass surveillance system, a blockchain platform, and an infection verification subsystem [10].

3.5.2 TELEMEDICINE AND REMOTE HEALTHCARE SYSTEMS

A preventative strategy that addresses the spread of predatory use of telemedicine is remote healthcare. To provide remote help linked to medical consultation qualifications, a medical chain, a platform built on an Ethereum and Hyper ledger foundation, has been used. The use of technology ensures the security and correct storage of all patient-doctor data generated during consultations. After completing the agreed-upon consent form for market inquiries, the technique enables the patient to safely share their information with researchers as a third party [10].

Another suggested solution, HealPoint, recommends the best doctors to a user (patient) based on particular criteria like location, expertise, and knowledge. Additionally, it enables remote medical consultations in some circumstances [56].

3.5.3 STOPPING THE SPREAD OF FAKE NEWS USING THE MIPASA PLATFORM

The COVID-19 disaster has made clear the crucial need for a safe, practical, trustworthy, accurate, and dependable solution that could repair non-scalable methods now in place for combating the COVID-19 outbreak. Decision-making for many different activities can be significantly changed by data connected to the COVID-19 verifiability process. One of the platforms for blockchain technology is called MiPasa, which offers a blockchain-based platform for combining, processing, and providing data connected to the spread of the COVID-19 infection from a variety of reliable sources, such as the WHO and accredited health associations and officials. Enabling data experts and community fitness management to exchange explanations to stop the epidemic's spread primarily helps governments recognize both individual mistakes and falsification. MiPasa, for instance, can assist in the anonymous, trustworthy, and simple identification of COVID-19 instances and viral hot spots by using data analytics on verified blockchain-based information. It is intended to operate as a fully secure system on top of the Hyperledger platform. MiPasa allows users and public health officials to upload contaminated cases to web-based interfaces and place them there.

To validate this, it examines data supplied by the WHO, for instance, to confirm that the uploaded information complies with the fundamental standards. If the information is verified, it is then given to the nationally selected national government and health officials [57].

3.5.4 COVID-19 TESTING CONFIDENTIALLY USING EPIOS

Throughout the COVID-19 period, there have been numerous reports of prejudice, discrimination, insults, and abuse, in which those who have the disease are blamed for spreading the pandemic and its prevalence. To prevent this bias, hospitals or laboratories should reserve the privacy of COVID-19-identified personalities. It is recommended that Epios assist in clandestine testing of people who have COVID-19 infection. It makes it simple for consumers to interact with labs that create and provide PCR test swabs. The suggested mechanism makes it impossible to pay the cost directly to the testing facilities. As an alternative, it mandates that the vendors of COVID-19 testing kits issue each kit's user a ticket. Additionally, it cryptographically protects the token (coupon) to assist the laboratories in determining the costs rather than following the customers who purchase PCR kits.

Additionally, it attempts to provide a mobile application that enables the anonymous purchase and submission of such kits to and from the PCR test workers in ways that are together.

The design also suggests safeguarding the anonymity of those who have been tested while providing COVID-19-relevant data to researchers, the government, and authorities, such as high-class COVID-19 revolution statistics [58].

3.5.5 USING AN ANONYMOUS CONTACT-TRACING-VIRI PLATFORM TO STOP THE SPREAD OF DISEASE

One of the goals of digital contact tracking is to limit the transmission of contagious diseases like COVID-19. User information privacy is impacted by discovering infected individuals and identifying infection hotspots. The primary technological changes in contact tracing platforms and resolutions, as previously indicated, might alter the adaptability and effectiveness of the suggested technologies for digital contact tracing. One of them is the cross-entity VIRI's (Virios Therapeutics, Inc.) platform, which has suggested an all-encompassing platform to tackle such research difficulties broadly. Additionally, it promises to defend the operator's data confidentiality.

BLE, with its ability to pinpoint the spread of COVID-19 infection at various locations, VIRI (Vireos Therapeutics, Inc.) was created to track the disease's extent across several geographic areas. It notifies a user through push notification each time they have had nearby interaction with a COVID-19-positive being. Based on the hazard scale, the system can inform the user about potentially fatal diseases in the next phase. For instance, VIRI can change a user's status from "cleared case attribute" to "probable COVID-19 case" after they have had the shortest interaction with an infected case.

The platform can be quickly integrated with current corporate solutions using open-source APIs. Additionally, VIRI verifies that the person is fully in control of their information, which is kept on their expedient namelessly utilizing blockchain technology and making use of its privacy-preserving features. Such can assist AI-based methods for pandemic COVID-19 forecasting [10, 58].

3.5.6 SELF-SOVEREIGN UNIQUENESS USING COVID-19 AND E-REZEPT SYSTEM

E-Rezept, a remote platform application founded on the idea of self-sovereign individuality, is used in the healthcare industry. Its primary goal is to enable instances to establish a purchase for pharmaceuticals remotely by providing proof in the form of the medications' unique IDs [59]. This technology is controllable and effortlessly integrates with current healthcare systems, unlike Medicalchain and HealPoint. COVID, which is built on Sovrin, a consent self-sovereign identification (SSI) network, is another example of a blockchain-based firm [10]. Law-abiding individuals can get rewards from the COVID platform in a responsible and trustworthy manner [60]. VeChain is a media application built on blockchain technology. It monitors vaccination development and ensures the accuracy of data about vaccine specifics [30].

3.6 A FEW BLOCKCHAIN CASES FOR THE COVID-19 PANDEMIC

3.6.1 HASHLOG

The Georgia-based health technology firm Acoer [61]'s initial endeavor was this. Distributed blockchain ledger technology may enable the hashlog blockchain solution, enabling the recording and data visualization of the coronavirus epidemic utilizing WHO and US CDC (United States Centers for Disease Control and Prevention) public data.

3.6.2 VECHAIN

It is a blockchain-based tool designed to track Chinese vaccine manufacturing. Distributed ledgers are used to record and maintain all operations associated with the manufacture of vaccines, including the components, codes, and packaging. Additionally, it offers a useful technique for lowering the danger of possible changes to vaccination information [1].

3.6.3 PHBC

With the help of this blockchain-based network, communities, and workplaces may be continuously and anonymously verified to be free of the fatal coronavirus COVID-19 and additional high-risk viruses. This blockchain-based platform's capacity to track the movements of uninfected people and prevent their return if they visit contaminated regions is a crucial component.

3.6.4 HYPERCHAIN

It is an order to propel contributions that were developed to help governments and health organizations supply donations to the country of China's sick. Using Hyperchain, which can attach up to millions of nodes and enable numerous individuals to get donated items and essential medical equipment from businesses, a lack of facilities during this outbreak can be remedied [1].

3.7 BLOCKCHAIN METHOD FOR COVID-19 PANDEMIC

Websites operated by the government, clinics, hospitals, and testing institutions use participating nodes in the blockchain net. The digital ledger also includes patient data, sample test results, treatment rank, and release summaries.

The patient is initially assessed and diagnosed based on the COVID-19 disease's precursor symptoms. After taking a sample from the patient, if the test results are positive, the patient is placed under quarantine for at least 14 days. The patient's care and monitoring are carried out at this time using a blockchain technology application. The patient subsequently goes through the healing process and is tested for COVID-19 once again. However, the patient is cleared, and a discharge statement is created if the sample result is unfavorable. The patient data are produced when a large-scale presentation is necessary; their privacy is safeguarded, and they are retained on file for potential usage. Blockchain technology ensures the correctness of the patient's recorded data.

According to the Organization for Economic Cooperation and Development (OECD), several industries, including supply chain, insurance, tourism, agriculture, construction, and automobiles, have completely shut down, causing the global economy to slow and expand at its slowest rate since 2009 (OECD Economic Outlook, Interim Report March 2020: Coronavirus: the world economy at risk, 2020) [1, 62].

3.8 LIMITATIONS OF BLOCKCHAIN TECHNOLOGY

It has been noted that BT has the following drawbacks, for example:

- Because each transaction requires considerable hardware resources, it consumes a lot of energy.
- Scalability is this technology's key flaw since validation takes some time, even after the majority of nodes have authorized the transactions.
- The complexity of blockchain technology and the requirement for a sizable user base are further drawbacks of this technology.

- Maintaining privacy is a big difficulty with this technology [1].

The limitations and advantages are given in Table 3.2 [41].

TABLE 3.2 Limitations and Advantages of Blockchain Technology [41]

Sl. No.	Advantages	Limitations
1.	While yet being accessible and secure, healthcare information. Real-time updates are made automatically to the information.	A security system should be installed to prevent the leakage of patient data.
2.	Efficiency gains and cost reductions.	Cost-effectiveness has not yet been established.
3.	There is no need to have faith in just one computer, database, or organization because the network processes the transactions.	Technical difficulties and regulatory problems.
4.	Enhanced security through dependable "phishing" protection and the safe-guarding of sensitive data.	Even though the data on the Blockchain may be de-identified and encrypted, there remains a danger of possible data breaches due to dispersed access.
5.	Enables interoperability to swiftly and effectively send the data to healthcare providers.	Smaller blockchain-based apps still raise certain questions regarding performance and scalability, which must be addressed.

3.9 CONCLUSION AND FUTURE DIRECTIONS

Here, we provide an overview of potential future research goals and prospects for utilizing blockchain technology to aid with the COVID-19 pandemic.

Although it has many wonderful features, blockchain still has security issues. Therefore, it should be thought to enhance blockchain by utilizing new security techniques.

For instance, a mining pool solution is described in Ref. [62] by tackling security bottleneck issues to improve mining process performance. In this case, data vulnerabilities in the blockchain's consensus procedures are addressed using security-defense techniques. Recipient-oriented transactions are advocated by Ref. [63] as a means of preventing blockchain double-spending offenses. Before adding the transaction to the block, it tries to get approval using the phrases "stealth address and master node." By confirming each transaction, the sender and the recipient of the transaction participate actively in the broadcast process in this situation [63].

To use the Blockchain as a role model for emergency healthcare services akin to the COVID-19 pandemic, it needs to be enhanced to function better from a variety of technological viewpoints. In the healthcare sector, for instance, scalability and lightweight blockchain implementation are crucial to reducing the amount of time needed for data verification and transaction latency. To speed up data exchange and reduce processing time, which results in robust data analysis for COVID-19, efficient mining techniques may be considered, together with optimizing verification operation time. Setting up local and private blockchain systems is another possible recommendation, which might help to lower the size of the Blockchain. Using such tools to track the illness in a given area to look for an active real-time reply.

Blockchain can be joined with additional technologies to provide appropriate presentation in deciding difficulties related to the COVID-19 epidemic. Construct a reliable healthcare architecture. For instance, the fundamentals of clever storage and excellent computation potential quirks that the cloud may help with. These characteristics might be used in addition to the Blockchain to provide better performance. Furthermore, drones are in favor of enhancing the epidemic's contactless surveillance. Moreover, using one effective technique to provide the necessary amenities to persons when all forms of transportation are prohibited is a quarantine.

This study examined possible applications for blockchain technology's properties in battling the COVID-19 virus. We chose instances of blockchain technology services that mostly focused on healthcare situations to demonstrate the critical function that blockchain technology may play during the COVID-19 crisis.

We looked at recently implemented systems that rely on blockchain technology to deliver a variety of facilities related to data privacy support, as an illustration, remote PM, digital contact tracing that is simple to do, and COVID-19 evaluation. Because of the extensive COVID-19 outbreak, we identified and categorized key research roadblocks and problems that prevent blockchain technology from being successfully applied in the healthcare industry.

Finally, in light of the COVID-19 pandemic, we make some recommendations about how to extend the usage of the Blockchain in the future. Blockchain applications offer a secure framework for gathering, storing, and disseminating vital data. Therefore, they may be utilized to reduce network latency. Thanks to the most recent integration of Blockchain with other cutting-edge technologies like Big Data, AI, and Cloud computing, a lethal ailment like COVID-19 may be successfully treated.

ACKNOWLEDGMENT

The authors are appreciative of the organization of Mohanlal Sukhadia University, Udaipur, Rajasthan, and Bhagwat University, Ajmer, Rajasthan, for their assistance.

CONFLICT OF INTEREST

There is no potential for a conflict of interest.

FUNDING

There is no funding issued.

KEYWORDS

- **blockchain**
- **COVID-19**
- **Google Scholar**
- **healthcare management**
- **medical supply chain**
- **MiPasa platform**
- **PubMed**
- **Scopus**
- **World Health Organization**

REFERENCES

1. Sharma, A., Bahl, S., Bagha, A. K., Javaid, M., Shukla, D. K., & Haleem, A. (2020). Blockchain technology and its applications to combat the COVID-19 pandemic. *Research on Biomedical Engineering*, 1–8.
2. Bansal, A., Garg, C., & Padappayil, R. P., (2020). Optimizing the implementation of COVID-19 "immunity certificates" using Blockchain. *Journal of Medical Systems*, *44*, 1, 2.

3. Bahl, S., Singh, R. P., Javaid, M., Khan, I. H., Vaishya, R., & Suman, R. (2020). Telemedicine technologies for confronting COVID-19 pandemic: A review. *Journal of Industrial Integration and Management*, *5*, 547–561.
4. Ghosh, A., Gupta, R., & Misra, A. (2020). Telemedicine for diabetes care in India during COVID-19 pandemic and national lockdown period: Guidelines for physicians. *Diabetes & Metabolic Syndrome: Clinical Research & Reviews*, *14*, 273–276.
5. Sharma, A., Bahl, S., Bagha, A. K., Javaid, M., Shukla, D. K., & Haleem, A. (2020). Multi-agent system applications to fight the COVID-19 pandemic. *Apollo Medicine*, *17*, 41.
6. Chang, M. C., & Park, D., (2020). How can Blockchain help people in the event of pandemics such as COVID-19? *Journal of Medical Systems*, *44*, 1, 2.
7. Khan, I., Haleem, A., & Javaid, M. (2020). Analyzing the COVID-19 pandemic through cases, deaths, and recoveries. *Journal of Oral Biology and Craniofacial Research*, *10*, 450–469.
8. Iyengar, K. P., Vaishya, R., Bahl, S., & Vaish, A., (2010). Impact of the coronavirus pandemic on the supply chain in healthcare. *British Journal of Healthcare Management*, *26*, 1.
9. Suman, R., Javaid, M., Haleem, A., Vaishya, R., Bahl, S., & Nandan, D. (2020). Sustainability of coronavirus on different surfaces. *Journal of Clinical and Experimental Hepatology*, *10*(4), 386–390.
10. Alsaed, Z., Khweiled, R., Hamad, M., Daraghmi, E., Cheikhrouhou, O., Alhakami, W., & Hamam, H., (2021). Role of blockchain technology in combating COVID-19 crisis. *Applied Sciences*, *11*, 12063.
11. Abd-Alrazaq, A. A., Alajlani, M., Alhuwail, D., Erbad, A., Giannicchi, A., Shah, Z., Hamdi, M., & Househ, M., (2021). Blockchain technologies to mitigate COVID-19 challenges: A scoping review. *Computer Methods and Programs in Biomedicine Update*, *1*, 100001.
12. Abu-Elezz, I., Hassan, A., Nazeemudeen, A., Househ, M., & Abd-Alrazaq, A., (2020). The benefits and threats of blockchain technology in healthcare: A scoping review. *International Journal of Medical Informatics*, *142*, 104246.
13. Monrat, A. A., Schelén, O., & Andersson, K., (2019). A survey of Blockchain from the perspectives of applications, challenges, and opportunities. *IEEE Access*, *7*, 117134–117151.
14. Fusco, A., Dicuonzo, G., Dell'Atti, V., & Tatullo, M., (2020). Blockchain in healthcare: Insights on COVID-19. *International Journal of Environmental Research and Public Health*, *17*, 7167.
15. Liao, C. H., (2020). Evaluating the social marketing success criteria in health promotion: A F-DEMATEL approach. *International Journal of Environmental Research and Public Health*, *17*, 6317.
16. Shen, B., Guo, J., & Yang, Y., (2019). MedChain: Efficient healthcare data sharing via Blockchain. *Applied Sciences*, *9*, 1207.
17. Xiao, Y., Zhang, N., Lou, W., & Hou, Y. T. (2020). A survey of distributed consensus protocols for blockchain networks. *IEEE Communications Surveys & Tutorials*, *22*, 1432–1465.
18. Zheng, Z., Xie, S., Dai, H., Chen, X., & Wang, H., (2017). An overview of blockchain technology: Architecture, consensus, and future trends. In: 2017 *IEEE International Congress on Big Data* (pp. 557–564).

19. Luu, L., Narayanan, V., Zheng, C., Baweja, K., Gilbert, S., & Saxena, P., (2016). A secure sharding protocol for open blockchains. In: *Proceedings of the 2016 ACM SIGSAC Conference on Computer and Communications Security* (pp. 17–30).
20. Min, X., Li, Q., Liu, L., & Cui, L., (2016). A permissioned blockchain framework for supporting instant transactions and dynamic block size. In: *2016 IEEE Trustcom/BigDataSE/ISPA* (pp. 90–96). IEEE.
21. Dennis, R., Owenson, G., & Aziz, B. (2016). A temporal blockchain: A formal analysis. In: *2016 International Conference on Collaboration Technologies and Systems (CTS)* (pp. 430–437). IEEE.
22. Xu, X., Pautasso, C., Zhu, L., Gramoli, V., Ponomarev, A., Tran, A. B., & Chen, S., (2016). The Blockchain is a software connector. In: *2016 13th Working IEEE/IFIP Conference on Software Architecture (WICSA)* (pp. 182–191). IEEE.
23. Bozic, N., Pujolle, G., & Secci, S., (2016). A tutorial on Blockchain and applications to secure network control planes. In: *2016 3rd Smart Cloud Networks & Systems (SCNS)* (pp. 1–8).
24. Otte, P., De Vos, M., & Pouwelse, J., (2020). TrustChain: A Sybil-resistant scalable blockchain. *Future Generation Computer Systems*, *107*, 770–780.
25. McGhin, T., Choo, K. K. R., Liu, C. Z., & He, D. (2019). Blockchain in healthcare applications: Research challenges and opportunities. *Journal of Network and Computer Applications*, *135*, 62–75.
26. Rasure, E., (2021). *Smart Contracts*. Available online: https://www.investopedia.com/terms/s/smart-contracts.asp (accessed on 4 December 2023).
27. Tricco, A. C., Lillie, E., Zarin, W., O'Brien, K. K., Colquhoun, H., Levac, D., Moher, D., et al., (2018). PRISMA extension for scoping reviews (PRISMA-ScR): Checklist and explanation. *Annals of Internal Medicine*, *169*, 467–473.
28. Bari, N., Qamar, U., & Khalid, A. (2021). Efficient contact tracing for pandemics using Blockchain. *Informatics in Medicine Unlocked*, *26*, 100742.
29. Casino, F., Dasaklis, T. K., & Patsakis, C., (2019). A systematic literature review of blockchain-based applications: Current status, classification, and open issues. *Telematics and Informatics*, *36*, 55–81.
30. Ahmad, R. W., Salah, K., Jayaraman, R., Yaqoob, I., Ellahham, S., & Omar, M., (2020). *Blockchain and COVID-19 Pandemic: Applications and Challenges* (pp. 1–19). IEEE TechRxiv.
31. Huang, Y., Bian, Y., Li, R., Zhao, J. L., & Shi, P. (2019). Smart contract security: A software lifecycle perspective. *IEEE Access, 7*, 150184–150202.
32. Di Angelo, M., & Salzer, G., (2019). A survey of tools for analyzing Ethereum smart contracts. In: *2019 IEEE International Conference on Decentralized Applications and Infrastructures (DAPPCON)* (pp. 69–78). IEEE.
33. Zaabar, B., Cheikhrouhou, O., Jamil, F., Ammi, M., & Abid, M., (2021). HealthBlock: A secure blockchain-based healthcare data management system. *Computer Networks*, *200*, 108500.
34. Huynh, T. T., Nguyen, T. D., & Tan, H., (2019). A survey on security and privacy issues of blockchain technology. In: *2019 International Conference on System Science and Engineering (ICSSE)* (pp. 362–367). IEEE.
35. Wood, G., (2014). Ethereum: A secure, decentralized generalized transaction ledger. *Ethereum Project Yellow Paper*, *151*, 1–32.

36. Debe, M., Salah, K., Rehman, M. H. U., & Svetinovic, D., (2019). IoT public fog nodes reputation system: A decentralized solution using Ethereum blockchain. *IEEE Access, 7*, 178082–178093.
37. Ting, D. S. W., Carin, L., Dzau, V., & Wong, T. Y., (2020). Digital technology and COVID-19. *Nature Medicine, 26*(4), 459–461.
38. Ramirez, L. L. J., & Beltrán, Á. N., (2020). *Blockchain Application in the Distribution Chain of the COVID-19 Vaccine: A Designing Understudy.* https://advance.sagepub.com/articles/preprint/Blockchain_application_in_the_distribution_chain_of_the_COVID-19_vaccine_a_designing_understudy/12274844.
39. Yong, B., Shen, J., Liu, X., Li, F., Chen, H., & Zhou, Q. (2020). An intelligent blockchain-based system for safe vaccine supply and supervision. *International Journal of Information Management, 52*, 102024.
40. Ahmed, N., Michelin, R. A., Xue, W., Ruj, S., Malaney, R., Kanhere, S. S., Seneviratne, A., et al., (2020). A survey of COVID-19 contact tracing apps. *IEEE Access, 8*, 134577–134601.
41. Chattu, V. K., Nanda, A., Chattu, S. K., Kadri, S. M., & Knight, A. W., (2019). The emerging role of blockchain technology applications in routine disease surveillance systems to strengthen global health security. *Big Data and Cognitive Computing, 3*, 25.
42. Eshan, B., Madhulika, B., Nautiyal, L., & Hooda, M., (2021). Deficiencies in blockchain technology and potential augmentation in cyber security. *Blockchain for Business: How It Works and Creates Value*, 251–293.
43. Kalla, A., Hewa, T., Mishra, R. A., Ylianttila, M., & Liyanage, M., (2020). The role of Blockchain to fight against COVID-19. *IEEE Engineering Management Review, 48*, 85–96.
44. Dai, H. N., Imran, M., & Haider, N., (2020). Blockchain-enabled internet of medical things to combat COVID-19. *IEEE Internet of Things Magazine, 3*, 52–57.
45. Sheffi, Y., (2003). Supply chain disruption management. In: *Presentation at the CMI Supply Chains Under Stress Conference, Adastral Park, Ipswich, United Kingdom.*
46. Editor's Desk, (2020). *Blockchain And Crypto Firm VeChain Utilized to Confirm Authenticity of Coronavirus KN95 Masks.* https://blockchainmagazine.net/blockchain-and-crypto-firm-vechain-utilized-to-confirm-authenticity-of-coronavirus-kn95-masks/.
47. ZIGURAT: Innovation and Technology Business School, (2020). *Blockchain in Healthcare: The Case of Coronavirus.* Available from: https://www.e-zigurat.com/innovation-school/blog/blockchain-in-healthcare/ (accessed on 4 December 2023).
48. Juma, H., Shaalan, K., & Kamel, I., (2019). A survey on using Blockchain in trade supply chain solutions. *IEEE Access, 7*, 184115–184132.
49. Gonczol, P., Katsikouli, P., Herskind, L., & Dragoni, N., (2020). Blockchain implementations and use cases for supply chains: A survey. *IEEE Access, 8*, 11856–11871.
50. Dimitrov, D. V., (2019). Blockchain applications for healthcare data management. *Healthcare Informatics Research, 25*, 51–56.
51. Duggal, M., (2020). *Blockchain and AI Amidst the Coronavirus Crisis: 'A Call to Arms.'* CryptoNewZ.
52. Kuo, L., (2020). *Fury in China as Footage Appears to Show Officials Taking Doctors' Face Masks.* The Guardian.
53. Lacina, L., (2020). *What's Needed Now to Protect Health Workers: WHO COVID-19 Briefing.* In: World Economic Forum.

54. Kuo, T. T., Kim, H. E., & Ohno-Machado, L., (2017). Blockchain distributed ledger technologies for biomedical and health care applications. *Journal of the American Medical Informatics Association*, *24*, 1211–1220.
55. Miller, S., (2020). *Building a Blockchain to Verify COVID-19 Data*. [Online].
56. Brett, C., (2020). *Telos Launches Epios Project for Anonymous COVID-19 Testing*. [Online].
57. Moss, A., Spelliscy, C., & Borthwick, J. (2020). *Demonstrating 15 Contact Tracing and Other Tools Built to Mitigate the Impact of COVID-19*. [Online].
58. El Sherif, A. (2020). *Spherity Contributes to Hackathon for Coronavirus Solutions*. [Online].
59. Saraf, C., & Sabadra, S., (2018). Blockchain platforms: A compendium. In: *2018 IEEE International Conference on Innovative Research and Development (ICIRD)* (pp. 1–6). IEEE.
60. Hedera, H., (2020). Acoer coronavirus tracker, powered by hedera hash graph, is now freely available to general public with added clinical trial data. *Hashgraph Hedera*, *11*, 1–6.
61. OECD Economic Outlook, (2020). *Interim Report March 2020: Coronavirus: The World Economy at Risk*. Organization for Economic Cooperation and Development (OECD).
62. Li, X., Jiang, P., Chen, T., Luo, X., & Wen, Q., (2020). A survey on the security of blockchain systems. *Future Generation Computer Systems*, *107*, 841–853.
63. Lee, H., Shin, M., Kim, K. S., Kang, Y., & Kim, J. (2018). "Recipient-Oriented Transaction for Preventing Double Spending Attacks in Private Blockchain," *2018 15th Annual IEEE International Conference on Sensing, Communication, and Networking (SECON),* Hong Kong, China, 2018, pp. 1–2, doi: 10.1109/SAHCN.2018.8397151.

CHAPTER 4

Opportunities and Challenges of Blockchain Technology in Disease Outbreak Tracking

GERA JEMIMAH,[1] B. MAHESHWARI,[1] G. S. N. KOTESWARA RAO,[2] N. RAGHAVENDRA NAVEEN,[3] SHAMS AAGHAZ,[2] A. V. S. S. S. GUPTA,[1] and SURYA KOVVASU[4]

[1]*Joginpally B.R. Pharmacy College, Yenkapally, Moinabad, Hyderabad, Telangana, India*

[2]*Department of Pharmacy, School of Medical and Allied Sciences, Galgotias University, Greater Noida, Uttar Pradesh, India*

[3]*Sri Adichunchanagiri College of Pharmacy, Adichunchanagiri University, B.G. Nagar, Karnataka, India*

[4]*Ambiopharm Inc., Beech Island, North Augusta, South Carolina, USA*

ABSTRACT

Globalization, growing population, and climate change have played an important role in bringing people close to each other and to animals, which led to the easy transmission of various infectious, communicable diseases and pandemics across the globe, making safer regions into non-safer zones and rapidly costing the lives of people.

Effective disease surveillance or tracking systems play an important role in the quick detection of outbreaks and prevention of the spread of epidemics and pandemics. It is a complex process that should be done for infectious and communicable diseases and pandemics, involving participation from many

Creating Smart Healthcare with Blockchain and Advanced Digital Technology.
Rishabha Malviya and Sonali Sundram (Eds.)

independent agencies reporting the data to a centralized information system at the national level through local health departments.

Globally, the information related to major diseases is coordinated by the leading agency, WHO, and International Health Regulations. Thus, effective tracking of outbreaks, epidemics, and pandemics helps in the early detection of the harm caused by them and their future transmission, so that efficient control and preventive measures are taken for their management by adopting appropriate medications and vaccination policies.

Traditional tracking systems are paper-based systems that remained a challenge to most governments due to the lack of appropriate mechanisms for timely detection of new infections and prediction of the risks due to these infections, as they led to the collection of data, which is inappropriate, redundant, incomplete, unscalable, easily alterable, and insecure. Thus, these systems posed a threat to data exchange and protection, integrity, and interoperability, leading to the spread of wrong information and creating unnecessary panic in the public. The COVID-19 pandemic has shown the importance of adapting digital technology by exposing the limitations of traditional healthcare systems in handling public health emergencies. Blockchain technology offers great potential in tracking outbreaks and pandemics by efficiently managing data through real-time disease surveillance by early identification of threats and reporting them to health authorities so that alerts will be sent to the public and preventive measures can be taken.

Blockchain technology has various applications in the healthcare sector, such as tracking or tracing diseases, outbreaks, and pandemics. It helps in the early detection of outbreaks and pandemics, alerting the people regarding the transmission of the disease and associated risks and fast-tracking drug delivery, thereby preventing massive casualties. Thus, blockchain technology offers various advantages over traditional systems in tracking diseases and pandemics due to its cost reduction, improved efficiency, and security in protecting confidential information related to the patient and providing versatility, interconnection, and accountability for easy data access.

Blockchain is a technology that can transform the healthcare sector in today's world, where there is a necessity for quality health facilities aided by advanced technologies. It can strengthen the resources of the countries by providing early warnings for diseases and pandemics, thereby reducing morbidity and mortality and helping in the reduction of delays associated with regulatory approvals.

4.1 INTRODUCTION

Throughout history, mankind has witnessed the disruption caused to the social and political lives and economy by the outbreak of infectious diseases like cholera, Ebola virus, yellow fever, Avian influenza, Nipah, Middle East respiratory syndrome (MERS), Zika virus, severe acute respiratory syndrome (SARS), flu, and H1N1, etc. These served as warning signals about future health emergencies and raised concerns about global health security. The recent global pandemic, COVID-19, has claimed the lives of millions of people across the world, posing a threat to their lives, amputated the global healthcare systems through forceful lockdowns and physical distancing, disrupting the supply chain of medicines, health equipment, and care to patients with various comorbid conditions. Due to globalization, transport across the nations has become more convenient, leading to high infection rates of disease across the world, making it more difficult to prevent outbreaks. This resulted in large-scale outbreaks of infectious diseases due to the ubiquitous nature of the microorganisms and created health emergencies. The COVID-19 pandemic also exposed the shortcomings in addressing these issues at a global level [1–3].

The efficacious way to control and suppress emergencies at the global level is to terminate the outbreak of infectious diseases and pandemics at its source, thereby simultaneously protecting the health of the population at the local as well as international levels [4, 5]. This requires cooperation from health, animal, defense, development, and other sectors by sharing the information obtained from the real-time disease surveillance systems so that the spread of infectious diseases can be detected and prevented instantaneously. Countries can avoid many outbreaks if health systems are strengthened and provided with sensitive real-time disease surveillance data, trained personnel, and effective coordination among various sectors so that threats can be identified early and reported for prompt response [6].

There is a dearth of accurate mechanisms to detect newly infected cases and anticipate the risk of coronavirus and other infections. Data tracking applications based on Bluetooth proximity and geo-location tracking functions have been used by many health sectors and government organizations for identifying the location, tracking the status of COVID-19 infected patients, and sharing the data, but these applications lacked integrity in maintaining the privacy of patients' data [7]. So, to prevent the widespread or outbreak of infectious diseases and pandemics, governments and healthcare systems should rely upon newer technology-empowered solutions that provide accurate and reliable data, like artificial intelligence (AI), machine learning (ML), internet of things (IoT), 3D printing, information communication technology (ICT), and blockchain technology (BCT) [8, 9].

The Ebola virus disease (EVD) outbreak has taught the necessity of technology-based strengthening of the infrastructure of real-time disease surveillance systems for the preparedness of a crisis [10]. Decentralization, transparency, and immutability features of blockchain technology can help in overcoming the challenges of traditional disease surveillance systems and can be exploited for early detection of outbreak threats and reporting them to healthcare authorities for preventive measures, management of supply chain, protection of privacy of data related to users, and to control the spread of misinformation during a crisis. Cooperation among hospitals, clinicians, researchers, and health service providers and exploration of the impact of blockchain technology in preventing outbreaks can help in the country's preparedness for future crisis management [6, 10].

4.2 TRACKING OF DISEASES USING TRADITIONAL SYSTEMS

4.2.1 DISEASE SURVEILLANCE SYSTEM

An efficient surveillance program of a disease plays a key role in providing warning signals in advance about future outbreak control and preventive measures for infectious diseases and pandemics. According to Last JM, infectious disease surveillance is a systematic, complex, ongoing collection, collation, and analysis of data, and timely propagation of the information for appropriate action to be taken, thereby identifying the root source [11]. All national health systems conduct surveillance for both infectious and chronic non-communicable diseases, where numerous independent agencies report to centralized information system.

Tracking/tracing of the contacts is a crucial step in traditional disease surveillance and reporting systems, where the flow of information is upwards from local to regional to state authorities and eventually to the center, i.e., vertical flow of information [2]. In the traditional system, tracking relies upon a paper-based system where a list of potential virus carriers who are in close contact with confirmed cases is stored over a period of time. Methods like calls, letters, and meeting the potential contacts directly (interview-based approach), are used to inform about the contact status [12]. Volunteers or healthcare professionals play a role in collecting the contact information by interviewing the patients, family members, and healthcare professionals or by medical records analysis and tracking or surveillance data [13].

To control pandemics like COVID-19, tracing the infected persons and their previous contacts, keeping records of infected persons, and controlling the dissemination are must because untimely tracing leads to data loss and the spread of false information. Storage of the data with integrity and immutability, and participation of various healthcare institutions in tracing, uploading, integration, and utilization of the infectious disease data are the essential requirements of an ideal infectious disease surveillance and reporting system [2].

4.2.2 LIMITATIONS OF TRADITIONAL SYSTEM

Though traditional disease surveillance systems are established platforms, they are associated with certain limitations like hierarchical upward reporting, management by superior level downwards, inability of peer-to-peer (P2P) data sharing, easy alteration, loss and hacking of data, insecure and loss of privacy of data, redundancy of data and unreliable traceability [2, 14]. These systems delay the information process and are considered incomplete, unorganized, and inaccurate. They are also laborious, costly, and one cannot identify the contact with unknown person. Inability of the public health agencies to receive and share the appropriate data at pandemic level and lack of interoperability with the use of inappropriate tools has led to the search of novel digital technologies that are capable of preventing future outbreaks at a faster pace [15–17].

4.2.3 MODERN SYSTEMS

COVID-19 pandemic has led the national government authorities to adapt and use more advanced digital disease surveillance systems for efficient control of infectious diseases and pandemics. These days, ML techniques are being used by many countries in the surveillance of diseases. COVID-19-related pandemics can be efficiently controlled with the institution of blockchain and other emerging technologies like AI, cloud computing, and Big Data. Blockchain, a decentralized technology, can efficiently replace or enhance the centralized systems that are already in operation [18, 19].

4.3 BLOCKCHAIN TECHNOLOGY IN HEALTHCARE

4.3.1 INTRODUCTION

Blockchain was invented in Japan by Satoshi Nakamoto in 2008 as a form of cryptocurrency system with the first digital currency called Bitcoin [18, 20]. Blockchain is a new disruptive, decentralized technology, a digital ledger with exclusive features like tamper-proof and confidential data infrastructure, inbuilt crypto security software, P2P networking system that altogether validate the transactions within the network, transparency, immutability, and traceability [3, 9, 21]. In short, it is a chain of blocks that are connected via a link. There is no third-party interference and owning by single entity. Therefore, it is secure and more efficient. It also prevents hacking and duplication of the data [19, 22, 23].

Blockchain technology helps in real-time sharing of information/transaction among the participating nodes in the chain. World Health Organization (WHO) can connect with health ministry of every country and even with regional hospitals of each country for sharing the real-time data, so that the world can be alerted about any novel communicable disease. Its hash function ensures the protection and privacy of infected patient's identity [24].

Blockchain technology consists of blocks, miners, and nodes, where multiple blocks form a chain, new block of chains can be created by miners and a blockchain copy will be maintained by electronic devices called nodes [9]. Relevant data will be collected from the participating nodes of blockchain to create raw data and converted into a large-scale data, subsequently [25]. As various participating nodes are uploading the information related to infectious disease, the time stamp function records the time of uploading very accurately. In blockchain technology, information need not be passed in a hierarchical manner, as every participating node can trace back to the root source in an easy manner. Therefore, blockchain technology can be a promising tool in disease direct reporting systems for the storage of disease information and tracing of root source [2].

Crowd-sourced data can be made user-centric data using blockchain technology [26]. Patients, diagnostic centers and clinical laboratories, hospitals, government, and healthcare institutions are the participating nodes of blockchain technology. Records of patient's medical history, test results, treatment plan and status, discharge summary, etc., are the documents that can be stored on the digital ledger with accuracy [9]. Various applications of blockchain are shown in Figure 4.1.

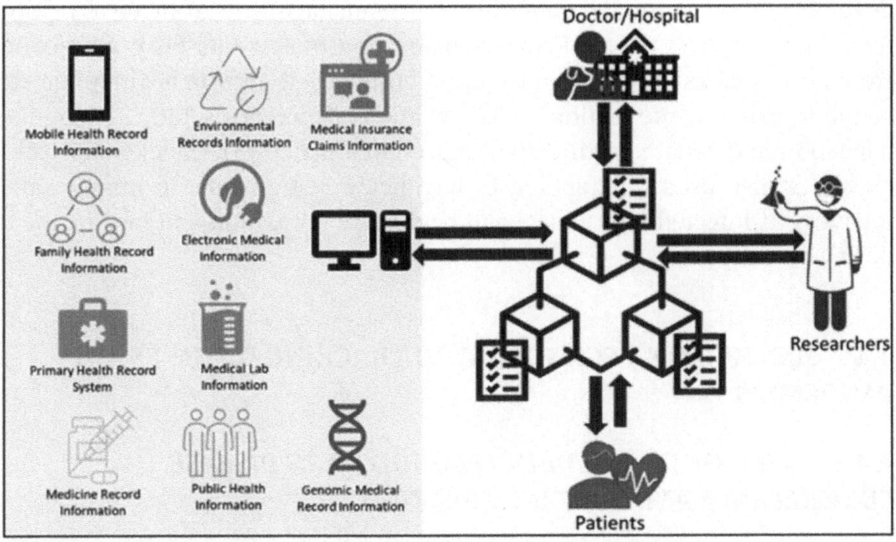

FIGURE 4.1 Blockchain-based applications in healthcare.
Source: Adapted from Ref. [60]

4.3.2 APPLICATIONS

The healthcare sector is one of the sectors that was hugely impacted by the COVID-19 pandemic and this sector can be transformed by exclusive features of blockchain technology [3]. Due to digital database and decentralized nature, blockchain technology plays a major role in healthcare sector in tracking of diseases (including COVID-19) and their spread, identification of high-risk patients and their movement and providing real-time data that is accessible to the public and health organizations globally [9]. Thus, this technology is useful in monitoring and treating potential patients at various stages with accuracy and efficacy and also preserves the information related to the patient [27].

The European Parliamentary Research Service (EPRS) considers blockchain to be a crucial technology in fighting COVID-19 and related pandemics [28]. This technology finds its applications in numerous fields of healthcare sector like tracking of outbreaks, tracking of donations, medical supply chain management (SCM), tracking of clinical drug trails, protection of user privacy [29], management of electronic medical records (EMRs), pandemic control and disease surveillance, monitoring of immunity or vaccination status, contact tracing, IoT (remote monitoring or mobile health), management of clinical trial research, processing of healthcare insurance claims, sharing of clinical research and medical data with healthcare collaborators, development of AI model, genomics, waste management of medical equipment and supplies, telemedicine, management of test kits [14], protection from cyberattacks, global monitoring of outbreaks to inform health policies, enabling privacy, prevention of falsification of diagnosis [30, 31], online education and secure certification and e-governance [3]. Blockchain technology is also used for tracking of healthcare instruments, to improve the recovery of infected individuals and healthcare protection and management during crisis [9].

4.4 BLOCKCHAIN TECHNOLOGY IN TRACKING DISEASES AND PANDEMICS

4.4.1 NEED OF BLOCKCHAIN TECHNOLOGY IN DISEASE SURVEILLANCE AND CONTACT TRACKING

Effective and appropriate disease surveillance needs availability of accurate data for the control of infectious diseases and prevention of the spread of pandemics. Public hospitals and clinical laboratories may give information related to spread of the infection, but the data obtained may not be reliable as it was collected in a traditional way. For efficient tracking of the source of an infectious disease, data has to be uploaded from multiple nodes, which is not possible with the traditional disease tracking systems. Quality of the healthcare system can be improved exponentially by sharing, maintaining privacy and securing the safety of data [32].

A proficient contact tracking and disease direct reporting system, which is capable of limiting the pandemic at the source, is instantly needed. Researchers and healthcare organizations are stressing on the fast, precise, and effective system that can cover large for monitoring and the control of infectious diseases [3, 9]. With smart contracts and consensus algorithm being desirable characteristics, blockchain is considered as a promising technology for the tracking of infectious diseases and related pandemics. Blockchain technology is a patient-centric platform rather than institution-centric and manages healthcare data by coordination of on-chain and off-chain events. This technology is also considered advantageous over other real-time and ML techniques in the surveillance of diseases. Contact tracing when combined with blockchain technology [33].

Therefore, as an emerging technology, blockchain can be efficiently applied to improve the storage of information and for tracking of the infectious diseases during their propagation. Thus, blockchain technology is considered as a powerful tool of disease surveillance and tracking system in providing real-time data [2].

4.4.2 REAL-TIME TRACKING THROUGH BLOCKCHAIN

Blockchain technology in public health initiative has ability to provide real-time disease surveillance, sharing and storage of secure data among national, state, and local health agencies and sending quick alerts after identifying the possible outbreaks or biological attacks, for suitable intervention. This surveillance system also helps in timely identification and reporting of infectious disease by aggregation of real-time data, rapid execution of necessary healthcare interventions and thus controls the spread of infectious diseases and pandemics. Combination of blockchain technology and AI can personalize the medication, treatments, and health recommendations on the basis of medical and hereditary history and other factors of the patient [6].

In Estonia, blockchain technology is being operated for the complete public health infrastructure. The UK, the USA, and Canada have also implemented real-time disease surveillance systems in various of their departments. In England and Canada, it is implemented in emergency departments' syndromic surveillance systems. European Antimicrobial Resistance Surveillance Network is another example of implementation of blockchain technology in real-time surveillance system [34]. Table 4.1 shows differences between traditional and blockchain-based real-time disease surveillance systems.

TABLE 4.1 Differences between Traditional and Blockchain-based Real-Time Disease Surveillance Systems

Sl. No.	Traditional System	Blockchain-based System
1.	Vertical flow of information	Horizontal flow of information
2.	Centralized surveillance system	Decentralized surveillance system
3.	Client-server database	Each node participates in administration
4.	Data is liable to hacking	Integrity and privacy of data is maintained
5.	Data is liable to alteration	Data is immutable
6.	Time consuming and laborious process	Quick and efficient process
7.	Use of paper-based contracts	Use of smart contracts

4.4.2.1 CONTACT TRACING

Contact tracing is an efficient tracking approach that can alert people exposed to infectious diseases, so that spread can be prevented by timely protection [35]. It is a process of identifying, assessing, and managing people who are in close contact with confirmed index case and then tracked and informed them about the risk, advised to get care and prior treatment so that further transmission of the infection can be prevented [17]. Contact tracing also plays a role in controlling epidemics and infections that are undetected due to asymptomatic nature. To minimize the outbreak and, if any person is confirmed to be infected, it is very important to perform tracing of the contacts for obtaining valuable information. Contact tracing approach has a history dated back to late 19th century, where UK has adopted this method in surveillance system for infectious disease like smallpox for notifying, isolating, disinfecting, and case finding by the medical officers [12].

A contact is a person who is in close association with the confirmed case and develops signs and symptoms after exposure. It is the responsibility of the public health officials to detect the contacts and notify to the center as well as the contact, thereby, manage and monitor them with regards to symptoms, treatment regimens and recovery during quarantine or self-isolation [12].

In the blockchain all blocks are connected in which data is stored and secured cryptographically. Each block has four components – hash of the block, transaction data, cryptographic hash of previous block and a time-stamp [12]. Update about the outbreak of infectious diseases and pandemics can be stored in each block at a particular time. Disease surveillance system becomes effective when blockchain technology is combined with AI and geographical information system (GIS). This combination of technology helps in investigation of epidemics, pandemics, SCM of drugs and vaccines [9, 36]. An example of blockchain-based contact tracing of COVID-19 is shown in Figure 4.2.

4.4.2.2 STORAGE OF THE DATA

Data collected by the process of contact tracing can be stored in two ways – on-chain and off-chain. On-chain storage is needed if data has to be transacted and for all the remaining data, off-chain can be employed.

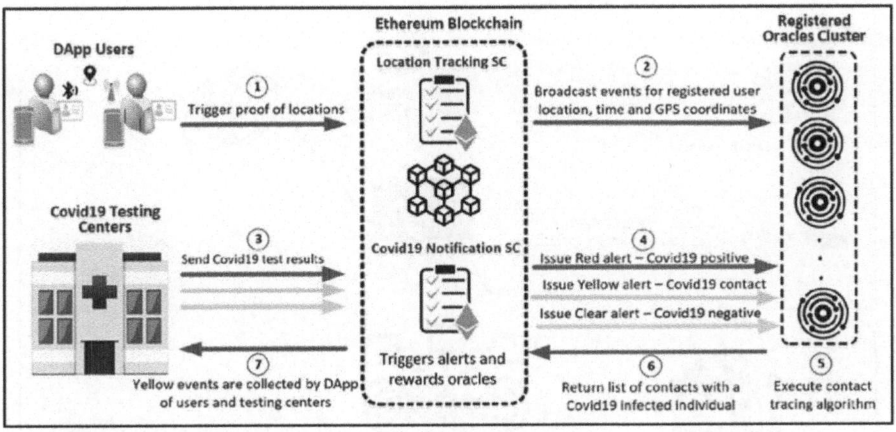

FIGURE 4.2 Blockchain based contact tracing of COVID-19.

Source: Adapted from Ref. [61]

4.4.2.3 PROPOSED MODELS OF CONTACT TRACING

4.4.2.3.1 Contact Tracing Combined with Blockchain Technology

There are three types of users in this model – contact tracer, patient, and administrator, which have access to the network with respect to their levels and are committed to policies concerning privacy and procedures related to safeguarding of personal data. All activities are performed according to smart contract – contact tracing records. Contacts are identified by conducting interview or investigation of the patient or care giver in a detailed way [35].

A list of people who are in close association with confirmed case will be prepared by contact tracer and once confirmed as contacts, they are notified and informed about self-quarantine, symptoms to watch for, self-reporting, testing and treatment options when health deteriorates, etc. After identifying the contacts by the hospital and other agencies, biodata related records are added to blockchain. Patient can access their medical records, self-monitor, and submit the symptoms so that contact tracer helps in monitoring their health. Information related to emergency or preventive messages will be sent to patient by contact tracer. Contacts information will be added by the patient, if he/she tests positive therefore contact tracer will send appropriate response quickly. Third party is not allowed to view the data; therefore, it is not misused and thus privacy is maintained [35]. Proposed framework for system design is shown in Figure 4.3.

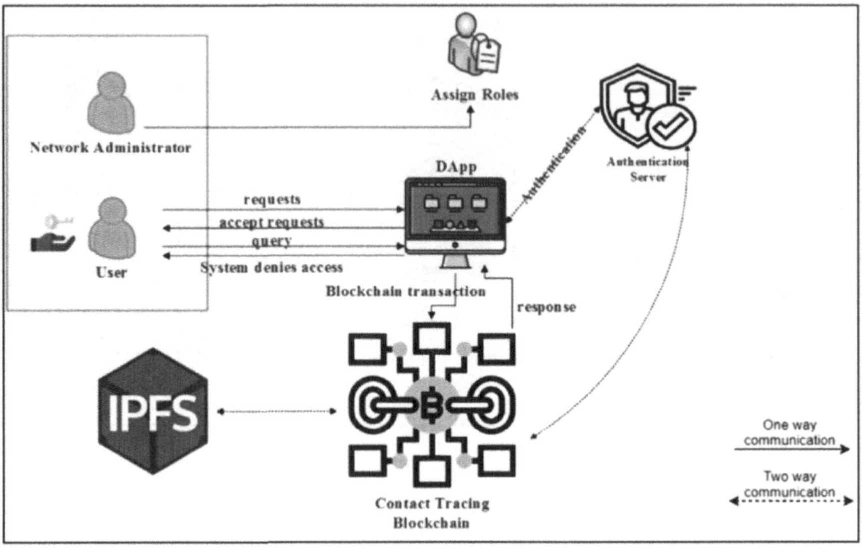

FIGURE 4.3 System design of proposed framework.

Source: Adapted from Ref. [35]

4.4.2.3.2 Contact Tracing Model Proposed by Peng Zhu et al.

According to this model, infectious disease tracing requires participation of three types on entities – health institutions, decision makers, and ordinary participants. Hospitals and CDCs of related regions act as health institution nodes that collect infectious case information, number of cases, checkup reports, and abnormal reports from different regions. The administration and national CDC are the decision makers, while researchers, healthcare experts, social groups, and the public act as ordinary participants [2].

Data related to infectious disease is generated and collected by regional hospitals and CDCs (originating points). Once the authenticity and effectiveness of the data is confirmed and agreed upon the consensus layer, the information to be stored is issued through P2P network in blockchain and thus stored and recorded in the data layer in a chain-wise manner [37]. Ordinary participants are destinations to receive the flow of information, and act as decision makers. Every participating entity has to register a node on the blockchain to get a unique ID consisting of public and private keys.

When there is an infectious disease outbreak, related information is collected by the nodes of local medical institutions and is stored in the blockchain after consensus and validation. This stored information can help in tracing, research analysis and for generation of early warning signals. If second hospital has information related to new disease, it will be uploaded and stored as hash in the blockchain. All the transaction data is uploaded in chronological order and therefore cannot be modified or altered. Once passes the consensus layer, updated information is recorded on the blockchain with current uploaded time (time stamp function of BCT). Finally, the information is delivered to all the participating nodes, which partake in uploading and storing of the data, thus responsible for horizontal transfer of disease information [2].

The final outcome will be obtained through DApp software. Consensus algorithm called PBFT (practical byzantine fault tolerance) is adopted to reach the consensus for all the participating nodes. Smart contracts will set the warning thresholds and send the alarms throughout the network. The entire process of infectious disease tracking is under the supervision of decision makers and highest CDCs. Risk of large-scale outbreak of pandemics can thus be reduced by sending early warning signals at initial stages [2].

4.4.2.3.3 Algorithmic Contact Tracing

Algorithmic contact tracing proposed is a digital epidemiological method that reduces transmission of virus most efficiently and automates the conventional tracing process, allows collection, aggregation, and analysis of contact data that is generated automatically, thus sends the early warning signals to prevent the outbreak. Immutability feature of blockchain can be disadvantageous in algorithmic contact tracing. Number of transactions executed per unit time, are also less when compared to traditional tracking systems. Therefore, this study concluded that depending on the question to be addressed in contact tracing one can opt either traditional system or algorithmic contact tracing [12].

4.4.2.3.4 Other Related Works

Chamola et al., explored the role of blockchain in epidemics of infectious diseases and in monitoring and management of coronavirus infected patients, but this is not empirical research [38]. According to Torky & Hassan, blockchain can be employed for automatic identification of patients infected with COVID-19 and determining the risk of its outbreak in the public. It can also be used for management of supply chain and follow-up of donations [39].

COVID-19 infected patients can also be identified from computed tomography (CT) slabs [40].

4.4.2.4 ROLE OF SMART CONTRACTS

These are the agreements executed without third-party intervention as a part of blockchain protocol. Being computerized transaction protocols, execute the terms of a contract. These are better alternatives to paper-based contracts and a complete solution, when combined with blockchain. They eliminate the delay in processing and there is no intervention by the third-party, therefore implemented by all stakeholders for rapid settlements. It is of low cost and prevents forgeries, thus saving millions of dollars [3, 12].

4.4.2.5 BCT APPLICATIONS AND PLATFORMS

Blockchain-based applications are commonly known as decentralized applications or DApps, which use smart contracts for operational management. Such smart contracts and DApps are developed by a famous blockchain protocol called Ethereum [41]. With the outbreak of COVID-19, many organizations have applied blockchain technology to find solutions for preventing the likelihood of outbreak of infectious diseases and pandemics in future (Table 4.2). They are as follows:

1. **COVID-19 Tracker App:** This is used for restoring the symptoms daily [42].
2. **NHS COVID-19:** This is a track and trace application that is concerned with user privacy and misuse of user's data [43].
3. **Contact Tracing by Google Apple:** This application protects identity and privacy of user, but privacy can be attacked, as the central server is used for searching contacts [44].
4. **Med Chain:** It is a permissioned type of blockchain technology proposed by Shen et al. to give the patients complete control of their medical records [45].
5. **Trace Together:** With this application developed in Singapore, potential virus carriers can be traced using Bluetooth low energy

(BLE), but the device of users has to be active all the time, therefore power of device is hugely consumed [46].

6. **Digital Health Passports:** These are proposed based on blockchain technology for providing immunity certification, response time reduction, unchangeable logs, and developed a solution that reduces the effect of infectious diseases and pandemics by providing timely responses [47].
7. **Go Data Software Applications:** This application is used for recording the symptoms of the contacted individuals and specifying possible COVID-19 clusters [12].
8. **Smartphone Contact Tracing Technology:** This technology helps in control and spread of infectious diseases and pandemics, minimizing quarantine restrictions and control of new cases, thus, helps in overcoming the crisis [48].
9. **Co-App DHS:** This is a blockchain based application built on Ethereum for tracking and automation of various processes that help in detection of COVID-19 at early stage. It is a platform that shares data end-to-end, helps in therapeutic development and deliver opinions and critical care support to self-isolated individuals and elderly people. This application follows private permissioned protocol and acts as additional support system to National Health Service (NHS). It allows users to own the information related to their COVID-19 test results, past health records and is interoperable with other DApps. Data of the test results can be directly shared to researcher and by using consensus, integrity of the data is verified. By using proof-of-authority (PoA) algorithm, the data is scaled up and the results are consolidated using K-means clustering model.

   Three types of the data are stored in the Co-App – confidential, transactional, and others. It also makes sure that the record of information/transactions pertaining to single patient is immutable [10].

   Independent existence, control of information, data usage transfer, confidentiality of data, limit purpose and protection are the characteristic features of this DApp. It also enables the users to request for COVID-19 test kit and health services. Using peer-to-peer connection, scientists can obtain the test results from the patients and provide appropriate guidance to them in terms of treatment regimen, self-isolation, etc. [10].

10. **Hashlog:** It helps in logging and visualization of outbreak data of coronavirus from CDC of USA and WHO. It was developed by Acoer, which is a health technology startup of Georgia [49].
11. **VeChain:** It is developed for monitoring production of vaccines and offers appropriate methods for reducing the risk of modifications to information related to vaccines. It was built in China [50].
12. **PHBC:** The prominent feature of this blockchain based platform is to trace the movement of uninfected person and aimed at continuous verification of communities and workplace, which are free from potentially risky viruses [9].
13. **Hyperchain:** It was developed by China to support government and health organizations in tracking of donation process [9].
14. **Healthchain:** It is a privacy preserving cross institution decentralized framework for disease classification designed by Kuo, Kim & Ohno-Machado [51] that primarily focuses on unification and sharing of data resources related to infectious diseases and dispense of early warning signals through smart contracts, but in addressing data storage and tracing issues.
15. **Self-Test and Tracing System of COVID-19 and Related Infectious Disease:** It is a low cost blockchain integrated with AI proposed by Mashamba et al. and is well established theoretically but lacked concrete models or methods [52].

TABLE 4.2 List of DApps and BCT-based Platforms

Sl. No.	DApps and BCT Platforms	Organization/Developer
1.	MedChain	Shen et al. [45]
2.	Trace together	Singapore
3.	Co-App DHS	Ethereum-based support to NHS
4.	Hashlog	Acoer
5.	VeChain, Hyperchain	China
6.	Health chain	Kuo et al. [51]
7.	MiPasa	WHO with IBM, Oracle, Microsoft
8.	P2P Mobile application design	Government organization
9.	Corona Warn app	Germany

4.4.3 ONGOING RESEARCH

4.4.3.1 MIPASA

It is a blockchain-based platform was launched in March 2020 by WHO to aid sharing of fully private information related to COVID-19 pandemic between individuals, state authorities, health institutions and enables self-reporting of data regarding infection times and locations by public health officials and individuals, thus prevents circulation of false information. It is built in partnership with IBM, Oracle, HACERA, and Microsoft [23].

4.4.3.2 P2P-MOBILE APPLICATION DESIGN

It is a blockchain-based application that supports users to measure the probability of COVID-19 outbreak, automatically and help in identifying the concealed infected sufferers by government officials [53].

4.4.3.3 ETHEREUM AND HYPERLEDGER-BASED MEDICAL CHAIN AND HEAL POINT

It is a platform related to telemedicine and remote healthcare systems that suggest relevant doctor to the patient [54, 55].

4.4.3.4 EPIOS

It is a private COVID-19 testing proposed the COVID-19 infection. It helps in contacting the labs that provide and prepare PCR kits and ticket will be given for each kit by the suppliers of the testing kit. These tokens or coupons are stored cryptographically in blockchain for tracking the users [56].

4.4.3.5 VIRI PLATFORM

It is an anonymous contact tracing platform that controls expansion of diseases. Disease scope in different regions can be traced by this platform and thus locate the spots where there is a growth of COVID-19 infection. If the user is in close contact with positive individual, it will be informed through notification by this application. Thus, this platform can play a role in predicting the pandemic globally [57].

4.4.3.6 COV-ID AND E-REZEPT SYSTEMS

E-Rezept is built on self-sovereign identification (SSI) concept. By showing their unique identifiers as evidence, they help the infected persons in remote purchasing of medications [58]. COV-ID is a blockchain based startup which is based on self-sovereign identity network called Sovrin [59].

China's health code system and German "Corona Warn app" are the other applications that employed blockchain technology.

4.5 LIMITATIONS OF BLOCKCHAIN TECHNOLOGY

Major challenge faced by blockchain technology is scalability. This is being solved using off-chain scaling mechanism of Interplanetary File System (IPFS) [12], Ethereum foundation by data partitioning, introduction of ZKSnarks and parallelization [62]. Other limitation of this technology is number of transactions per second (TPS). Being a technology-centric platform, it is subjected to challenges like implementation barriers, high cost, social acceptance, adoption by users, privacy of patient data and its security and transparency [35].

Data is also prone to attack by cyber criminals, lack of proper user testing and user-behavior research and potential conflict of interest. As a small number of nodes are involved, this technology faces challenges related to governance. Further, storing large scale data is also impractical. Blockchain technology is still not widely accepted and used, therefore, subjected to vigorous scrutiny and challenges [10].

4.6 CONCLUSION

Outbreak of Ebola virus, SARS, MERS, H1N1 and the related infectious diseases and epidemics in the past made the government and healthcare organizations realize the ability of novel digital technologies in offering suitable solutions to unknown challenges in public health [3]. With the recent COVID-19 pandemic, barriers pertaining to entry and acceptance of novel innovative technologies in healthcare have been lowered, favoring implementation of these technologies [14].

Blockchain is a decentralized technology which has the ability to replace or alter or augment the existing centralized disease surveillance systems. This technology finds enormous scope in the healthcare sector, research, and clinical care and can help in critical decision making at the times of crisis. This technology secures global health by strengthening the abilities of the countries in detecting the infections that pose a threat to public health and provides surveillance of early warnings of epidemics and pandemics and thus turns down the mortality, morbidity, and economic costs [14].

Decentralization, immutability, and transparency features of blockchain technology help in real-time data surveillance across the nation, which can be widened to other nations and thus ensuring global health security through global surveillance and collaboration among various countries [6]. Beyond contact tracing, blockchain technology can also provide remarkable benefits in various sectors of public healthcare. Preparedness and response strategies can be improved, spread, and outbreak of pandemics and infectious diseases can be prevented by refined solutions, protection of user privacy, management of medical supplies, tracking of donations, etc. [10]. Countries like India, Pakistan, and Africa can benefit from the implementation of this digital technology, which offers simplified warning signals for prevention of the outbreak [34].

Blockchain-based applications and platforms can block the epidemics and pandemics by early detection, tracking of drug trials at a faster pace and mainly by alerting about the possible outbreaks [23]. Real-time information can be shared between participating nodes in the chain in an immutable way.

From the literature review, it was evident that blockchain technology was introduced as a probable technology that helps in control of the infection at its source, so that a possible outbreak can be prevented. It also aids in restraining the misinformation related to pandemics.

Destructive outbreaks of infectious diseases can be prevented effectively when blockchain is combined with AI and other emerging technologies. Based on the research work done so far, this technology offers wider applications in the healthcare sector both during and after the pandemics [14]. Finding the solutions to the challenges faced by blockchain technology and developing a wider understanding, literacy, and target-specific research can make this technology an ideal disease surveillance platform for infectious diseases and outbreaks. We need to look back at the existing infrastructure for combating the outbreaks, thereby improving the adaptability of this technology and regulations associated with it, so that another pandemic like COVID-19 may not be faced in the future [23].

KEYWORDS

- **blockchain technology**
- **contact tracing**
- **disease surveillance**
- **heal point**
- **Hyperledger-based medical chain**
- **real-time tracking**
- **traditional system**

REFERENCES

1. Chattu, V. K., Kumar, R., Kumary, S., Kajal, F., & David, J. K., (2018). Nipah virus epidemic in southern India and emphasizing "one health" approach to ensure global health security. *Journal of Family Medicine and Primary Care*, *7*, 275.
2. Peng, Z., Jian, H., Yue, Z., & Xiaotong, L., (2021). Enhancing traceability of infectious diseases: A blockchain-based approach. *Information Processing and Management*, *58*, 102570.
3. Zaina, A., Raghad, K., Mousab, H., Eman, D., Omar, C., Wajdi, A., & Habib, H., (2021). Role of blockchain technology in combating COVID-19 crisis. *Applied Sciences*. doi: 10.3390/app112412063.
4. Cordes, K. M., Cookson, S. T., Boyd, A. T., Hardy, C., Malik, M. R., Mala, P., El Tahir, K., et al., (2017). Real-time surveillance in emergencies using the early warning alert and response network. *Emerging Infectious Diseases*, *23*(1), S131.
5. Baldominos, A., Ogul, H., Colomo-Palacios, R., Sanz-Moreno, J., & G´omez-Pulido, J. M., (2020). Infection prediction using physiological and social data in social environments. *Information Processing and Management*, *57*(3). doi: 10.1016/j.ipm.2020.102213.
6. Vijay, K. C., Anjali, N., Soosanna, K. C., Syed, M. K., & Andy, W. K., (2019). The emerging role of blockchain technology applications in routine disease surveillance systems to strengthen global health security. *Big Data and Cognitive Computing*, *3*(25), 1–10s. doi: 10.3390/bdcc3020025.
7. Marbouh, D., Abbasi, T., Maasmi, F., Omar, I. A., Debe, M. S., Salah, K., Jayaraman, R., & Ellahham, S., (2020). Blockchain for COVID-19: Review, opportunities, and a trusted tracking system. *Arabian Journal for Science and Engineering*, *45*, 9895–9911.

8. AKalla, A., Hewa, T., Mishra, R. A., Ylianttila, M., & Liyanage, M., (2020). The role of blockchain to fight against COVID-19. *IEEE Engineering Management Review*, *48*, 85–96.
9. Abhishek, S., Shashi, B., Ashok, K. B., Mohd, J., Dinesh, K. S., & Abid, H., (2022). Blockchain technology and its applications to combat COVID-19 pandemic. *Research on Biomedical Engineering*, *38*, 173–180.
10. Sohag, S., & Farabi, S., (2020). High-level design and rapid implementation of a clinical and non-clinical blockchain-based data sharing platform for COVID-19 containment. *Frontiers in Blockchain*, *3*, 1–14. doi: 10.3389/fbloc.2020.553257.
11. Last, J. M., (2001). *Dictionary of Epidemiology* (4th edn., p. 61). Oxford University Press: New York, NY, USA.
12. Lamport, L., Shostak, R., & Pease, M., (1982). The byzantine generals problem. *ACM Transactions on Programming Languages and Systems, 4*(3), 382–401. doi: 10.1145/357172.357176.
13. Dai, H. N., Imran, M., & Haider, N., (2020). Blockchain-enabled internet of medical things to combat COVID-19. *IEEE Internet of Things Magazine*, *3*, 52–57.
14. Wei, Y. N., Tien-En, T., Prasanth, V. H, M., Andrew, H. S., F., Khung-Keong, Y., Dean, H., Fuji, S. S. F., et al., (2021). Blockchain applications in health care for COVID-19 and beyond: A systematic review. *The Lancet*, 3, e819–e829.
15. Dimitrov, D. V., (2019). Blockchain applications for healthcare data management. *Healthcare Informatics Research, 25*(1), 51–56. doi: 10.4258/hir.2019.25.1.51.
16. Armbruster, B., & Brandeau, M. L., (2007). Contact tracing to control infectious disease: When enough is enough. *Health Care Management Science*, *10*(4), 341–355. doi: 10.1007/s10729-007-9027-6.
17. Arriagada, B. G., Gilthorpe, M., & Müller, V. C., (2020). The ethical imperatives of the COVID-19 pandemic: A review from data ethics. *Veritas*, *46*, 13–35. doi: 10.4067/s0718927320200002000013.
18. Mello, M. M., & Wang, C. J., (2020). Ethics, and governance for digital disease surveillance. *Science*, *368*(6494), 951–954. doi: 10.1126/science.abb9045.
19. Rahouti, M., Xiong, K., & Ghani, N., (2018). Bitcoin concepts, threats, and machine-learning security solutions. *IEEE Access*, *6*, 67189–67205.
20. Abu-Elezz, I., Hassan, A., Nazeemudeen, A., Househ, M., & Abd-Alrazaq, A., (2020). The benefits, and threats of blockchain technology in healthcare: A scoping review. *International Journal of Medical Informatics*, *142*, 104246.
21. Yuan, R., Xia, Y., Bin, C. H. B., Zang, B. Y., & Xie, J., (2018). ShadowEth: Private smart contract on public blockchain. *Journal of Computer Science and Technology*, *33*(3), 542–556. doi: 10.1007/s11390-018-1839-y.
22. Hussien, H. M., Yasin, S. M., Udzir, S. N. I., Zaidan, A. A., & Zaidan, B. B., (2019). A systematic review for enabling of develop a blockchain technology in healthcare application: Taxonomy, substantially analysis, motivations, challenges, recommendations, and future direction. *Journal of Medical Systems*, *43*(10), 320. doi: 10.1007/s10916-019-1445-8.
23. Ahmed, B., (2020). *Blockchain Technology and COVID-19*. Technology Digital World. https://www.bbvaopenmind.com/en/technology/digital-world/blockchain-technology-and-covid-19/ (accessed on 4 December 2023).

24. Xu, H., Zhang, L., Onireti, O., Fang, Y., Buchanan, W. B., & Imran, M. A., (2020). *Beep Trace: Blockchain-Enabled Privacy-Preserving Contact Tracing for COVID-19 Pandemic and Beyond.* arXiv. doi: 101109/JIOT.2020.3025953.
25. Iyengar, K. P., Vaishya, R., Bahl, S., & Vaish, A., (2020). Impact of the coronavirus pandemic on the supply chain in healthcare. *British Journal of Healthcare Management, 26*, 1–4. doi: 10.12968/bjhc.2020.0047.
26. Yue, X.,Wang, H., Jin, D., Li, M., & Jiang, W., (2016). Healthcare data gateways: Found healthcare intelligence on blockchain with novel privacy risk control. *Journal of Medical Systems, 40*, 218. doi: 10.1007/s10916-016-0574-6.
27. Papadopoulos, T., Baltas, K. N., & Balta, M. E., (2020). The use of digital technologies by small and medium enterprises during COVID-19: Implications for theory and practice. *International Journal of Information Management.* doi: 10.1016/j.ijinfomgt.2020.102192.
28. Kassab, M. H., DeFranco, J., Malas, T., Laplante, P., Destefanis, G., & Neto, V. V. G., (2019). Exploring research in blockchain for healthcare and a roadmap for the future. *IEEE Transactions on Emerging Topics in Computing, 9*, 1835–1852.
29. De, R., Pandey, N., & Pal, A., (2020). Impact of digital surge during COVID-19 pandemic: A viewpoint on research and practice. *International Journal of Information Management, 55.* doi: 10.1016/j.ijinfomgt.2020.102171.
30. Arifeen, M., Al Mamun, M., Kaiser, M. S., & Mahmud, M., (2020). *Blockchain-Enable Contact Tracing for Preserving User Privacy During COVID-19 Outbreak.* Preprints. doi: 10.20944/preprints202007.0502.v1.
31. Marbouh, D., Abbasi, T., Maasmi, F., Omar, I. A., Debe, M. S., & Salah, K., (2020). Blockchain for COVID-19: Review, opportunities, and a trusted tracking system. *Arab Journal of Science and Engineering, 12*, 1–17. doi: 10.1007/s13369-020-04950-4.
32. Bansal, A., Garg, C., & Padappayil, R. P., (2020). Optimizing the implementation of COVID-19 "immunity certificates" using blockchain. *Journal of Medical Systems, 44*, 140. doi: 10.1007/s10916-020-01616-4.
33. George, R. V., Harsh, H. O., Ray, P., & Babu, A. K., (2019). Food quality traceability prototype for restaurants using blockchain and food quality data index. *Journal of Cleaner Production, 240.* doi: 10.1016/j.jclepro.2019.118021.
34. Sudip, B., Amarjeet, S., & Md Mahbub, H., (2019). Strengthening public health surveillance through blockchain technology. *AIMS Public Health, 6*(3), 326–333.
35. Nida, B., Usman, Q., & Ayesha, K., (2021). Efficient contact tracing for pandemics using blockchain. *Informatics in Medicine Unlocked, 26*, 100742.
36. Christodoulou, K., Christodoulou, P., Zinonos, Z., Carayannis, E. G., & Chatzichristofis, S. A., (2020). Health information exchange with blockchain amid COVID-19 like pandemics. In: *6th International Conference on Distributed Computing in Sensor Systems (DCOSS)* (p. 412–417). doi: 10.1109/DCOSS49796.2020.00071.
37. França, A. S. L., Amato, N. J., Gonçalves, R. F., & Almeida, C. M. V. B., (2020). Proposing the use of blockchain to improve the solid waste management in small municipalities. *Journal of Cleaner Production, 2*, 44. doi: 10.1016/j.jclepro.2019.118529.
38. Chamola, V., Hassija, V., Gupta, V., & Guizani, M., (2020). A comprehensive review of the COVID-19 pandemic and the role of IoT, drones, AI, blockchain, and 5G in managing its impact. *IEEE Access, 8*, 90225–90265. doi: 10.1109/ACCESS.2020.2992341.

39. Nguyen, D. C., Ding, M., Pathirana, P. N., & Seneviratne, A., (2021). Blockchain and AI-based solutions to combat coronavirus (COVID-19)-like epidemics: A Survey. *IEEE Access*, *9*, 95730–95753.
40. Braithwaite, I., Callender, T., Bullock, M., & Aldridge, R. W., (2020). Automated and partly automated contact tracing: A systematic review to inform the control of COVID-19. *The Lancet Digital Health*, *2*, e607–e621.
41. Bogner, A., Chanson, M., & Meeuw, A., (2016). A decentralized sharing app running a smart contract on the Ethereum blockchain. In *Proceedings of the 6th International Conference on the Internet of Things – IoT'16 (New York, NY)* (pp. 177, 178). doi: 10.1145/2991561.2998465.
42. Spector, T., (2020). *New Symptom Tracking App Aims to Slow Spread of Coronavirus*. Available online at: https://medicalxpress.com/news/2020-03-symptom-tracking-app-aims-coronavirus.html (accessed on 4 December 2023).
43. Levy, I., (2020). *The Security Behind the NHS Contact Tracing App* (pp. 1–14). Available: https://www.ncsc.gov.uk/blog-post/security-behind-nhs-contact-tracing-app (accessed on 4 December 2023).
44. Mozur, P., Zhong, R., & Krolik, A., (2020). *In Coronavirus Fight, China Gives Citizens a Color Code, with Red Flags*. New York, NY. Available: https://www.nytimes.com/2020/03/01/business/china-coronavirus-surveillance.html (accessed on 4 December 2023).
45. Shen, B., Guo, J., & Yang, Y., (2019). MedChain: Efficient healthcare data sharing via blockchain. *Applied Sciences, 9*, 1207.
46. Bay, J., Kek, J., Tan, A., Hau, C. S., Yongquan, L., Tan, J., & Quy, T. A., (2020). *BlueTrace: A Privacy-Preserving Protocol for Community-Driven Contact Tracing Across Borders, 9*.
47. Garg, L., Chukwu, E., Nasser, N., Chakraborty, C., & Garg, G., (2020). Anonymity preserving IoT-based COVID-19 and other infectious disease contact tracing model. *IEEE Access*, *8*, 159402–159414. doi: 10.1109/access.2020.3020513.
48. Douceur, J. R., (2002). The sybil attack. In: *Proceedings of the 1st International Workshop on Peer-to-Peer Systems* (pp. 251–260). Springer.
49. Hashgraph, H., (2020). *Acoer Coronavirus Tracker, Powered by Hedera Hashgraph, Now Freely Available to General Public with Aided Clinical Trial Data*. Available: https://hedera.com/blog/acoer-coronavirus-tracker-powered-by-hedera-hashgraph-now-freely-available-to-general-public-with-added-clinical-trial-data (accessed on 4 December 2023).
50. Nasdaq, (2018). *VeChain Announces Blcokchain Vaccine Tracing Solution for China*. Available: https://www.nasdaq.com/articles/vechain-announces-blockchain-vaccine-tracing-solution-china-2018-08-16 (accessed on 4 December 2023).
51. Kuo, T. T., Kim, H. E., & Ohno-Machado, L., (2017). Blockchain distributed ledger technologies for biomedical and health care applications. *Journal of the American Medical Informatics Association*, *24*(6), 1211–1220. doi: 10.1093/jamia/ocx068.
52. Mashamba-Thompson, T. P., & Crayton, E. D., (2020). Blockchain and artificial intelligence technology for novel coronavirus disease-19 self-testing. *Diagnostics*, *10*(4), 19. doi: 10.3390/diagnostics10040198.
53. Nguyen, D. C., Ding, M., Pathirana, P. N., & Seneviratne, A., (2021). Blockchain and AI-based solutions to combat coronavirus (COVID-19)-like epidemics: A survey. *IEEE Access*, *9*, 95730–95753.

54. Healpoint Whitepaper 1.1, (2021). Available: https://healpoint.io/whitepaper.pdf (accessed on 4 December 2023).
55. Kumar, M., & Chand, S. (2021). MedHypChain: A patient-centered interoperability hyperledger-based medical healthcare system: Regulation in COVID-19 pandemic. *J Netw Comput Appl.* Apr 1;179:102975. doi: 10.1016/j.jnca.2021.102975. Epub 2021 Jan 13. PMID: 34173429; PMCID: PMC7805409.
56. Moss, A., Spelliscy, C., & Borthwick, J., (2020). *Demonstrating 15 Contact Tracing and Other Tools Built to Mitigate the Impact of COVID-19.* Available: https://techcrunch.com/ (accessed on 4 December 2023).
57. El Sherif, A., (2020). *Spherity contributes to #WirVsVirus Hackathon for Corona-Virus Solutions.* https://medium.com/spherity/spherity-contributes-to-wirvsvirus-hackathon-for-corona-virus-solutions-3c59b1557fdf (accessed on 4 December 2023).
58. Mandrino, J., (2020). *VeChain Announces Blockchain Vaccine Tracing Solution for China.* Available: https://www.nasdaq.com/articles/vechain-announcesblockchain-%0Avaccine-tracing-solution-china-2018-08-16 (accessed on 4 December 2023).
59. Bez, M., Fornari, G., & Vardanega, T., (2019). The scalability challenge of Ethereum: An initial quantitative analysis. In: *2019 IEEE International Conference on Service-Oriented System Engineering (SOSE) (San Francisco East Bay, CA)* (pp. 167–176). doi: 10.1109/SOSE.2019.00031.
60. Pravin, P., Neeraj, P., Sameer, S., Thierry, O. E., & Madhusudan, S., (2022). eHealthChain—A blockchain-based personal health information management system. *Annals of Telecommunications*, *77*, 33–45. doi: 10.1007/s12243-021-00868-6.
61. Haya, R. H., Khaleed, S., Raja, J., Ibrar, Y., Mohammed, O., & Samer, E., (2021). COVID-19 contact tracing using blockchain. *IEEE Access*, *9*, 62956–62971.
62. John Kolb, Moustafa AbdelBaky, Randy H. Katz, & David E. Culler. (2020). Core Concepts, Challenges, and Future Directions in Blockchain: A Centralized Tutorial. *ACM Comput.* Surv. *53*, 1, Article 9 (January 2021), 39 pp. https://doi.org/10.1145/3366370.

CHAPTER 5

Blockchain Role in Medical Supply Chain Management

SHASHIMALA TIWARI

Specialist-FRU, India Health Action Trust, Uttar Pradesh Technical Support Unit, Lucknow, Uttar Pradesh, India

ABSTRACT

The strategy to control the flow of resources, goods, information, and services throughout the process of converting raw inputs into complete outputs for end users is known as supply chain management (SCM). The only obstacles that plague the sector are shifting consumer demands and security concerns; the traditional supply chain is struggling to stay relevant. Both issues are serious; however, they can be resolved with blockchain technology. Blockchain was created as a secure open ledger for recording digital transactions that are administered by a peer-to-peer (P2P) network. Blockchain can be viewed as a condensed form of the internet, in which computers communicate directly with one another rather than through a central server. The purpose of their connection is to store data and perform transactions with it. Blockchain-based new ways to deal with making and dispersing items like drugs offer the possibility to follow the entire lifecycle of medications down to a solitary portion. A blockchain is a distributed dataset of registers or a public record of all transactions or digital events that have been achieved and divided between participating parties. Pharmaceutical supply monitoring, like patient records, is fraught with difficulties. As a result, constructing a permission blockchain with known participants is a viable option. The sheer complexity of such a project, which would require several organizations to appreciate the mutual benefits of adopting ledger

Creating Smart Healthcare with Blockchain and Advanced Digital Technology.
Rishabha Malviya and Sonali Sundram (Eds.)

systems into their supply chain processes, is arguably the biggest barrier. The most difficult issue is trust: every party who joins a blockchain must have complete faith in the other members. Furthermore, because this technological installation necessitates complete transparency and a shift in internal insurance operations, a major investment in staff training will be necessary. Blockchain helps in allowing steady and cost-efficient transfer of products and refining traceability of products, organization between the consumers, partners, and financial aid.

5.1 INTRODUCTION

The medical care store network is going to embrace it perhaps speedier than different industries due to a few explicit difficulties which are hard to address with the real advancements and which could be better covered by blockchain technology. But prior to moving into a few additional substantial models in the medical services record network, we want first to see some basic [1]. A blockchain is basically a distributed database of registers or a public record of all transactions or digital events that have been accomplished and divided between participating parties. Every transaction in the community record is verified by the agreement of a majority of the members of the organization [1].

The blockchain's essential component is to coordinate data, information, and content in a way that ensures data isn't duplicated, but at the same time is reliable, accurate, up-to-date, and quickly verified [1]. Blockchain-based work procedure for health services requests. At first, all the records from medical devices, labs, web-based entertainment, and various other sources are consolidated and create essential data that is automatically filled in proportion to big data [3]. This data is the fundamental element of the whole blockchain-based health services, and it is the primary part which forms the first layer of the load [3].

In rundown blockchains:

- Offer a coordinated method for organizing and storing information on the web;
- Are continually developing internet-based data sets;
- Are continuously assembling and keeping up with records;
- Typically manage exchanges;
- Permit clients to trade data or money with each other or the application program interface and proficiently without the mediator.

5.2 KEY PRINCIPLES OF BLOCKCHAIN TECHNOLOGY

The five essentials' standards hidden the blockchain innovation are:

1. **Appropriated Database:** Everyone on a blockchain approaches the whole data set and its finished history with practically no go-between controlling it [1].
2. **Shared Transmission:** Correspondence happens straightforwardly among peers and not through a focal hub. Every hub store and advance data to any remaining hubs.
3. **Straightforwardness:** Each and every exchange and its related worth are apparent to anybody with admittance to that blockchain.
4. **Irreversibility of Data:** When an interchange is placed in the data set in this way approved, the records can't be modified because they are connected to each exchange record that preceded them. The recording on the data set is super durable, sequentially requested and accessible to all others in that blockchain [1].
5. **Computational Logic:** The advanced idea of the record permits blockchain exchanges to be customized and attached to computational rationale. Clients can arrange calculations and rules to set off consequently exchanges between nodes [1].

5.3 BLOCKCHAIN IN HEALTHCARE SUPPLY CHAIN

Blockchain-based new ways to deal with making and dispersing items like drugs offer the possibility to follow the entire lifecycle of medications down to a solitary portion. Various innovation and drug organizations are now chipping away at inventive arrangements that consolidate computerized stamping of drug items with blockchain innovation to give a way to safely and dependably track items all through their whole lifecycle [1].

In order to create a comprehensive medical care engineering that is divided into four parts, blockchain innovation is located at the center of the basic information layer, which is considered to be the main structure. There are several components at each blockchain step, such as conventions and agreement calculations [3].

The drug production network is one feature of the pharma scene that could profit from the one-of-a-kind qualities and key standards of the blockchain innovation recorded earlier [1].

The production network in the drug business is mind-boggling, with drugs passing from assembling to merchants, repackages, and wholesalers prior to arriving at the retailer and clients. There is next to no ability to see all through this inventory network to follow authenticity [1]. Companies are now working with blockchain innovation to bring honesty, recognizability, and straightforwardness to that worldwide production network. The presentation of blockchain in such a case can receive a few rewards here. Medications can be labeled with standardized tags and whenever they are examined, their records can be kept on a blockchain in non-alterable and secure computerized blocks.

These records will be refreshed progressively as the medications are moved from one substance to the others in the production network. Parties with approved admittance, including patients, can check the records whenever. The permanent idea of blockchain gives drug recognizability from maker to client and permits individuals to check to assume the framework is compromised somewhere [1].

Furthermore, and aside from guaranteeing item honesty and being hostile to duplicating endeavors, blockchain innovation can assist with beating the monetary issues looked at by more modest retailers and administrators along the production network by getting and robotizing installments between trusted parties [1].

Cold chain the board is another significant angle which can be upheld and examined through blockchain innovation in the relationship with temperature following devices [1]. This carries us to a subsequent remark about gadget the board through blockchain innovation, which is one more significant subject for medical care, and which would be tended to in a different article about clinical gadgets the executives as well as wearables and other injectables which are prospering in the health-tech space and which should be gotten as well [1].

5.4 SUPPLY CHAIN MANAGEMENT (SCM)

Supply chain management (SCM) is the method to deal with dealing with the progression of assets, products, data, and administrations all through the technique of changing over crude contributions to finish yields for end shoppers [2].

The whole system holds seven vital components, to be specific: Preparation, Manufacture, Inventory, Goods Return, Data, Source, and Shipping. The parts are utilized to assemble the basic design of an association. Since the parts go about as the business' forthcoming, it sneaks up all of a sudden in space [2].

The main problems that encompass the business are inconsistent purchaser needs and security concerns; the standard production network is confronting troubles to support its importance. The two issues are critical however can be tackled with the assistance of blockchain innovation [2].

5.5 OBSTACLES IN THE SUPPLY CHAIN MANAGEMENT (SCM) SECTOR

A portion of the unmistakable issues looked at in SCM are as per the following:

1. **Absence of a Worldwide Record:** Regardless of the worldwide market being interlocked, most organizations don't share their data set. This prompts correspondence obstructions between firms, assisting exploiters [2].
2. **Low-Quality Traceability:** Following resources are troublesome in supply chain management notwithstanding proposing progressed cycles and gear. This prompts the exploiters to supplant unique items with fakes [2].
3. **Pointless Costs:** As the information is kept bound to associations, each firm spends assets gathering similar information separately. This prompts a superfluous ascent in its application program interface and efforts [2].
4. **Long Assessments:** Evaluating a resource's quality in the supply chain management cycle is troublesome because of its length. Since there is no viable gamble in the executive's framework included, the business is confronted with dreary consequences [2].
5. **Solitary Consumer Needs:** Staying aware of the most recent shopper needs is troublesome, yet going to practical lengths to counter them is even tougher [2].

5.6 BLOCKCHAIN-BASED HEALTHCARE USES

Blockchain innovation is rethinking information demonstration and administration conveyed in much medical care uses. This is mostly due to its compliance and ability to separate, safeguard, and distribute clinical information and services in an exceptional way [2]. The forefront of various ongoing developments in the medical services sector is blockchain innovation.

Theoretically, data sources, blockchain inventions, medical care presentations, and partners are organized into four layers that coordinate emerging blockchain-based medical care advancements (Figure 5.1).

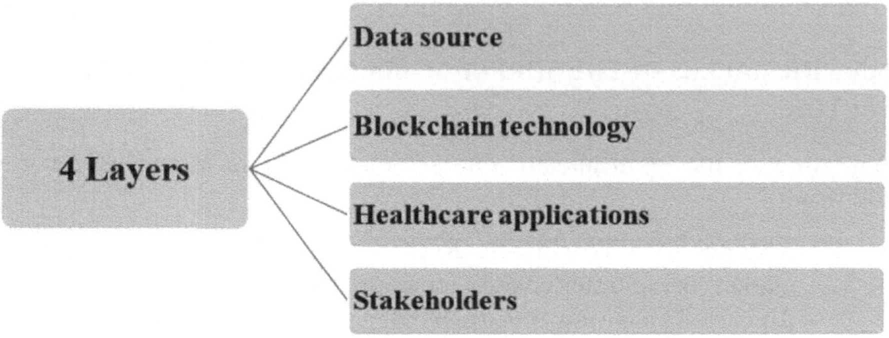

FIGURE 5.1 Four layers of blockchain use.

The essential parts of the blockchain are savvy agreements, marks, wallets, incidents, participation, and computerized assets. For communication with different assignments and structures, or even across many organizations, many conventions could be utilized. This might incorporate, for example, peer-to-peer, concentrated, dispersed, and dispersed. Policymakers could pursue a decision either open, isolated, or even combine in light of the scope of requirements they need to fulfill [2].

The following step is to guarantee that the requests are compatible with the full framework when the stage is created using blockchain innovation. Applications for healthcare powered by blockchain can be categorized into three broad categories. Right off the bat, information the executives, including worldwide logical information sharing for innovative work (research and development), information the board, information capacity and electronic health records (EHRs) [3].

The inferior addresses SCM uses, containing medical preliminaries and drugs. At long last, the second-rate class covers the IoMT, including a conversion of medical services internet of things (IoT) and clinical appliances, healthcare IoT foundation and information safety, and AI.

Lastly, at the highest point of the order comes the partner coating, which comprises gatherings that are profiting from blockchain-based medical care uses like commercial customers, technologists, and patients. The essential worries of customers at this layer are to share, process, and manage information deprived of imperiling its safety and privacy [3] (Figure 5.2).

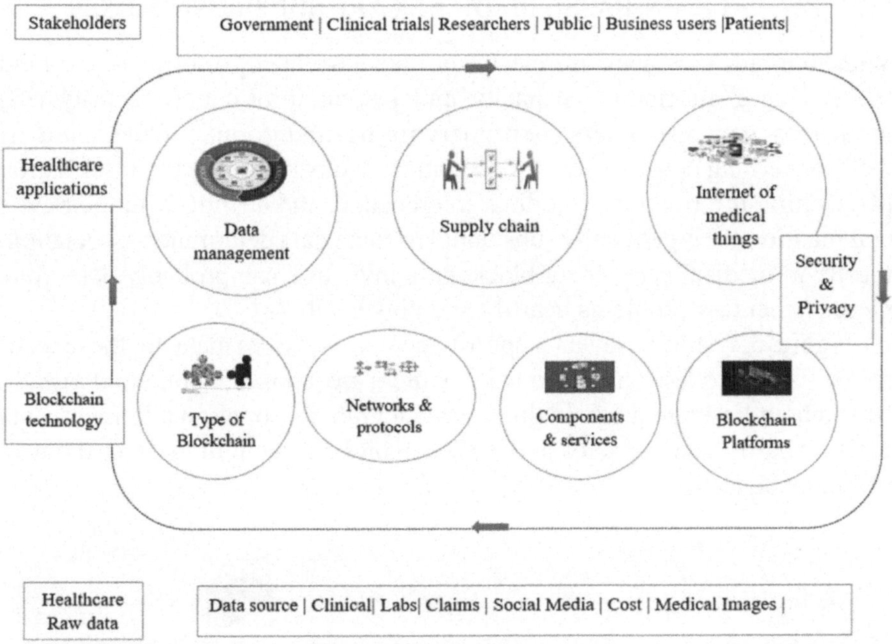

FIGURE 5.2 Workflow of medical care applications.

A workflow for medical care applications founded on blockchain. The workflow is made up of four key layers: stakeholders, blockchain technology (BCT), healthcare applications, and raw data from the healthcare industry. As a decentralized technology, the blockchain allows a variety of stakeholders to profit from healthcare applications [3] (Figure 5.3).

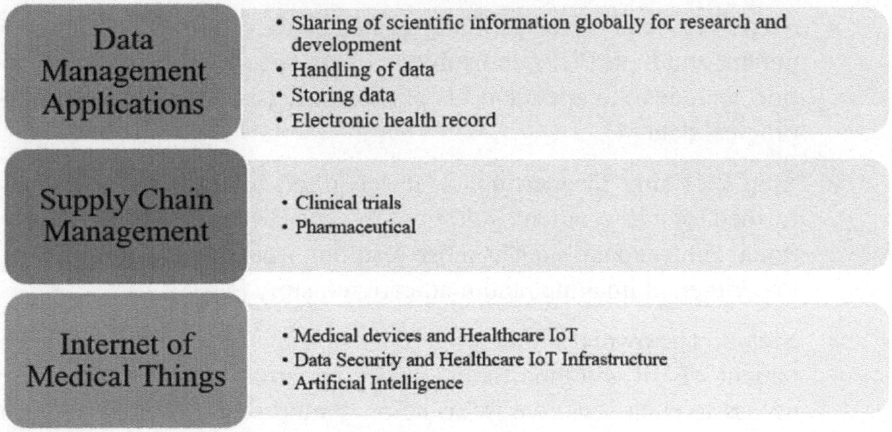

FIGURE 5.3 Blockchain supply workflow.

5.7 BLOCKCHAIN-BASED MEDICAL CARE SUPERVISION USES

With the advancement in electronic health-related information, cloud medical care information capacity and patient information security (IS) guidelines, new open doors are primary for health information the board, as well concerning patients' comfort to contact and part their health information [4]. Getting information, hoarding, interchange, and dealing with their even combination are gigantically substantial to some data determined association, mostly in medical care where blockchain invention can probably determine these elementary problems heartily and powerfully [4].

Figure 5.4 shows seven steps of medical services data in the executive's work process in blockchain, which are spoken about underneath. Blockchain-based requests in this class integrate information allotment, data on the board, data capacity and EHRs, which are communicated about in restraints beneath:

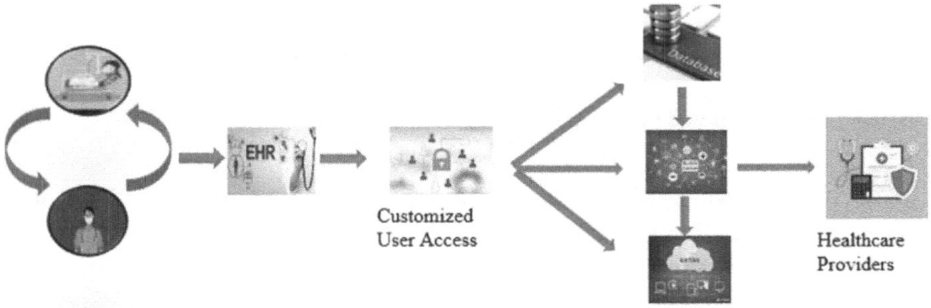

FIGURE 5.4 Medical services data on the executive's work process.

- **Step 1:** Principal information is created by the association between a patient and their PCPs and subject matter specialists. This information includes therapeutical history, present issues and other physiological data [4].
- **Step 2:** Using the pertinent data acquired in Step 1, an EHR is formed for every patient. Additionally recorded in the EHR are additional clinical data, such as those resulting from nursing carefulness, experimental imaging, and medication history [5].
- **Step 3:** The owner of this property is the exclusive recipient of each patient's EHR and modified admission control. Parties who require access to such sensitive information should send a written request

for permission to the owner of the EHR, who will then decide who gets access [5].

- **Steps 4, 5, and 6:** These steps are crucial for the data set, blockchain, and distributed storage at the heart of the entire interaction. Data set and dispersed storage store the registers in a circulated method and a blockchain gives outrageous safeguard to assurance tweaked valid client access [5].
- **Step 7:** The final step involves gaining access to healthcare providers such as temporary facilities, neighborhood care centers, and emergency clinics. These providers will be authorized by the business owner. For instance, your medical record will be accessible and open on your phone and approved through a circulated record, such as a blockchain, independent of where you are treated in the world [5]. Medical service providers will continuously update this record over time.

5.8 WORLDWIDE SYSTEMATIC DATA DISTRIBUTION

Distribution of medical services and clinical information is one fundamental and crucial stage to work on the nature of medical services providers and make the healthcare system more intelligent [9]. Publishing medical records could occur among individuals. For example, a patient who needs to share his medical history with a doctor at their first meeting [6]. Moreover, the distribution could occur between a patient and a partner, such as a patient sharing his medical history with an insurance agency or a research center. Even the information could be shared across borders [7]. However, the practical aspect of the current healthcare systems has several limitations. One limitation is that patients rarely have access to their health records [8].

To improve the connection and collaboration with the healthcare industry, blockchain technology could play a pivotal role, enabling and establishing an efficient distribution mechanism for electronic health information. This is considered one of the most crucial contributions of blockchain-based healthcare [9]. Below, we describe some of the contributions made in this regard. Castaldo and Cinque [7] proposed a cataloging system to facilitate and improve the exchange of electronic health information across different countries in Europe in the most reliable way by using a secure blockchain. The given solution ensures control and shares the user's data easily without compromising privacy. It provides an excellent way to enhance the intelligence of healthcare systems while keeping patient data confidential. Additionally, Vishal Patel [10] introduced a framework for cross-domain image distribution using blockchain technology as a distributed data supply to create a record of radiological examinations and manage image access through customized user permission.

In a similar study, Fan et al. [11] developed a Medical Block framework based on blockchain technology to address data management and data sharing issues in an electronic medical records system and improve clinical information distribution. Patients can access the EMRs of different hospitals through the Medical Block framework by avoiding the previous medical data being fragmented into multiple databases. Furthermore, data sharing and collaborations using blockchain could help hospitals gain a better understanding of patients' medical history prior to the appointment.

A hierarchical location distribution plan based on blockchain technology. The goal was to achieve security-preserving location distribution by blockchain for telecare medical information systems. They define the necessary requirements for location privacy preservation, variability, hierarchical security protection, and anonymity, by using the Merkle tree and order-preserving encryption [12].

An efficient meeting-based healthcare data sharing based on blockchain. Medical Chain uses a survey chain structure approach to verify the integrity of a shared clinical IoT data stream. The evaluation results demonstrate that Medical Chain can achieve higher efficiency and meet the security requirements of healthcare data sharing [13].

5.8.1 DATA MANAGEMENT

Data security and privacy are consistently abused, whether intentionally or by unauthorized users, even though many businesses, particularly healthcare organizations, are the amount of data collected in this period or others like the IoT is increasing substantially [14]. Many institutions have suffered a significant loss in wealth and reputation as a result. Health data users play a variety of responsibilities, and access to the data should be controlled by the credentials assigned to each function. Blockchain technology can be used to seamlessly ensure this kind of access. The blockchain technologies that have been created for this purpose are described below.

Medical Record [56] is a decentralized electronic medical record (EMR) management system in which smart contracts are used to execute data agreements and operations, which are stored in the blockchain. Patients receive comprehensive, unchangeable medical data and services from medical records, which collaborate with suppliers' entire health data for data auditing, authentication, confidentiality, and exchange.

To allay users' worries about their lack of ability to regulate uploaded ledgers, Zhu et al. [15] developed a method for providing manageable blockchain data management in the cloud situation. They included a unique trust authority node in their model so that consumers may stop any potentially dangerous acts even in the event of a mainstream attack.

Additional work by Genestier et al. [16] offered a novel concept for overhauling consent management in the healthcare system, focusing on giving users complete authority over all health record data via blockchain. However, neither an access control system nor an authorization design is used in their execution.

5.8.2 STORAGE OF DATA (APPLICATIONS BASED ON CLOUD)

Each deal is recorded in blocks on a decentralized storage system in a blockchain based on the healthcare industry. EHRs, which are regarded as the foundation of a massive distributed medical storage, are used in the medical care system to organize patient medical data [17]. Where security is a top priority, the latter could be kept on-site or in the cloud. In order to support a lot of information technology (IT) infrastructure, cloud storage is primarily made up of several loading devices associated with a huge volume. One illustration of such IT infrastructure is a healthcare system built on the blockchain. Fast transmission, good allocation, large store volume, simple access, and energetic relationship are all benefits of cloud storage technology [18].

To accomplish accountability, integrity, and security, the major goal of this study is to maintain private medical care data on the blockchain by creating a set of safety standards. However, Bock Cloud—a novel word coined by Kaur et al.—describes the combination of blockchain technology and a cloud environment. Utilizing the cloud is intended to preserve data disseminated and secure under one roof without including other parties. The study addressed issues with the need for collaboration and policy creation among healthcare service providers, public health groups, and governments.

Digital Health Record Because customary medical records are kept on paper, it is difficult to follow the progression of a patient's health over time [22]. Additionally, they are susceptible to inaccurate data, which occasionally leads to patients receiving mistreatment. By introducing EHRs, IT gave the chance to reduce this work. The quality of care was greatly improved by medical practices thanks to electronic access to health records [23]. EHR also makes it possible for increasing levels of preventative treatment and better disease management. Additionally, the digital record offers improved decision-support features and increased caregiver communication. As a result, the healthcare industry is beginning to recognize its importance [24].

Blockchain technology has been the topic of numerous studies to secure, distribute, and preserve EHR data both within and between institutions. By creating protected cloud storage for patients' private medical records, a blockchain architecture for secure health data sharing [25]. This framework uses digital documentation with access control privileges to its owners' data to handle medical data. By using cloud encryption underneath the chain, this is stored. Guo et al. [26] described an attribute-based signature system that makes use of blockchain technology and different authorities to ensure and validate EHRs in a similar study. Group message broadcasts are made easier, and collusion attacks may be resisted.

Wang & Song [18] suggested a secure cloud-based EHR system. Other methods are employed in addition to blockchain to assure the accuracy and traceability of medical facilities. Ro et al. [55] have lectured on several issues connected to the unification of scattered health records and the access management of stakeholders from healthcare providers, whereas the aforementioned three research have mostly concentrated on the cryptographic elements of securing EHR blocks.

Private health record, a circulated paradigm for assimilating personal health records (PHRs) that combines organizational semantic interoperability with up-to-date visualization of various PHR formats, was proposed as a solution to these two problems. PHR employs an equivalent database to store PHR in blocks. Last but not least, Hussein et al. [27] created a framework based on genetic algorithms and separate wavelet transforms for protecting medical records utilizing blockchain technology. To create the required user security key, the suggested solution makes use of a modified cryptographic hash generator [28].

5.8.3 USE CASES IN HEALTHCARE

Managing Information Health Education: The blockchain's main application is as a system for tracking Bitcoin transactions, but this system might also be applied to education [32, 33]. The transfer of skills and knowledge from various sources is the foundation of education. It makes the supposition that everyone who is involved is trustworthy. Regulating bodies find it difficult to keep tabs on how knowledge is changing in medical education as online learning grows in popularity [34, 35]. Blockchain technology may help health professions educators recover the value of instruction and the informative impact on several groups of students, according to Funk et al. [34].

Additionally, it can aid in developing the relative worth of educational interferences. Any organization that uses blockchain technology will also be capable to issue certification on their own, directly, and without the need for a middleman. The management of medical libraries may also be impacted by blockchain in several ways, including the gathering, preservation, and sharing of reliable information by producing time-stamped, verifiable versions of journal articles [36]. We can guarantee that the knowledge is safe and unaltered by using blockchain in healthcare. For instance, using blockchain technology to store educational data in records would make it simple for health educators to monitor their influence when their learners eventually become instructors themselves.

Additionally, it will make it simple to keep track of the most popular and successful learning modules. Additionally, certification could be given to the appropriate people without the assistance of a third party. These concepts illustrate the potential advantages blockchain technology can have for health education. Enrolment Data Management: Administrative enrollment data is produced as a result of enrolling members in health insurance plans, meeting eligibility requirements, and maintaining credentialing records [37].

Manual data management has a long history, which necessitates a laborious process of verifying qualifications, credentials, and eligibility. The entire enrollment process is slowed down by this onerous administrative effort, which creates a barrier to a productive healthcare system.

However, this data might be saved in a blockchain and quickly checked against valid sources and pertinent records. An administrative assistant could profit from this in the quest for greater enrollment process efficiency through streamlined procedures, eligibility checks, network administration, and coordination. Security: Due to its significance in overcoming the security concerns of the EHR in Healthcare, blockchain technology has experienced a significant surge in the health industry [38]. EHRs have the probability to enhance healthcare delivery [39].

When an analytical result, like an MRI scan, is saved in the EHR system, it is produced [40]. As a result, the safety of such digital data is of extreme importance, and blockchain is presently being used to make sure the safety and security of healthcare data [53]. Blockchain technology is important for maintaining the importance of information and lowering loading costs for data administration in healthcare. Blockchain technology continues to be essential to the future of company data management because of its special capacity to secure digital information.

5.8.4 SUPPLY CHAIN MANAGEMENT (SCM)

Supply chain management (SCM) is intended to incorporate the industry's greatest practices to simplify the full delivery process, from ordering to supply [41, 42]. SCM is a difficult concept in the healthcare industry because there is an inherent danger of supply chain process compromise that could have a negative influence on patient safety due to dispersed ordering settings for medical supplies, medications, and other resources [43, 44]. A World Health Organization (WHO) study found that unsuitable dose of counterfeit medications purchased from unreliable sources results in the deaths of over 1,00,000 persons in Africa. In addition to product and drug counterfeiting, a healthcare facility's incomplete product registry and packaging mistakes may completely disrupt the SCM [46].

Blockchain is a very important monitoring technique for getting a handle on the entire process of moving pharmaceuticals and medical supplies [47]. Additionally, the blockchain's distributed ledger enables medical professionals and healthcare regulators to verify and validate the credentials of vendors [48].

Blockchain technology has a lot of potential in this area for building a reliable network of suppliers that enables healthcare managers to protect patients from shady vendors. Additionally, blockchain technology promises major improvements in the transaction, fraud prevention, data provenance, and demand forecasting (Figure 5.5).

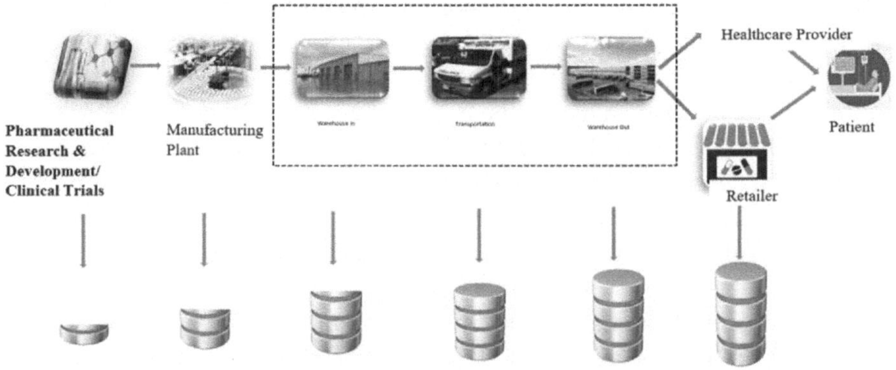

FIGURE 5.5 Supply chain distribution flow.

- **Step 1:** When a novel drug or method of treatment is developed, it creates a barrier requiring patent protection and a protracted clinical testing process. As a type of transaction, this data is entered into the digital ledger.
- **Step 2:** The patent is transferred to the industrial facility for mass construction after the clinical trial is deemed successful. Each product has a distinct identity that is linked to a different block in the blockchain, as well as other pertinent data.
- **Step 3:** Following the completion of huge production and wrapping, medications are assembled in a warehouse in preparation for circulation. The blockchain contains data like time, lot number, barcode, and expiration date.
- **Step 4:** The blockchain also stores transportation-related information, such as the amount of time it takes to travel between warehouses (IN), the authorized agent, and further details.
- **Step 5:** Medical and drug supplies are often distributed to healthcare professionals or retailers by a 3rd party distribution linkage. This is accomplished by using a warehouse (OUT) for every 3rd party, from which all distribution endpoints are connected. The blockchain has also been updated with a different transaction.
- **Step 6:** In order to authenticate and avoid counterfeit, care suppliers such as hospitals must submit information such as lot number, product owner, batch number, and expiration date. The blockchain also includes this.
- **Step 7:** A store follows the same procedures as Step 6 in this step.
- **Step 8:** Since the blockchain supply chain provides prospective customers with transparent information for verification, patients are urged to assess authenticity at every stage.

5.8.5 CLINICAL TRIALS

Patient enrollment, data exchange, and personal data privacy are only a few of the difficulties clinical trials in healthcare must overcome [49, 50]. These problems may be solved by blockchain technology. It offers safe, transparent, and reproducible methods for exchanging clinical trial data [50,

51]. To address trust loss and modify data openness in clinical trials, Smart agreements on a private Ethereum network. The purpose of this work was to strengthen the scientific validity of clinical trial findings, which could be compromised by problems like incomplete information and selective reporting [52]. Shae and Ts artificial intelligence (AI) designed four novel system components on top of the conventional blockchain to grow the capacity of clinical trials and the accuracy of medicine [53].

A unique information management architecture based on approval blockchain technology employing keen contracts was proposed by Choudhury et al. in a different study [54]. Their blockchain proof-of-concept protocol features smart contract enrollment and is based on time-stamped consent gathering [51].

5.8.6 PHARMACOLOGICAL DATA MANAGEMENT

Pharmaceutical companies are constantly working to both create new medicines for a variety of conditions and raise the standard of existing ones. Such medications must go through a protracted process to ensure their safety, efficacy, statistical validity, and patent protection. Clinical trials typically take a significant portion of the time during this lengthy process, which typically lasts from discovery to commercialization [55].

Because of the lack of security and privacy, a lengthy process like this is susceptible to drug recalls and counterfeiting [56]. The use of blockchain technology through the entire pharmaceutical industry could remove this barrier. Using blockchain's distributed ledger, we might protect anonymity and guarantee security by making sure that each trial event is documented in the tamper-proof blockchain nodes. To make sure that the completely pharmaceutical conform to the conservation of patent security, a private blockchain could be deployed [57, 58]. Approximately 60% of pharmaceutical businesses are working on or conducting experiments with blockchain, according to recent research [59], which illustrates the promise of technology in this sector.

The threats posed to the general public and consumers by counterfeit medications are significant and widespread [60, 61]. The objective was to make it easier to trace fake medications. The approach prevents traditional drug supply chain fraud, which is a serious problem for some Asian nations [60].

A Gcoin blockchain was proposed by Tseng et al. [62] as the foundation of the drug data movement to provide clear drug transaction data. Manufacturers, wholesalers, merchants, pharmacies, hospitals, and customers all share in this. Drug supply chain oversight may result from the documenting of drug transactions instead of the regulation (government audits). Moreover, the examination and inspection classical of drug supply chain regulation could be replaced by a surveillance net approach [62].

5.9 ROUTINE CASES IN SUPPLY CHAIN MANAGEMENT (SCM)

5.9.1 ENTITLEMENTS AND PRESENTING MANAGEMENT

The medical billing procedure is a crucial aspect of the healthcare industry. This is so that proper service delivery can never be guaranteed in the absence of billing [66]. The entire billing process might be complicated because some payments are either totally paid for by the patient or by their health insurance plan [67].

Excessive billing is one of the biggest problems with medical billing since there is little communication and no confidence between patients, doctors, and insurance companies. The abuse of claims and billing in the healthcare industry can be stopped or at least reduced by employing a transparent system that benefits all parties. Blockchain technology can guarantee a transparent system that keeps everyone involved in the entire process and eliminates uncertainty between them [66].

5.9.2 QUALITY CONTROL

A medicine is deemed to be an imitation if it contains unsuitable elements and is sold to conceal or simulate its validity, background, or even effectiveness [68, 69]. Additionally, counterfeit goods and medications have a substantial impact on SCM [70].

Their presentation in the pharmacological sector is a modest aspect that significantly undermines the effectiveness, sincerity, and solid profitability of a specific healthcare business [71]. Customers frequently don't know the precise origins of the goods they buy and consume in a global market [72]. Around the world, this kind of medicine poses a serious hazard to life since it is harmful to the patient [73].

Additionally, this poses a risk to the standing of the original pharmaceutical firms, prompting them to spend a significant amount of money on defense [68]. A study discovered that methods like spectroscopy and chromatography, which identify active substances and analyze the makeup of image samples, are useful for spotting fake goods [73].

They have several limits, though, as they rely on electromechanical equipment, which raised the overhead expense. Having the information of pharmaceutical manufacturers, containing product serial numbers and package numbers, on the blockchain would be one way to address these issues, allowing pharmaceutical firms, drug manufacturers, and consumers to connect to the blockchain and confirm the accuracy of the data. This procedure confirms low-cost product registration, medicine following, and anti-counterfeiting measures.

5.10 INTERNET OF MEDICAL THINGS (IOMT)

The growth of health and medical information systems depends on the internet of medical things (IoMTs) systems [74]. IoMTs technology enables real-time data collection, processing, and sharing over the Internet for medical devices including wearables, body scanners, and heart monitors.

With the development of AI, for instance, healthcare providers can now take an image using the IoMTs paradigm, spot worrisome cells or even cancerous portions, and communicate this information with people who have the legal right to access it. The progress in the IoT for healthcare and smart medical devices in the field of AI is mostly covered in the following topics (Figure 5.6).

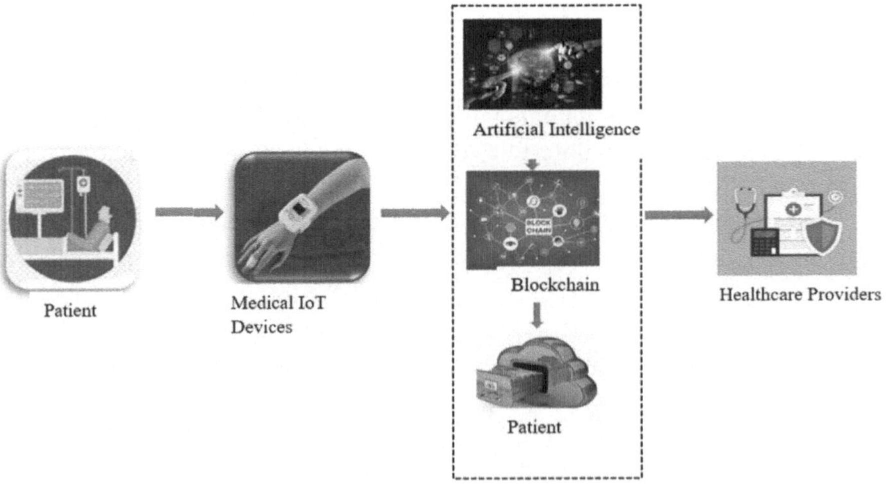

FIGURE 5.6 Internet of medical things functions in blockchain.

- **Step 1:** Internet of medical things, the patient serves as the sole data basis.
- **Step 2:** Medical internet of things devices is typically either intimately involved or remotely monitoring patients' bodies, producing a significant amount of data.
- **Step 3:** Blocks are used to collect the data generated in step 2 in step 3. Blockchain will benefit from AI to develop intellectual virtual agents, which can automatically generate new ledgers. Decentralized AI systems could assist blockchains to attain the best level of safety in cases involving delicate health information when safety is the top importance [75].
- **Step 4:** Healthcare workers are the final users who request access to a reliable delivery of care that has been approved by the owner.

5.11 HEALTHCARE INTERNET OF THINGS (IOT) AND MEDICAL DEVICES

Internet of things (IoT) is a grouping of calculating plans that may interchange data across a network utilizing the Internet protocol without involving any human-machine contact. The IoT plays a key function in the healthcare system as a result of such a potent seamless contact [76]. The IoMTs currently revolve around wearable and medical technology [77]. Wireless body-area network (WBAN) methods are a substantial component of the IoMTs in the healthcare division. In particular, in the medical and healthcare sectors for distant monitoring of physiological parameters, WBANs are emerging as a crucial enabling technology [78–81].

IoT devices, for instance, can be used to notify people of upcoming calories burned, appointments, changes in blood pressure, and much more [82, 83]. The work that is currently being done to assimilate blockchain with the IoMTs is reviewed in the discussion that follows. Blockchain smart contracts were used by Griggs et al. [84] to create a system for secure real-time patient observation and medical involvement. The study suggests incorporating blockchain to carry out smart contracts that assess data gathered by a patient's IoT medical equipment based on personalized threshold values. In order to solve the issue of logging data transfer transactions in an IoT healthcare system, this is done.

A decentralized big data source is used to supply and subsequently part of healthcare organizations, communities, and individuals utilizing blockchain in Rahman et al.'s [85] intelligent dyslexia analytics solution, cellular multimedia during dyslexia testing, health information is recorded and kept in a decentralized big data source. This data can then be united for additional clinical study and statistical analysis. IoT and blockchain technology were combined to generate structural health monitoring by Jo et al. [86]. They put forth a revolutionary approach that, by splitting them into edge and core networks, activates locally centralized and globally decentralized distribution. As a result, it improves the blockchain system's efficiency and scalability.

The main difficulty with this paradigm is maintaining security while transferring data between pervasive social network nodes. The authors created two protocols to solve this issue. The purpose of this scheme was to create a smartphone application-based mobile health scheme for cognitive behavioral treatment for sleeplessness [87].

5.12 HEALTHCARE INTERNET OF THINGS (IOT) INFRASTRUCTURE AND DATA SECURITY

The medical care information and communication technology (ICT) framework comprised of a huge number and IoT gadgets, including terminals, sensor, symptomatic instruments, remote passages, and so on. This framework empowers numerous medical care frameworks, for example, wearable gadgets and remote checking administrations to communicate and share information about the patient's basic circumstances with parental figures. Throughout the transmission cycle, information navigates through obscure correspondence organizations which may be powerless against safety and protection breaks [88]. To report the previously declared safety encounters in medical care IoT, scientists are investigating different procedures to shield clients' information from the illegal entrance. The creators likewise recommended a mist registering engineering that surveys weaknesses of existing and recently added equipment into the medical care IoT utilizing OpenVAS structure [89].

The review proposes the expansion of a safeguarding coat against figuring out by return situated programming and check adding procedures. Albeit the safety insurance of embedded clinical gadgets and devices is very much aided in this review, heterogeneous innovations are expected to incorporate a combined proficiency, yet to the detriment of expanded intricacy to the entire framework [90].

A different extent of collected tactile traffic is taken care of into two recognition subsystems: anomaly identification (ADSs) and Misuse location for better execution. Curiously, when the extent of change builds the framework completes well, and it shows the most noteworthy exactness as far as Sensitivity and Specificity when tangible information extent on abuse recognition is 0:25%. This cycle demonstrates an expanded recognized rate [91].

Notwithstanding, the above price of this new analysis is the twofold recently projected model. As oneself driving the independent vehicle is forming an ongoing conveyance framework steadily, its utilization in medical services is imperative, particularly, in the medical services SCM. Aloqaily et al. [93] acquainted an interruption discovery component with oppose assault like Denial of Service, Probe, Remote to the client, and so on [92].

The creators proposed a profound conviction network for information aspect decrease, and a choice tree involving ID3 calculation for interruption order. The discovery precision of the frameworks is 99.92%, which is very high; notwithstanding, the bogus negative rate is 1.53%. The outcome implies around three interruption assaults could enter the framework for each 200 client meetings. With an end goal to lessen the safety weakness of radio frequency identification in medical care IoT framework, Catarinucciet et al. [94] proposed a shrewd emergency clinic framework that comprises of mixture detecting network taking advantage of compelled application convention, IoT savvy passage, and a UI to give outsiders the capacity to engage patients with health checking framework [95].

The future design is a mix of Wireless and blockchain networks which can be utilized for medical care administrations, yet a legitimate execution of such an enormous and complex organization might open possible restrictions; for instance, computational above streamlining of blockchain may be troublesome [95, 96]. Esposito et al. [97] investigated medical services' IS and protection by presenting various types of information structures in the blockchain.

A nearby PC is utilized as a Miner and various IoT gadgets are bunched together to such an extent that one is chosen as a group head to decrease access check utilizing strategy header. Likewise, this research utilized a common intersection network where numerous information proprietors are allowed to embed information into the blocks which are constrained by a single administrator. Be that as it may, this might prompt the absence of dependability among clients [98, 99].

A few security and security weaknesses in the ebb and flow IoT environment were recognized for additional examination including insurance during refreshing programming of billions of IoT gadgets (medical services, for example) where blockchain could be utilized to upgrade security [100]. As indicated by the above conversation, we can derive that albeit ordinary security frameworks give improved security, complete carefully designed frameworks can't be guaranteed. Blockchain is viewed by quite a few people as a possible arrangement among other cutting-edge advancements to be carried out in a little and medium-scale medical services IoT frameworks [101].

5.13 MAN-MADE BRAINPOWER

Blockchain advances get progressively strong and more powerful, as they turn into combined with AI in different genuine word medical services arrangements [102]. AI and profound learning are the super driving elements for AI space, which is likewise tenaciously working on the headway of robotization. The capacity of a machine to organize or predict designs precisely increases as we feed it more information [103]. Kuo & Ohno-Machado [104] presented the ModelChain system in light of blockchain innovation. This system uses a secluded blockchain to empower various foundations to add health information to prepare an AI model further develop care without unveiling their health registers [104]. Such a system builds the safety and strength of the dispersed protection safeguarding medical care prescient demonstrating across various establishments. Wang et al. [105] planned a blockchain-based equal medical services framework (PHS), including counterfeit frameworks, computational trials and equal execution (ACP). The ACP zeroed in mostly on addressing a patient's determination, condition, and treatment process [106].

5.14 CASES USE FOR BLOCKCHAIN ON THE INTERNET OF MEDICAL THINGS (IOMTS)

Absence of Normalization: The speed increase of the medical care industry towards embracing best-in-class IoMTs innovation is colossal. Notwithstanding medical care suppliers on-premises, clinical gadgets, the IoMTs opens the office of clinical benefits to be gotten to pervasively to perpetually direct patients. This is likewise the structure blocks of telehealth observation requests as remote gadgets are related to catching bio-signals. Consequently, the carefully designed transmission of clinical information is extremely significant [107]. This issue results from the high heterogeneity in correspondence conventions, clinical gadgets and stages, which could be named as the absence of normalization among IoMTs producers. In this manner, safeguarding such factor normalized transmission medium is troublesome in the ongoing point of view [108, 109].

5.15 CONCLUSION

Blockchain innovation is supposed to reform the medical care environment. Not just the cycle will be straightforward and safe, yet additionally, the nature of medical services will be expanded at a lower cost. The patients will reserve the option to conclude who can and can't get to their information and for what reason. For sure, the assumption for a person's protection shifts starting with one country and then onto the next because of the government policies.

Thusly, future investigation on the regulation, standardization, and crossline health data recovery approaches together with preservation and use goal is properly dire. Hence, there is a requirement for inventive systems and calculations to limit the mining delays. Specifically, the pertinence of blockchain to address belief corruption and to reinforce information transparency on the medical trials. A few specialists propose the utilization of blockchain to work on the scientific validity of findings from medical trials, which could be subverted by issues like missing information and selective publication. We additionally talked about the issue of tracking medications; obviously, blockchain innovation will be an imperative apparatus for pharmacists and medical services providers to properly and timely verify the flow of authentic medications and their delivery to the patients. At last, we introduced the utilization of blockchain in IoMT. These systems generate data consistently and can be subject to malicious attacks while in communication at different levels of the underlying communication network. In this chapter, we talked about a few exploratory studies that propose to modify secure systems using blockchain technology to ensure the integrity of health information. The primary issue that we accept needs attention from specialists is the way the blockchain will work in complex and diverse communication systems. The IoMTs delivery system will utilize communication networks owned by different service providers with different data access regulation policies. We likewise suggest further examination of innovative solutions that promote blockchain as a support that allows various parties (organizations, devices, users, etc.) of the IoMTs paradigm to access essential reliable blockchain infrastructures.

KEYWORDS

- **blockchain**
- **data security**
- **internet of medical things**
- **pharmaceutical sector**
- **quality control**
- **supply chain management**

REFERENCES

1. Philippe, G., (2019). *Blockchain in the Healthcare Supply Chain*. https://www.linkedin.com/pulse/blockchain-healthcare-supply-chain-philippe-%E8%8F%B2%E5%8A%9B%E6%B5%A6-gerwill/.
2. Lalit, B., (2021). *The Role of Blockchain in Supply Chain Management.* https://www.c-sharpcorner.com/article/the-role-of-blockchain-in-supply-chain-management/.
3. Saraf, C., & Sabadra, S., (2018). Blockchain platforms: A compendium. In: *Proceedings of the 2018 IEEE International Conference on Innovative Research and Development (ICIRD)* (pp. 1–6). Bangkok, Thailand.
4. Dimitrov, D. V., (2019). Blockchain applications for healthcare data management. *Healthc. Inform. Res., 25*, 51–56.
5. Panesar, A., (2019). *Machine Learning and Artificial Intelligence for Healthcare: Big Data for Improved Health Outcomes*. Springer: Emeryville, CA, USA.
6. Frost, J. H., & Massagli, M. P., (2008). Social uses of personal health information within PatientsLikeMe, an online patient community: What can happen when patients have access to one another's data? *J. Med. Internet Res., 10*, e15.
7. Castaldo, L., & Cinque, V., (2018). Blockchain-based logging for the cross-border exchange of e-health data in Europe. In: *International ISCIS Security Workshop* (pp. 46–56). Springer: Cham, Switzerland.
8. Hien, D. T. T., Hien, D. H., & Pham, V. H., (2018). A survey on opportunities and challenges of blockchain technology adoption for revolutionary innovation. In: *Proceedings of the ACM Ninth International Symposium on Information and Communication Technology, Danang City, Vietnam* (pp. 200–207).

9. Liang, X., Zhao, J., Shetty, S., Liu, J., & Li, D., (2017). Integrating blockchain for data sharing and collaboration in mobile healthcare applications. In: *Proceedings of the 2017 IEEE 28th Annual International Symposium on Personal, Indoor, and Mobile Radio Communications (PIMRC), Montreal, QC, Canada* (pp. 1–5).
10. Patel, V., (2018). A framework for secure and decentralized sharing of medical imaging data via blockchain consensus. *Health Inform. J.*
11. Fan, K., Wang, S., Ren, Y., Li, H., & Yang, Y., (2018). Medblock: Efficient and secure medical data sharing via blockchain. *J. Med. Syst., 42*, 136.
12. Ji, Y., Zhang, J., Ma, J., Yang, C., & Yao, X., (2018). BMPLS: Blockchain-based multi-level privacy-preserving location sharing scheme for telecare medical information systems. *J. Med. Syst., 42*, 147.
13. Shen, B., Guo, J., & Yang, Y., (2019). MedChain: Efficient healthcare data sharing via blockchain. *Appl. Sci., 9,* 1207.
14. Vo, H. T., Kundu, A., & Mohania, M. K., (2018). *Research Directions in Blockchain Data Management and Analytics* (pp. 445–448). EDBT: Lisbon, Portugal.
15. Zhu, L., Wu, Y., Gai, K., & Choo, K. K. R., (2019). Controllable and trustworthy blockchain-based cloud data management. *Future Gen. Comput. Syst., 91*, 527–535.
16. Genestier, P., Zouarhi, S., Limeux, P., Excoffier, D., Prola, A., Sandon, S., & Temerson, J. M., (2017). Blockchain for consent management in the e-health environment: A nugget for privacy and security challenges. *J. Int. Soc. Telemed. eHealth, 5*, GKR-e24.
17. Zhang, R., & Liu, L., (2010). Security models and requirements for healthcare application clouds. In: *Proceedings of the 2010 IEEE 3rd International Conference on Cloud Computing, Miami, FL, USA* (pp. 268–275).
18. Wang, H., & Song, Y., (2018). Secure cloud-based electronic health record system using attribute-based cryptosystem and blockchain. *J. Med. Syst., 42*, 152.
19. Al Omar, A., Bhuiyan, M. Z. A., Basu, A., Kiyomoto, S., & Rahman, M. S., (2019). Privacy-friendly platform for healthcare data in cloud based on blockchain environment. *Future Gen. Comput. Syst., 95*, 511–521.
20. Kaur, H., Alam, M. A., Jameel, R., Mourya, A. K., & Chang, V., (2018). A proposed solution and future direction for blockchain-based heterogeneous Medicare data in cloud environment. *J. Med. Syst., 42*, 156.
21. Li, X., Huang, X., Li, C., Yu, R., & Shu, L., (2019). EdgeCare: Leveraging edge computing for collaborative data management in mobile healthcare systems. *IEEE Access, 7*, 22011–22025.
22. Wang, S. J., Middleton, B., Prosser, L. A., Bardon, C. G., Spurr, C. D., Carchidi, P. J., Kittler, A. F., et al., (2003). A cost-benefit analysis of electronic medical records in primary care. *Am. J. Med., 114*, 397–403.
23. Miller, R. H., & Sim, I., (2004). Physicians' use of electronic medical records: Barriers and solutions. *Health Affairs, 23*, 116–126.
24. Terry, A. L., Thorpe, C. F., Giles, G., Brown, J. B., Harris, S. B., Reid, G. J., Thind, A., & Stewart, M., (2008). Implementing electronic health records: Key factors in primary care. *Can. Fam. Phys., 54*, 730–736.
25. Chen, Y., Ding, S., Xu, Z., Zheng, H., & Yang, S., (2018). Blockchain-based medical records secure storage and medical service framework. *J. Med. Syst., 43*, 5. [CrossRef].
26. Guo, R., Shi, H., Zhao, Q., & Zheng, D., (2018). Secure attribute-based signature scheme with multiple authorities for blockchain in electronic health records systems. *IEEE Access, 776*, 1–12. [CrossRef].

27. Hussein, A. F., Arun, K. N., Ramirez-Gonzalez, G., Abdulhay, E., Tavares, J. M. R., & De Albuquerque, V. H. C., (2018). A medical records managing and securing blockchain based system supported by a genetic algorithm and discrete wavelet transform. *Cognit. Syst. Res., 52*, 1–11. [CrossRef].
28. Rivest, R., (1992). *The MD5 Message-Digest Algorithm*. Technical Report; RFC Editor: Marina Del Rey, CA, USA. [CrossRef].
29. Yang, J., Onik, M. M. H., Lee, N. Y., Ahmed, M., & Kim, C. S., (2019). Proof-of-familiarity: A privacy-preserved blockchain scheme for collaborative medical decision-making. *Appl. Sci., 9*, 1370.
30. Zhang, X., & Poslad, S., (2018). Blockchain support for flexible queries with granular access control to electronic medical records (EMR). In: *Proceedings of the 2018 IEEE International Conference on Communications (ICC), Kansas City, MO, USA* (pp. 1–6).
31. Zhang, X., Poslad, S., & Ma, Z., (2018). Block-based access control for blockchain-based electronic medical records (EMRs) query in eHealth. In: *Proceedings of the 2018 IEEE Global Communications Conference (GLOBECOM), Abu Dhabi, UAE* (pp. 1–7).
32. Sharples, M., & Domingue, J., (2016). The blockchain and kudos: A distributed system for educational record, reputation, and reward. In: *European Conference on Technology Enhanced Learning; Springer: Cham, Switzerland* (pp. 490–496).
33. Devine, P., (2015). Blockchain learning: Can crypto-currency methods be appropriated to enhance online learning? In: *Proceedings of the ALT Online Winter Conference, Manchester, UK.*
34. Funk, E., Riddell, J., Ankel, F., & Cabrera, D., (2018). Blockchain technology: A data framework to improve validity, trust, and accountability of information exchange in health professions education. *Acad. Med., 93*, 1791–1794.
35. Benna, I. I., (2019). Optimizing health, education, and governance delivery through blockchain. In: *Optimizing Regional Development Through Transformative Urbanization* (pp. 24–47). IGI Global: Hershey, PA, USA.
36. Hoy, M. B., (2017). An introduction to the blockchain and its implications for libraries and medicine. *Med. Ref. Serv. Q., 36*, 273–279.
37. Iezzoni, L. I., (1997). Assessing quality using administrative data. *Ann. Internal Med., 127*, 666–674.
38. Alonso, S. G., Arambarri, J., López-Coronado, M., & De La Torre, D. I., (2019). Proposing new Blockchain challenges in e-Health. *J. Med. Syst., 43*, 64.
39. desroches, C. M., Campbell, E. G., Rao, S. R., Donelan, K., Ferris, T. G., Jha, A., Kaushal, R., Levy, D. E., Rosenbaum, S., Shields, A. E., et al., (2008). Electronic health records in ambulatory care—A national survey of physicians. *N. Engl. J. Med., 359*, 50–60.
40. Bahga, A., & Madisetti, V. K., (2013). A cloud-based approach for interoperable electronic health records (electronic health records). *IEEE J. Biomed. Health Inform., 17*, 894–906.
41. Lee, S. M., Lee, D., & Schniederjans, M. J., (2011). Supply chain innovation and organizational performance in the healthcare industry. *Int. J. Oper. Prod. Manag., 31*, 1193–1214.
42. Dehgani, R., & Jafari, N. N., (2019). The impact of information technology and communication systems on the agility of supply chain management systems. *Kybernetes.*
43. Kim, C., & Kim, H. J., (2019). A study on healthcare supply chain management efficiency: Using bootstrap data envelopment analysis. *Health Care Manag. Sci.,* 1–15.

44. Clauson, K. A., Breeden, E. A., Davidson, C., & Mackey, T. K., (2018). *Leveraging Blockchain Technology to Enhance Supply Chain Management in Healthcare.* Blockchain Healthc. Today.
45. World Health Organization, (2017). *WHO Global Surveillance and Monitoring System for Substandard and Falsified Medical Products*. World Health Organization: Geneva, Switzerland.
46. Jayaraman, R., AlHammadi, F., & Simsekler, M. C. E., (2018). Managing product recalls in healthcare supply chain. In: *Proceedings of the 2018 IEEE International Conference on Industrial Engineering and Engineering Management (IEEM), Bangkok* (pp. 293–297).
47. Dujak, D., & Sajter, D., (2019). Blockchain applications in supply chain. In: *SMART Supply Network* (pp. 21–46). Springer: Cham, Switzerland.
48. Narayanaswami, C., Nooyi, R., Raghavan, S. G., & Viswanathan, R., (2019). Blockchain anchored supply chain automation. *IBM J. Res. Dev.*
49. Isojarvi, J., Wood, H., Lefebvre, C., & Glanville, J., (2018). Challenges of identifying unpublished data from clinical trials: Getting the best out of clinical trials registers and other novel sources. *Res. Synth. Methods, 9*, 561–578.
50. Benchoufi, M., & Ravaud, P., (2017). Blockchain technology for improving clinical research quality. *Trials, 18*, 335.
51. Benchoufi, M., Porcher, R., & Ravaud, P., (2017). Blockchain protocols in clinical trials: Transparency and traceability of consent. *F1000Research, 6,* 66.
52. Nugent, T., Upton, D., & Cimpoesu, M., (2016). Improving data transparency in clinical trials using blockchain smart contracts. *F1000Research, 5*, 2541.
53. Shae, Z., & Tsai, J. J., (2017). On the design of a blockchain platform for clinical trial and precision medicine. In: *Proceedings of the 2017 IEEE 37th International Conference on Distributed Computing Systems (ICDCS), Atlanta, GA* (pp. 1972–1980).
54. Choudhury, O., Fairoza, N., Sylla, I., & Das, A. (2019). *A Blockchain Framework for Managing and Monitoring Data in Multi-Site Clinical Trials.* arXiv 2019, arXiv:1902.03975.
55. Schöner, M. M., Kourouklis, D., Sandner, P., Gonzalez, E., & Förster, J., (2017). *Blockchain Technology in the Pharmaceutical Industry.* Frankfurt School Blockchain Center: Frankfurt, Germany.
56. Marucheck, A., Greis, N., Mena, C., & Cai, L., (2011). Product safety and security in the global supply chain: Issues, challenges, and research opportunities. *J. Oper. Manag., 29*, 707–720.
57. Xu, X., Lu, Q., Liu, Y., Zhu, L., Yao, H., & Vasilakos, A. V., (2019). Designing blockchain-based applications a case study for imported product traceability. *Future Gen. Comput. Syst., 92*, 399–406.
58. Westerkamp, M., Victor, F., & Kupper, A., (2019). Tracing manufacturing processes using blockchain-based token compositions. *Dig. Commun. Netw.* In press.
59. *60 of Pharma Companies Using or Trying Blockchain Survey*. Available online: https://pharmaphorum.com/news/60-of-pharma-companies-using-or-trying-blockchain-survey/ (accessed on 4 December 2023).
60. Sylim, P., Liu, F., Marcelo, A., & Fontelo, P., (2018). Blockchain technology for detecting falsified and substandard drugs in distribution: Pharmaceutical supply chain intervention. *JMIR Res. Protoc., 7*, e10163.

61. Mackey, T. K., & Liang, B. A., (2011). The global counterfeit drug trade: Patient safety and public health risks. *J. Pharm. Sci., 100*, 4571–4579.
62. Tseng, J. H., Liao, Y. C., Chong, B., & Liao, S. W., (2018). Governance on the drug supply chain via Gcoin blockchain. *Int. J. Environ. Res. Public Health, 15*, 1055.
63. Toyoda, K., Mathiopoulos, P. T., Sasase, I., & Ohtsuki, T., (2017). A novel blockchain-based product ownership management system (POMS) for anti-counterfeits in the post supply chain. *IEEE Access, 5,* 17465–17477.
64. Sidorov, M., Ong, M. T., Sridharan, R. V., Nakamura, J., Ohmura, R., & Khor, J. H., (2019). Ultralightweight mutual authentication radio frequency identification protocol for blockchain enabled supply chains. *IEEE Access, 7*, 7273–7285.
65. Pun, H., Swaminathan, J. M., & Hou, P., (2018). *Blockchain Adoption for Combating Deceptive Counterfeits*. SSRN: New York, NY, USA.
66. Dhillon, V., Metcalf, D., & Hooper, M., (2017). *Blockchain Enabled Applications: Understand the Blockchain Ecosystem and How to Make It Work for You*. Springer: Emeryville, CA, USA.
67. *Course 2: The Medical Billing Process*. Available online: https://www.medicalbillingandcodingonline.com/medical-coding-for-billers/ (accessed on 4 December 2023).
68. *Counterfeit Medications*. Available online: https://en.wikipedia.org/wiki/Counterfeit_medications (accessed on 4 December 2023).
69. Deisingh, A. K., (2005). Pharmaceutical counterfeiting. *Analyst, 130*, 271–279.
70. Zhu, Q., & Kouhizadeh, M., (2019). Blockchain technology, supply chain information, and strategic product deletion management. *IEEE Eng. Manag. Rev., 47*, 36–44.
71. Plotnikov, V., & Kuznetsova, V., (2018). The prospects for the use of digital technology "blockchain" in the pharmaceutical market. In: *MATEC Web of Conferences* (Vol. 193, p. 02029). EDP Sciences: Ho Chi Minh, Vietnam.
72. Montecchi, M., Plangger, K., & Etter, M., (2019). It's real, trust me! Establishing supply chain provenance using blockchain. *Bus. Horiz*. In press.
73. Kumar, R., Agarwal, A., & Shubhankar, B., (2018). Counterfeit drug detection: Recent strategies and analytical perspectives. *Int. J. Pharma Res. Health Sci., 6*, 2351–2358.
74. Chiuchisan, I., Costin, H. N., & Geman, O., (2014). Adopting the internet of things technologies in health care systems. In: *Proceedings of the 2014 International Conference and Exposition on Electrical and Power Engineering (EPE), Iasi, Romania* (pp. 532–535).
75. *Decentralized AI: Blockchain's Bright Future*. Available online: https://espeoblockchain.com/blog/decentralized-ai-benefits/ (accessed on 4 December 2023).
76. Moosavi, S. R., Gia, T. N., Rahmani, A. M., Nigussie, E., Virtanen, S., Isoaho, J., & Tenhunen, H., (2015). SEA: A secure and efficient authentication and authorization architecture for IoT-based healthcare using smart gateways. *Procedia Comput. Sci., 52*, 452–459. [CrossRef].
77. Haghi, M., Thurow, K., & Stoll, R., (2017). Wearable devices in medical internet of things: Scientific research and commercially available devices. *Healthc. Inform. Res., 23*, 4–15.
78. Yuce, M. R., (2010). Implementation of wireless body area networks for healthcare systems. *Sens. Actuators Phys., 162*, 116–129.
79. Crosby, G. V., Ghosh, T., Murimi, R., & Chin, C. A., (2012). Wireless body area networks for healthcare: A survey. *Int. J. Ad Hoc Sens. Ubiquitous Comput., 3,* 1.

80. Rani, A. A. V., & Baburaj, E., (2019). Secure and intelligent architecture for cloud-based healthcare applications in wireless body sensor networks. *Int. J. Biomed. Eng. Technol., 29*, 186–199.
81. Elhayatmy, G., Dey, N., & Ashour, A. S., (2018). Internet of things based wireless body area network in healthcare. In: *Internet of Things and Big Data Analytics Toward Next-Generation Intelligence; Springer: Cham, Switzerland* (pp. 3–20).
82. Zanjal, S. V., & Talmale, G. R., (2016). Medicine reminder and monitoring system for secure health using IoT. *Procedia Comput. Sci., 78*, 471–476.
83. Dimitrov, D. V., (2016). Medical internet of things and big data in healthcare. *Healthc. Inform. Res., 22*, 156–163.
84. Griggs, K. N., Ossipova, O., Kohlios, C. P., Baccarini, A. N., Howson, E. A., & Hayajneh, T., (2018). Healthcare blockchain system using smart contracts for secure automated remote patient monitoring. *J. Med. Syst., 42*, 130.
85. Rahman, M. A., Hassanain, E., Rashid, M. M., Barnes, S. J., & Hossain, M. S., (2018). Spatial blockchain-based secure mass screening framework for children with dyslexia. *IEEE Access, 6*, 61876–61885.
86. Jo, B., Khan, R., & Lee, Y. S., (2018). Hybrid blockchain and internet-of-things network for underground structure health monitoring. *Sensors, 18*, 4268.
87. Ichikawa, D., Kashiyama, M., & Ueno, T., (2017). Tamper-resistant mobile health using blockchain technology. *JMIR mHealth uHealth, 5*, e111.
88. *3 Phishing Hacks Breach 20,000 Catawba Valley Patient Records*. Available online: https://www.healthcareitnews.com/news/3-phishing-hacks-breach-20000-catawba-valley-patient-records (accessed on 4 December 2023).
89. Nikoloudakis, Y., Pallis, E., Mastorakis, G., Mavromoustakis, C. X., Skianis, C., & Markakis, E. K., (2019). Vulnerability assessment as a service for fog-centric information and communication technology ecosystems: A healthcare use case. *Peer-to-Peer Netw. Appl.*, 1–9.
90. Nausheen, F., & Begum, S. H., (2018). Healthcare IoT: Benefits, vulnerabilities, and solutions. In: *Proceedings of the 2018 IEEE 2nd International Conference on Inventive Systems and Control (ICISC), Coimbatore, India* (pp. 517–522).
91. Otoum, S., Kantarci, B., & Mouftah, H., (2018). Adaptively supervised and intrusion-aware data aggregation for wireless sensor clusters in critical infrastructures. In: *Proceedings of the 2018 IEEE International Conference on Communications (ICC), Kansas City, MO, USA* (pp. 1–6).
92. Otoum, S., Kantarci, B., & Mouftah, H. T., (2019). On the feasibility of deep learning in sensor network intrusion detection. *IEEE Netw. Lett.*
93. Aloqaily, M., Otoum, S., Al Ridhawi, I., & Jararweh, Y., (2019). An intrusion detection system for connected vehicles in smart cities. *Ad. Hoc. Netw*. In press.
94. Catarinucci, L., De Donno, D., Mainetti, L., Palano, L., Patrono, L., Stefanizzi, M. L., & Tarricone, L., (2015). An IoT-aware architecture for smart healthcare systems. *IEEE Internet Things J., 2*, 515–526.
95. Saia, R. (2018). *Internet of Entities (IoE): A Blockchain-based Distributed Paradigm to Security*. arXiv 2018, arXiv:1808.08809.
96. Saia, R., Carta, S., Recupero, D., & Fenu, G., (2019). Internet of entities (IoE): A blockchain-based distributed paradigm for data exchange between wireless-based devices. In: *Proceedings of the 8th International Conference on Sensor Networks (SENSORNETS 2019), Prague, Cxech Republic.*

97. Esposito, C., De Santis, A., Tortora, G., Chang, H., & Choo, K. K. R., (2018). Blockchain: A panacea for healthcare cloud-based data security and privacy? *IEEE Cloud Comput., 5*, 31–37.
98. Dorri, A., Kanhere, S. S., & Jurdak, R. (2016). *Blockchain in Internet of Things: Challenges and Solutions*. arXiv 2016, arXiv:1608.05187.
99. Dorri, A., Kanhere, S. S., & Jurdak, R., (2017). Towards an optimized blockchain for IoT. In: *Proceedings of the ACM Second International Conference on Internet-of-Things Design and Implementation, Pittsburgh, PA, USA* (pp. 173–178).
100. Khan, M. A., & Salah, K., (2018). Internet of things security: Review, blockchain solutions, and open challenges. *Future Gen. Comput. Syst., 82*, 395–411.
101. *Top 10 Biggest Healthcare Data Breaches of All Time*. Available online: https://www.healthcareitnews.com/news/3-phishing-hacks-breach-20000-catawba-valley-patient-records (accessed on 4 December 2023).
102. Boulos, M. N. K., Wilson, J. T., & Clauson, K. A., (2018). Geospatial blockchain: Promises, challenges, and scenarios in health and healthcare. *Int. J. Health Geogr., 17*, 25.
103. Mamoshina, P., Ojomoko, L., Yanovich, Y., Ostrovski, A., Botezatu, A., Prikhodko, P., Izumchenko, E.,Aliper, A., Romantsov, K., Zhebrak, A., et al., (2018). Converging blockchain and next-generation artificial intelligence technologies to decentralize and accelerate biomedical research and healthcare. *Oncotarget, 9*, 5665.
104. Kuo, T. T., & Ohno-Machado, L. (2018). *ModelChain: Decentralized Privacy-Preserving Healthcare Predictive Modeling Framework on Private Blockchain Networks*. arXiv 2018, arXiv:1802.01746.
105. Wang, S., Wang, J., Wang, X., Qiu, T., Yuan, Y., Ouyang, L., Guo, Y., & Wang, F. Y., (2018). Blockchain-powered parallel healthcare systems based on the ACP approach. *IEEE Trans. Comput. Soc. Syst., 5*, 942–950.
106. Qiu, J., Liang, X., Shetty, S., & Bowden, D., (2018). Towards secure and smart healthcare in smart cities using blockchain. In: *Proceedings of the 2018 IEEE International Smart Cities Conference (ISC2), Kansas City, MO, USA* (pp. 1–4).
107. Pirbhulal, S., Wu, W., & Li, G., (2018). A biometric security model for wearable healthcare. In: *Proceedings of the 2018 IEEE International Conference on Data Mining Workshops (ICDMW), Singapore* (pp. 136–143).
108. *Internet of Medical Things (IoMT)—The Future of Healthcare*. Available online: https://igniteoutsourcing.com/healthcare/internet-of-medical-things-iomt-examples/ (accessed on 4 December 2023).
109. Tiwari, S., (2022). *Bioinformatics Tools, and Big Data Analytics for Patient Care* (p. 240). In Routledge Taylor & Franchis Group.
110. Zheng, Z., Xie, S., Dai, H., Chen, X., & Wang, H., (2017). An overview of blockchain technology: Architecture, consensus, and future trends. In: *Proceedings of the 2017 IEEE International Congress on Big Data (BigData Congress), Honolulu, HI, USA* (pp. 557–564).
111. Gatteschi, V., Lamberti, F., Demartini, C., Pranteda, C., & Santamaría, V., (2018). Blockchain and smart contracts for insurance: Is the technology mature enough? *Future Internet, 10*, 20.

CHAPTER 6

Impact of Blockchain on Drug Traceability

MANDEEP SINGH, RUHUL AMIN CHOUDHURY, and VASUDEVA KILARU

Department of Student Research and Project, Lovely Professional University, Jalandhar, Punjab, India

ABSTRACT

Counterfeit drugs permeate the drug supply chain very often. It is very crucial to build a robust system that ensures no scope for counterfeit drugs in the drug supply chain. In this chapter, we focus on the review of literature on drug traceability in the healthcare supply chain. We also consider discussing the advantages and disadvantages of existing blockchain-based and non-blockchain-based solutions for drug traceability. Moreover, we also briefly introduce the concept and history of blockchain as decentralized ledger technology to enhance digital life and currency. More particularly, we discuss the application of blockchain technology in the supply chain of drugs. We discuss the implementation and execution details of blockchain to enhance the security of the supply chain, drastically reducing the probability of counterfeit drugs permeating the supply chain. The chapter also focuses on a clear presentation of implementation details and results upon testing the proposed method on the real-world supply chain. A critical analysis of the standard of working for DApp, one of the blockchain-based technology applications, presented in the previous literature is presented. The chapter concludes with the ideas that turned into working products, and future scope for enhancing the existing methods with other technologies such as AI (artificial intelligence) are mentioned to encourage further research. It is stated that blockchain can revolutionize the domain of the healthcare supply chain using decentralized ledger technology.

Creating Smart Healthcare with Blockchain and Advanced Digital Technology.
Rishabha Malviya and Sonali Sundram (Eds.)

6.1 INTRODUCTION

Counterfeit drugs are fraudulently produced, mislabeled, and prescribed concerning identity/brand similar to a genuine product to permeate the healthcare supply chain quickly [1, 2]. The supply chain of healthcare is one of the most complex networks of independent bodies, unlike other supply chains which contain semi-independent entities, such as raw material suppliers, drug scientists or labs, manufacturers, distributors, hospitals, patients, and pharmacies. Tracking drug supply in such a complex network may not be feasible since the scope for counterfeit drugs to permeate the healthcare supply chain is huge. Some of the potential inefficiencies are largely highlighted during the COVID-19 pandemic [3]. The independence between the individual entities in a supply chain aggravates the challenge of mitigating counterfeit drugs.

Counterfeit drugs are a class of drugs in medicine which are fake and sometimes harmful to human health, also leading to economic loss. Drugs with an improper amount of active pharmaceutical ingredient (API) or no API, contamination, incorrect API, low-quality API, repackaged expired products, or produced under substandard conditions are generally considered to be counterfeit drugs [4, 5]. Mitigating counterfeit drugs in the healthcare supply chain is essential to prevent economic loss. Counterfeit drugs lead to heavy annual economic loss in the pharmaceutical industry along with adverse human life loss. The US pharmaceutical industry has faced a $200 billion annual economic loss due to counterfeit medicines [6, 7]. According to the World Health Organization (WHO), the inefficiency to trace counterfeit medicines is the major cause of death in developing nations, and most of the victims are children [8, 9].

A healthcare supply chain, or more precisely a drug supply chain, consists of individual entities such as an API supplier who is in charge of supplying the raw materials, a producer who has been given the go-ahead by a governing authority like the US Food and Drug Administration (US FDA) responsible for packing drugs into a Lot or sending drugs for packaging, and transport to primary distributors. The primary distributor is responsible for distributing the lots to pharmacies or secondary distributors based on the demand and size of the lots. The secondary distributors, in the case of large lots, transfer lots to the pharmacies. At last, the pharmacies dispense the medicines to patients based on the doctor's prescription [10]. In some cases, the transportation of lots or drugs between the individual entities of the supply chain is carried out by a third-party logistics service provider like

FedEx, otherwise, distributors carry lots using only their own vehicles. The chain of healthcare supply is shown in Figure 6.1.

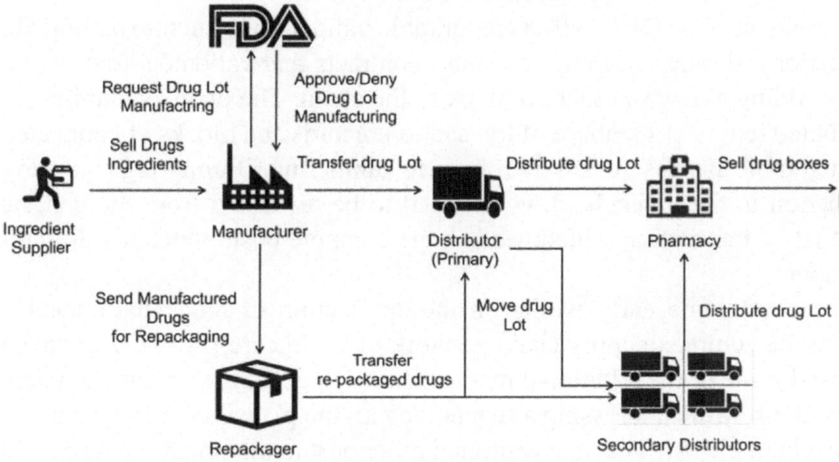

FIGURE 6.1 Healthcare supply chain.
Source: Adapted from Ref. [5]

A specialized drug tracking and tracing mechanism is essential to mitigate counterfeit drugs permeating the healthcare blockchain. Many public healthcare organizations, and drug regulatory bodies such as DSCSA, and WHO have emphasized building IT solutions to track and trace drugs, whenever the position or environment of the drug changes in the supply chain, as an integral system or mechanism of the pharmaceutical supply chain that ensures quality and authenticity of drug supply tracking. In recent times, the Chinese and US governments are mandated to enhance the tracking and tracing of drugs in the supply chain.

The fundamental concept of blockchain technology is an architecture for a blockchain resembling a linked list (unlike a linked list, the nodes are blocked and mutable only forward in chronological order where each node has its own set of the local copy of the nodes/data blocks in the chain, blocks of the longest chain, starting from the genesis block, called the distributed ledger technology (DLT) [11, 12]. Blockchain, in simple terms, is a novel model of application development for tracking and tracing any virtual asset that has value. Each transaction on the virtual asset such as a change of ownership or/and change of value is stored as a new block that's chained to the existing blockchain network [13]. After the successful implementation of the data structure within the Bitcoin application, many real-world applications have been developed in diverse domains, such as the IoT [14], e-Government [15] like Digi-locker, and e-document management like LaTeX [16, 17]. These applications are heavily benefited by the key ideas of blockchain, such as DLT, self-cryptographic validations structure among the transactions, through hashes, i.e., smart contracts that validate a transaction before adding a new transaction block to the chain. The open availability of distributed ledger or database of transaction records and blocks of connected cryptographic hashes makes it robust to tampering. Tampering with any transaction in the blockchain would need to be reworked from the genesis to the latest transaction which needs huge compute cost; hence it's difficult to tamper.

There are some early works on the application of blockchain specifically to the complex supply chain network of healthcare [5, 18]. They have proposed some of the additional mechanisms that generalize to the complete supply chain while addressing a few among all the plausible problems in the supply chain [5, 18]. They concentrated more on supplier, manufacturer, and wholesaler as being the stakeholders while identified and prioritized every individual entity of the supply chain including the pharmacies as stakeholders unlike those considered in the work [18]. The primary contributions of the research are the work proposed a new design of smart contracts or hashes that can handle transactions between participants in the pharmaceutical supply chain was proposed as part of a blockchain-based solution for the industry [5]. This solution offers accessibility, immutability, traceability, and security of data provenance for drugs, presenting a tested smart contract with defined principles and analyzing the performance of the proposed blockchain solution feasibility.

6.2 OVERVIEW OF BLOCKCHAIN

Some of the early literature on blockchain defined the technology behind the bitcoin as a data structure similar to a linked list where nodes are self-cryptographically linked through hashes, i.e., "chain of blocks" [11]. Blockchain was introduced as a peer-to-peer (P2P) version of maintaining any virtual asset that has value and under transactions such as change of ownership or state. Blockchain technology is based on a distributed ledger system of database that stores blocks chained chronologically. These blocks store information regarding any transaction on the virtual asset. As mentioned in the Introduction, these blocks are chained or linked through hashing (cryptographically) that ensuring the immutability of transactions and the DLT enables participants to have a local copy of the database of transactions making blockchain a hash-based proof-of-work (PoW) [19–21]. The blockchain data structure is represented in Figure 6.2.

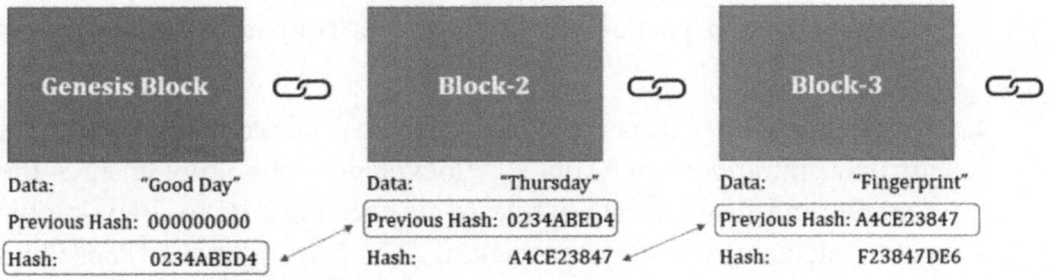

FIGURE 6.2 Blockchain data structure.

Source: Adapted from Ref. [21]

Blockchain technology has developed in the last decades and is almost exploding. The evolution of blockchain with its wide range of application domains can categorize its development into four key stages [22]:

1. **Blockchain 1.0:** 1.0 is the initial stage of blockchain introduced in 2008 [11]. The first stage majorly focused on applications of blockchain in digital currencies maintained and validated using cryptographic hashes or contracts. Blockchain 1.0 was mainly introduced to reduce the cost of intermediaries and improve security [22, 23].
2. **Blockchain 2.0:** 2.0 was majorly focused on designing smart contracts, introduced in 2013. A smart contract is a set of instructions that are automatically executed to validate any transaction, chaining the information of the transaction as a block into the chain [24, 25]. These smart contracts are used as agreements between the participants of the transactions in the network blockchain. Through smart contracts, the networks of blockchain enable the idea of a decentralized system requiring no third party to monitor the transactions except the participants in the blockchain network, who monitor the transactions through smart contracts and distributed-cum-centralized ledger. Smart contracts improve the automation of validating transactions, reducing human error or third-party security vulnerabilities [22]. One of the most famous practical examples of blockchain implementing smart contracts is Ethereum [26].

3. **Blockchain 3.0:** 3.0 was introduced in 2015, mainly focusing on the application in the development of decentralized web applications and computing services [27]. The applications are developed on a decentralized system on an open-source platform [28]. 3.0 has introduced the notion of cryptographic tokens, which are valued assets that each participant holds to perform transactions in the network [29].
4. **Blockchain 4.0:** 4.0 is the convergence of blockchain systems and artificial intelligence (AI) [13]. Blockchain technology ensures the security and flow of data, while AI utilizes the data to draw intelligent conclusions or decision-making. The convergence of these two hyped technologies unveils the idea of Trustworthy AI and Intelligent Distributed systems. Blockchain and AI are very complementing technologies that boost the efficacy of one another. In other words, blockchain ensure secure data making the AI system's predictions trustworthy since blockchain brings trust in data [30].

Based on the characteristics of blockchain applications, the major types are [13, 27]. A public blockchain or open blockchain is a permissionless blockchain network that allows everyone to take part in transactions [32, 33]. All the participants in the open blockchain are anonymous and are permitted to view the transaction log prior to their first transaction. All open blockchain networks are operated at a cost of privacy. Some of the popular examples of public blockchains are Bitcoin, Litecoin, and Ethereum [32]. The privacy blockchain is confined to authenticated participants who are permitted to make transactions. The permissioned blockchain is a closed network, allowing authenticated individuals or groups to join and make transactions. The very popular example of privacy blockchains is Hyperledger Fabric [32], Ripple [33] and other business blockchain platforms of software companies. A few partially defined fundamental types of blockchain technology are consortium and permissioned blockchains. Permissioned blockchains are partially public blockchain networks in which authorized individuals are invited to make or monitor the transactions in the network. These networks are restricted to participants who are invited by the organization monitoring the network. Consortium blockchains are semi-centralized blockchain networks that are controlled by a small group of validation nodes with predefined features such as smart contracts. According to IBM [13], Consortium based blockchains are a class of blockchain-based applications managed by organizations internally with customers or confined/authorized users who share the responsibility. The participants could be other organizations or direct customers with shared responsibility as hosts.

The smart contracts or agreements in blockchain technology which validate the new transactions before adding the data blocks into the chain are designed based on a consensus algorithm among the community of blockchain. The consensus algorithm is defined to represent the state of a distributed ledger. Consensus ensures the standard of a block before adding new transaction data into the networks while also preserving the character of the chain to be compatible and extensible. The features such as PoW (introduced in 2008 [11]), proof-of-importance (PoI), proof-of-stake (PoS), delegated-proof-of-state (DPoS), proof-of-activity (PoA), proof-of-burn (PoB), and proof-of-deposit (PoD) [27] are the ideal features of the consensus algorithm.

6.3 RELATED WORK

In this section, we cover a complete overview of efforts which were focused on addressing the problem of traceability in the supply chain, especially in the healthcare system. The efforts made in the field of drug traceability are briefly explained, categorizing the efforts into blockchain-based and non-blockchain-based.

6.3.1 NON-BLOCKCHAIN-BASED WORKS

In a supply chain, the product or component considered to be tracked and recorded timely are generally attributed as traceable resource units (TRUs). TRUs are generally the main product/service in a supply chain, and sometimes, the intermediate stages and their states are also considered for tracking to ensure the efficient tracking of the main TRU. Fundamentally, the TRUs are tracked in multiple phases, mainly there are two folds involved, one is to maintain the history transaction and the other is to track the product or TRU in real-time. In order to track and understand the transaction that happens in the supply chain over time during the lifetime of TRU, some of the published and followed mechanism has already been proven to be effective to mitigate the challenge of counterfeit drugs permeating the supply chain. Various techniques leveraged and designed to track the real-time position of the TRU were effective in identifying and distinguishing TRUs. Most of the mechanisms followed are designed to record the transactions and attributes.

Some of the current and recent advancements in approaching the problem of mitigating counterfeit drugs are, initially, the identifying technologies of barcodes and RFID tags. Data is collected using wireless sensor networks (WSN), and product information is collected using electronic product codes (EPC) that enhance the mechanism of real-time tracking of TRUs [35]. GS1 standard barcodes containing unique serialized product identifier is used for smart tracking along with lot production and expiration details. Each entity or stakeholder poses a unique record of TRU's possession, which an end customer can verify authenticity through a centralized database in a real-time synchronized data network or (GDSN) through a web app or mobile app. In general, these products or TRUs can be tracked using a barcode that encodes the data regarding the authenticity at warehouses, pharmacies or others. Data-Matrix tracking systems are one of the recent ideas to track the product in a supply chain by maintaining a data matrix that stores the details of each drug including the stakeholders and their unique IDs [28]. This system of tracking enables users to monitor or understand the complete details of the drug in the market.

NFC (near field communication) product tags, which were proposed in the recent past, have achieved high standards of tracking in terms of visibility and authenticity across the pharmaceutical supply chain. Much like the earlier methods, NFC-based tags allow users to access the complete details of a drug through a mobile application, but NFC tags also enhance the visibility, authenticity, and reliability of drug tracking through a key value registered to the drug in addition to the tag on the drug or product. A few other methods have also been based on maintaining a centralized database which had a vulnerability to being tampered and a few other methods had issues in scalability and interpretability [36–38].

6.3.2 *BLOCKCHAIN-BASED METHODS FOR DRUG TRACING AND TRACKING*

Since most of the traditional methods proposed had a serious vulnerability of security and tampering of the data due to centralized maintenance of data. In contrast, all the blockchain-based product traceability mechanism guarantees security, transparency, verifiable, and traceability. Blockchain is a DLT, that uses the complex ideas of distributed databases or computing to effectively enhance security by reducing the control to intermediaries that prevent the data from tampering.

Oftentimes, transparency in the supply chain is misunderstood as the traceability of the drug or product. Understanding the transparency in the network reveals that transparency refers to how open the network between the participants is. In other words, transparency refers to how well the stakeholders such as pharmacies and manufacturers know the other participants at various stages. While traceability deals with the minute level of information on the drugs and their position in the supply chain and how timely the changes are being updated to the participants on the network.

6.4 APPLICATION OF BLOCKCHAIN IN DRUG TRACEABILITY

According to JP Morgan Chase and EY [34], In the long run, blockchain enables a transformation of operating models across industries. It also mentions, "Just as the internet upended how we share information, blockchain has the potential to revolutionize how we exchange value, transfer ownership and verify transactions."

Figure 6.3 represents blockchain architecture for drug traceability. In the literature, the standard architecture of employing the blockchain networks in drug tracking and tracing was explained by various internal mechanisms followed by the systems, i.e., interactions between the stakeholders and the smart contracts, which are crucial to validate any transaction in the chain [5]. DApp (decentralized application) was proposed to leverage the advantages of blockchain into the application and use the resources, including smart contracts and decentralized storage by users to perform tasks. The DApp was deployed using an API (application programming interface), which is Infura, JSON RPC, and Web3. The participants initiate the transaction through pre-authorized protocols or functions to use resources such as smart contracts, and decentralized databases (DDBs) to effectively track and trace the drugs in the blockchain. The transactions are stored in time-stamped logs and IPFS hashes.

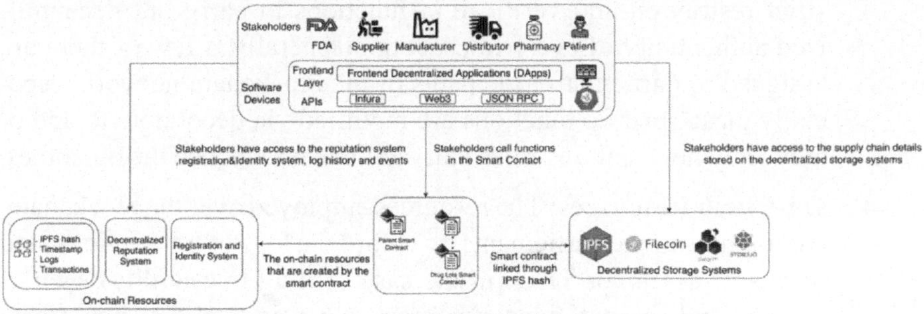

FIGURE 6.3 Blockchain architecture for drug traceability.

Source: Adapted from Ref. [5]

The key ideas in the DApp architecture proposed in the chapter consist of the following terminologies:

1. **Stakeholders or Participants:** These include regulatory agencies such as US FDA, and other direct participants such as API providers, manufacturers, pharmacies, distributors, and patients. The direct participants and regulatory bodies are responsible to carry out particular tasks and are provided with access to use the on-chain resources including decentralized storage, time-stamped history of logs of transactions, and smart contractions. Additionally, the stakeholders also possess access to view the IPFS details of drug lots, images, and other fine details recorded in the DDB.
2. **Decentralized Storage System (IPFS [39]):** It offers off-chain storage for supplying or aiding chain transactions data that guarantees security, and integrity of the stored data with reduced vulnerabilities to tampering with the data. The integrity of the data that can be stored can be assured by maintaining unique hashes to every file uploaded on the decentralized storage. Each unique hash of files is recorded as a transaction between the stakeholder or product and the DDB. The unique hashes recorded on the DDB to every transaction or modification in the files ensure the security of files and modifications since any changes through tampering produces a hash deviating from the recorded.
3. **Ethereum Smart Contract:** Smart contracts are a set of virtual agreements that participants abide by while performing transactions on the blockchain network that automatically validates any new transaction on the chain and registers the data to the corresponding transaction on to the chain resources. Smart contracts employ strict restriction and verification functions to carry out decentralized authenticity of every transaction. Generally, a few of them are assigned to particular participants of the blockchain network, especially these specific functions are modified via decorators to add or avoid any new features/rules that facilitate or enhance the outcomes.
4. **On-Chain Resources:** The resources employed over the blockchain, common to all the participants, to record the logs of transactions, and details of assets, or TRU (in the case of drug traceability) such as storage, and computational resources to run and validate new transactions using smart contracts. Compute and storage are also utilized to deploy an identification system to link the Ethereum address of

the participants to human interpretable form and for hashing the participant's credentials.

The system proposed in the study is a blockchain-based solution to tackle counterfeit drugs, preventing the supply chain [5]. The proposed system was efficient enough in mitigating the counterfeit drugs in the market, however, the proposed method doesn't claim it efficient to track the TRU or drug throughout the supply chain. For the same, various ideas were drafted with the necessary equipment such as GPS, temperature sensors, and other barcodes.

6.5 IMPLEMENTATION OF THE PROPOSED METHOD

The method proposed in the study was implemented using Ethereum, ethers being the currency of transactions in the blockchain [5]. The smart contracts are coded up in Solidity language, which is compiled and tested in Remix web IDE. The code is publicly open source on the GitHub repository (https://github.com/DrugTraceability/DrugTraceability/blob/master/Code).

The flow of the method starts from the manufacturer when he requests the FDA for initiating the manufacturing process of the drug lot and updates the details about the drug lot over the blockchain decentralized ledger open to all the participants. Using the IPFS, the images and details of the manufactured and packaged drug lot are updated on the ledger and communicated between the participants. The updates via hashes enable the participants to timely track the history of the drug. However, as discussed earlier, real-time tracking is not proposed. The images of packaged lots are updated and left to distributors. The relationship and the guidelines of the interaction are maintained through the Ethereum smart contracts. The interaction is briefly conveyed in Figure 6.4.

The first verified participant of the network, i.e., the manufacturer, deploys the smart contract with all the details of the drug lot. In a method, the approval of the FDA for initiating the manufacturing of the drug lot is not authorized through smart contracts with assumed to be done through the manual process [5]. Whenever a drug lot is manufactured, an event is triggered to all the participants on the blockchain, however, the primary distributed will get access to some special functions to initiate or transact with the manufacturer to buy the lot and distribute to the secondary distributors or pharmacies. Additionally, the drug lot image can be uploaded to IPFS by the manufacturer for the participants to access after the manufacturing. After a newly manufactured lot is announced for sale by the manufacturer to the primary distributor, through a set of functions, the primary distributor can

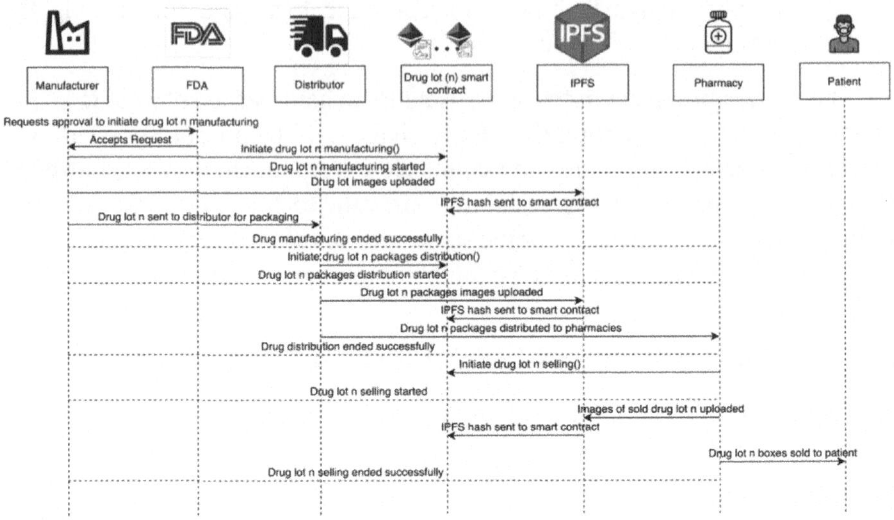

FIGURE 6.4 Interaction between the participants in the method proposed by Ahmad Musamih et al.

Source: Adapted from Ref. [5]

place or request the order of a drug lot, which the manufacturer can accept and initiate the sale. Any processed change of ownership is tracked and logged in the list of transactions. All the details of the lot are synchronized into the ledger. The details of the drug lot are mostly mapped to an encrypted code while a few other details such as the owner's name are not hashed since the owner of the drug lot is a single entity. The functions that any participant can access at any point in time are accessed through smart contracts based on the position, owner, and state of the drug lot. Details of the drug lot are uploaded into the IPFS in hashed code in a one-on-one relationship. Functions like lot Details are accessed by the buyers on the blockchain, and functions like GrantSale are accessed by the sellers by the smart contract to perform a transaction by initiating functions. Some of the functions build to execute the transaction by the participants on the blockchain:

i. **Creating a Lot:** Used to initiate the lot after FDA approval to the manufacturer.

ii. **Grant Lot Sale:** Used to raise an event to notify and sell the lot available for sale.

iii. **Buying Lot:** A function to buy the lot from the seller, executed to record the buy transaction.

iv. **Buying Lot Boxes:** A function to buy the boxes if in case, the buyers request for part of the drug lot to sell.

6.6 TRACEABILITY ANALYSIS OF THE PROPOSED SOLUTIONS

In order to use and leverage the advantages of the blockchain in efficiently tracing the drugs, i.e., the authenticity of the drug lot, any change in the state, or ownership should trigger an event that is stored in the ledger. A QR code is used to replace the hash or more specifically the Ethereum address of the drug log to simplify the method of scanning and verifying the authenticity of the drug. The DApp interacts with nodes of Ethereum using a local node or remote node using web3j. The JSON-RPC is used, i.e., infura or Ethereum node to map hashes of the lot encoded or encrypted. The mappings of the different drug lots, functions, and events are stored in the ledger for future reference.

The functions such as lotSold, imageuploaded, lotManufactured, and newOwner are made accessed and initiated by the smart contracts based on the transactions that happen to allow the participants to perform the actions to proceed in the blockchain.

The Ethereum network distributes the information among the participating entities. Each entity in the network will have its duplicate copy of the ledger that is immutable and synchronized to all the entities in subject to any change in the details or ownership of the drug lot. The methods since ensuring security through immutability, decentralized security system and sophisticated smart contracts that turn out to be effective in healthcare applications, especially the drug traceability through the use of Infura or Ethereum node, web3j interface, and FSON-RPC for mapping of the hashes.

The cost analysis of the method concluded that the method has an estimated expenditure of 2.8 GWEI based on the ETH or Ethereum gas station [40]. Table 6.1 presents the cost analysis of the method.

TABLE 6.1 Comparing the Resource Cost of the Method in ETH Gas and US Dollars

Function Caller	Function Name	Transaction Gas	Execution Gas	Cost in USD
SC owner	grantSale	29,745	8,473	0.00845
Buyer	buyBox	62,305	40,841	0.0228
Buyer	buyLot	40,845	19,573	0.01334
SC owner	IoT details	1,07,356	83,844	0.04226

Based on the security analysis of the method, it is concluded that the integrity of the data and transactions is maintained due to the immutable ledger technology that only registers the logs of transactions in one way. The accountability of the transaction is possible since the functions are stored using the Ethereum address. Authorization, availability, and non-reproduction of the transaction (due to cryptographic encryption). MITM attacks are prevented due to the assigned private key to the original data, and which needs to be confirmed via signing through the key. However, the standard of security received by using the features of Remix online editor to test and debug. Additionally, SmartCheck is used to further enhance the bug-free report in validation. The Oyente tool was used using Linux to analyze the code to rule out hidden vulnerabilities.

6.7 LIMITATION OF THE METHOD

1. **Immutability:** Being an advantage of blockchain also has some negative challenges, such as the inability to change or modify any transaction that was recorded incorrectly due to human error. The immutability can be addressed to an extent using simulated annealing. The idea of simulated annealing can allow the change of a block for the stipulated period with a high rate of ease and throughout increments of blocks in the blockchain, the rate of ease to change the registered block or log of the transaction is decreased. This is the hypothesis that would work effectively for problems based on the nature of the solution and its promising results from other problems.
2. **Data Privacy:** It is both the strength and the weakness of the method. A few participants would like to erase their data from the permanent storage in the blockchain on-chain resource. To an extent, the problem can also be solved using the idea of simulated annealing, i.e., allowing the deletion of data for a stipulated period and restricting the action of deletion later on.
3. **Scalability:** It is another important issue of the blockchain-based solution for the supply chain [5]. The major drawback is the huge compute demand by the method to the participants. The cost of executing a function or the smart contracts requires various Ethereum nodes as analyzed in Ref. [31]. The only solution to reduce the compute cost is again to implement the method with centralized storage and compute services on-chain, making the method a semi-centralized but fully immutable ledger technology.

4. **Interoperability and Efficiency:** The development of smart contracts has a significant impact on the blockchain solution's effectiveness. The consensus algorithm also impacts the efficiency of the whole blockchain-based solution since 90% of the compute power and storage required in the solution via blockchain is to execute the smart contracts and store the transaction log on the decentralized ledger.

6.8 CONCLUSION

The research in the domain of application of blockchain to the supply chain, especially to try to mitigate the fake/counterfeit products in the market, is exploding. With the introduction of robust mechanisms and applications, the ability of blockchain is advancing towards solving the drawbacks. In this chapter, we started the introduction to the importance of solving a drug traceability problem and eradicating it with the review of blockchain technology and its evolution. We further covered the review of existing methods, both non-blockchain-based and blockchain. Later on, we also discussed the advantages and disadvantages of existing methods. After that, we elaborated on the successful methodologies among the proposed ideas. From that, we moved on to propose the theoretical notion of a novel idea, combining robust blockchain technology with AI. In conclusion, we additionally presented our views on the scope of the future development of existing methods to solve the problem of drug traceability.

Some of the possible areas of research to eliminate the drawbacks mentioned in the chapter would be to introduce a new state variable mechanism. When the drug's value changes, notify the participants through an observer pattern. Aid smart contract validation using AI systems to automate the process of validating a transaction before adding it into the ledger of the blockchain (IBM's research on intelligent contracts replacing smart contracts). AI can also be employed to generate the novel hash function that usually takes long years to hand design the state-of-the-art bug-free and secure functions.

ACKNOWLEDGMENT

The research for the chapter titled "Impact of Blockchain on Drug Traceability" is supported by Lovely Professional University. All the technical equipment support, financial support, and scientific support are due to Lovely

Professional University. Much research literature is reviewed for completing the research work on the topic. Online resources and published domains in a similar field have influenced the view and research on the topic. We are grateful to the online repository of literature on the topic of blockchain influence on medicine and the healthcare supply chain.

KEYWORDS

- **artificial intelligence**
- **blockchain**
- **drug supply chain**
- **drug tracing**
- **medicine**
- **online resources**

REFERENCES

1. Chambliss, W., Carroll, W., Yelvigi, M., et al., (2012). "Role of the pharmacist in preventing distribution of counterfeit medications. *J. Am. Pharm. Assoc., 52*(2), 195–199.
2. Ziance, R. J., (2008). "Roles for pharmacy in combating counterfeit drugs. *J. Am. Pharm. Assoc., 48*, e71–e88.
3. *"Shortage of Personal Protective Equipment Endangering Health Workers Worldwide"* https://tinyurl.com/v5qauvp (accessed on 4 December 2023).
4. Toscan P. (2013). *The Dangerous World of Counterfeit Prescription Drugs*. Available: https://www.cnbc.com/2011/10/04/the-dangerous-world-of-counterfeit-prescription-drugs.html". (accessed on 4 December 2023).
5. Ahmad, M., Khaled, S., Raja, J., Junaid, A., Mazin, D., Al-Hammadi, Y., & Samer, E. (2013) *A Blockchain-based Approach for Drug Traceability in Healthcare Supply Chain.* https://www.middleeastmedicalportal.com/a-blockchain-based-approach-for-drug-traceability-in-healthcare-supply-chain/ (accessed on 4 December 2023).
6. Funding, H. R., (2017). *20 Shocking Counterfeit Drugs Statistics*. Available: https://healthresearchfunding.org/20-shocking-counterfeit-drugs-statistics/ (accessed on 4 December 2023).
7. Blackstone, E. A., Fuhr, J. P. Jr., & Pociask, S., (2014). The health and economic effects of counterfeit drugs. *Am. Health Drug Benefits, 7*, 216–224.
8. Daniela, B. C. L., (2017). *1 in 10 Medical Products in Developing Countries is Substandard or Falsified.* Available: https://www.who.int/news/

item/28-11-2017-1-in-10-medical-products-in-developing-countries-is-substandard-or-falsified (accessed on 4 December 2023).
9. The Guardian, (2017). *10% of Drugs in Poor Countries Are Fake, Says WHO*. Available: https://www.theguardian.com/global-development/2017/nov/28/10-of-drugs-in-poor-countries-are-fake-says-who (accessed on 4 December 2023).
10. U.S. Food and Drug Administration, (2016). *A Drug Supply Chain Example*. Available: https://www.fda.gov/drugs/drug-shortages/graphic-drug-supply-chain-example (accessed on 4 December 2023).
11. Nakamoto, S., (2008). *Bitcoin: A Peer-to-Peer Electronic Cash System* (p. 21260). Decentralized business review. Available online: https://www.debr.io/article/21260-bitcoin-a-peer-to-peer-electronic-cash-system (accessed on 4 December 2023).
12. Andrychowicz, M., Dziembowski, S., Malinowski, D., & Mazurek, L., (2015). On the malleability of bitcoin transactions. In: *The Proceedings of Financial Cryptography and Data Security* (pp. 1–18).
13. IBM Research Group. IBM Research. https://www.ibm.com/blogs/client-voices/build-trust-ai-blockchain-technology/ (accessed on 4 December 2023).
14. Suliman, A., Husain, Z., Abououf, M., Alblooshi, M., & Khaled, S., (2019). Monetization of IoT data using smart contracts. *IET Networks, 8*(1), 32–37.
15. Khan, K. M., Arshad, J., & Khan, M. M., (2020). Simulation of transaction malleability attack for blockchain-based e-voting. *Computers & Electrical Engineering, 83*, 106583.
16. Nizamuddin, N., Salah, K., Azad, M. A., Arshad, J., & Rehman, M. H., (2019). "Decentralized document version control using Ethereum blockchain and IPFS. *Computers & Electrical Engineering, 76*, 183–197.
17. Leslie, L. (2022). *LaTeX Document Management Administration. 12*(8), 3723; https://doi.org/10.3390/app12083723. https://www.latex-project.org/ (accessed on 4 December 2023).
18. Muniandy, M., & Ong, T. E. G., (2019). Implementation of pharmaceutical drug traceability using blockchain technology. *Inti. Journal. 2019*, 035. eISSN:2600-7920.
19. Thwin, T. T., & Vasupongayya, S., (2019). Blockchain-based access control model to preserve privacy for personal health record systems. *Secur. Commun. Networks, 2019*, 8315614.
20. Morkunas, V. J., Paschen, J., & Boon, E., (2019). How blockchain technologies impact your business model. *Bus. Horiz., 62*, 295–306.
21. Zhaoyuan, H., & Paul, T. (2023). Blockchain applications in forestry: A systematic literature review. *Applied Sciences.*
22. Angelis, J., & Da Silva, E. R., (2019). Blockchain adoption: A value driver perspective. *Bus. Horiz., 62*, 307–314.
23. Swan, M., (2015). *Blockchain: Blueprint for a New Economy*. O'Reilly Media, Inc.: Newton, MA, USA.
24. Dinh, T. T. A., Liu, R., Zhang, M., Chen, G., Ooi, B. C., & Wang, J., (2018). Untangling blockchain: A data processing view of blockchain systems. *IEEE Trans. Knowl. Data Eng., 30*, 1366–1385.
25. Bao, J., He, D., Luo, M., & Choo, K. K. R., (2020). A survey of blockchain applications in the energy sector. *IEEE Syst. J., 15*, 3370–3381.
26. Ethereum Foundation. (2023). *Ethereum Blockchain Technology*. ethereuem.org (accessed on 4 December 2023).

27. Ismail, L., & Materwala, H., (2019). A review of blockchain architecture and consensus protocols: Use cases, challenges, and solutions. *Symmetry, 11*, 1198.
28. Raval, S., (2016). *Decentralized Applications: Harnessing Bitcoin's Blockchain Technology.* O'Reilly Media, Inc.: Newton, MA, USA.
29. Xu, M., Chen, X., & Kou, G., (2019). A systematic review of blockchain. *Financ. Innov., 5*, 27. [CrossRef].
30. *IBM Blockchain and Trustworthy AI.* IBM Research. research.ibm.com/ (accessed on 4 December 2023).
31. Datta, S., & Sinha, D., (2021). BESDDFFS: Blockchain and EdgeDrone based secured data delivery for forest fire surveillance. *Peer Peer Netw. Appl., 14*, 3688–3717.
32. Morkunas, V. J., Paschen, J., & Boon, E., (2019). How blockchain technologies impact your business model. *Bus. Horiz., 62*, 295–306.
33. Hölbl, M., Kompara, M., Kamišali´c, A., & Nemec, Z. L., (2018). A systematic review of the use of blockchain in healthcare. *Symmetry, 10*, 470.
34. Morgan, J. P. *JP Morgan on the Blockchain.* https://www.jpmorgan.com/onyx/blockchain-launch (accessed on 4 December 2023).
35. Buterin, V., (2014). *A Next-Generation Smart Contract and Decentralized Application Platform* (Vol. 3, pp. 1–36). White Pap.
36. *Litecoin – Open-Source P2P Digital Currency*. Available online: https://litecoin.org/ (accessed on 4 December 2023).
37. Zheng, Z., Xie, S., Dai, H. N., Chen, X., & Wang, H., (2018). Blockchain challenges and opportunities: A survey. *Int. J. Web Grid Serv., 14*, 352–375.
38. Mallett, R., Hagen-Zanker, J., Slater, R., & Duvendack, M., (2012). The benefits and challenges of using systematic reviews in international development research. *J. Dev. Eff., 4*, 445–455.
39. Datta, S., Kumar, S., Sinha, D., & Das, A. K., (2021). BSSFFS: Blockchain-based sybil-secured smart forest fire surveillance. *J. Ambient Intell. Humaniz. Comput., 12*, 1–32.
40. Eth Gas Station. Available: https://ethgasstation.info/ (accessed on 4 December 2023).

CHAPTER 7

Patient Selection and Treatment Strategies Using Computational Machine Analysis

ANJALI GUPTA,[1] NEHA SHARMA,[2] and PAVAN KUMAR ARYA PADARTHI[3]

[1]*Parexel International Pvt. Ltd., Chandigarh, India*

[2]*Department of Pharmacy, School of Medical and Allied Sciences, Galgotias University, Greater Noida, Uttar Pradesh, India*

[3]*University of Hertfordshire, Luton, United Kingdom*

ABSTRACT

In a short time frame, several scientific domains have quickly shifted toward data-driven models. In some cases, this strategy has been made possible by simultaneous advancements in data collecting and the creation of networked system technologies. As a result of the advancement of communication as well as sensor technologies, big data, or massive data that are hard to record, retain, and analyze with standard database management systems, has now been collected in a number of industries recently. Because of technological advancements, it is expected that the usage of big data will open up new investigation directions. It is also anticipated that the utilization of big data-sets in the healthcare sector would lead to the creation of new knowledge and improvements in the outcomes of diagnosis and treatment. In addition, AI adoption in healthcare has been extensively explored, yet, due to a variety of issues, it has not been widely deployed. A lot of research has been done on the adoption of AI in healthcare, but for a variety of reasons, it hasn't been widely used. The daily explosion of data produced by billions of smart

Creating Smart Healthcare with Blockchain and Advanced Digital Technology.
Rishabha Malviya and Sonali Sundram (Eds.)

devices is currently the most challenging data-related concern that needs to be addressed. To deal with the growing volume of data in healthcare applications, difficulties must be solved, such as a lack of standardized tools, efficient algorithms, and a sufficient number of qualified data scientists. As a result, research into deep learning (DL) models and how they apply to e-healthcare is becoming more and more popular. Intelligent agents are systems that behave intelligently. They act in a way that they believe is appropriate for their goals and circumstances, are adaptable to changing environments and goals, learn from experience, and make decisions that are reasonable given their limited sensory perception and computational power. The study of the creation of intelligent agents is known as computational intelligence. There are many advantages of using computational intelligence models to maintain and advance healthcare. Among the rapidly expanding uses of computational intelligence in healthcare are intelligent synthetic characters, man-machine interfaces, menu generators, user acceptance analysis, photo archiving, and communication systems. The issues of computational analysis in therapeutic drugs are covered in this chapter, along with data mining analysis, big data interpretation, and patient selection.

7.1 INTRODUCTION

The concept of data has become ingrained in every aspect of our daily lives as a result of the routine collection, storage, processing, and analysis of enormous amounts of data. This trait is cross-disciplinary and applies to fields including machine learning (ML), engineering, economics, and medicine. Over the past few decades, the possible applications of such amounts of the dataset, known as Big Data, for improving individual care, patient care, and public health have gained momentum over the past few decades [1].

The term "Big Data" describes how data today's data is frequently too big, complex, and varies very rapidly to be stored, analyzed, and converted into value using prior technology. Big data is driven by technology trends: business activities are increasingly being conducted digitally, and consumers are producing more data on their own, such as in social networks, where petabytes of data may be processed in the cloud at a lesser amount of time and price when big data processing techniques are used [2].

Big Data is frequently used in the healthcare industry to describe a vast volume of data from E-health records, administrative claims, clinical trials, wearable technology, social networks, and personal genetics services. Modern analysis techniques developed to address huge data concerns are referred to as predictive analytics. Data mining, ML, and predictive modeling are some of these statistical techniques. Several aspects of medication management, including the diagnosis of complicated cases as well as those most at risk for non-compliance with prescription instructions or adverse effects, have benefited from the application of predictive analytics utilizing big data [3].

The globe has been struggling to find the right solutions to the problems of population aging and a shortage of medical personnel. According to estimates from the World Health Organization (WHO), there are around 60 million medical professionals needed worldwide and 43 million of them exist [4]. By 2030, these numbers will have risen to 82 million and 67 million, significantly. The proportion of medical shortages will decrease. However, a shortage of more than 15 million medical personnel is unthinkable, necessitating some creative solutions. The exponential increase of online devices has made it possible to gather big data on health-related aspects like oxygen saturation level, blood pressure, heart rate, electromyogram (EMG), blood glucose level, galvanic skin reaction (GSR), mechanomyogram (MMG), wrist pulse signal, body temperature, electrocardiogram (ECG), magnetoencephalogram (MEG), electrooculography (EOG), and electroencephalogram (EEG) [5]. In the healthcare industry, big data is intimidating because of its sheer amount, variety of datasets, as well as management deadlines [6]. The increasing utilization of telehealth will put the storage space for patient's data to further testing, as well as the creative usage of Google Glass by doctors, would increase the behavioral as well as social components of the big dataset [7]. E-medical records (EMRs) are known for facilitating the flow of healthcare and including a wealth of information like patient characteristics, medical, and genetic data. Data analytics can be utilized to organize and retrieve this data. Therefore, the idea of "big data" can be used [3]. A variety of data analytics approaches are used to evaluate the data and establish smart healthcare apps [5]. This chapter will go through the analysis of data mining, big data interpretation, patient selection, and computational analysis in therapeutic medications and their challenges.

7.2 ANALYSIS OF DATA MINING

Analysis of data mining is a type of ML method where a software system evaluates a huge amount of information to construct an algorithm. To test a hypothesis, conventional statistics are used. Data mining is advantageous since it uses both Naive Bayes and decision tree methods to create automated algorithms [8].

7.2.1 NEED FOR DATA MINING

Data mining research refers to the process of studying vast volumes of the dataset using deep learning (DL) rather than traditional data analysis in order to develop a useful algorithm. Though data mining is essential in applied medicine for predicting variables that cause a lot of discovery and a massive production by finding hidden variables that have never been monitored and accounted for before using traditional statistical approaches [8]. Employing Rapid I to evaluate our findings revealed significant aspects for each medical state. As a result, making such technologies helpful for biomedical researchers is a key issue in biomedical data mining. The utilization of data mining in treatment seems to be critical for predicting attributes that lead to illness progression and death [9]. The world is mostly unaware of data mining as a career. Almost all of the time, individuals are completely unaware that it is taking place. Involuntary or unexpected acts are worth explaining in our lives, but which we rarely notice. When we sign up for a supermarket purchasing card, use a credit card, or access the Internet, we generate daily data. Pattern markers of human activities, behaviors, purchase time, and even actions can be found within those data sets. Companies may use data mining to find and identify trends, allowing them to make smarter decisions and better serve their consumers. Physicians and medical researchers are in the same boat. Since the fundamental problem of biomedical technology is to make such platforms usable for biomedical researchers, data mining will have an impact on scientific understanding. Data mining is significant in applied medicine because it can anticipate factors that standard statistical methods can't. In a simplified way, data mining is the method of extracting hidden vital content (intriguing trends) from massive databases electronically, timesaving, cost, and work while also allowing for significant scientific discovery [10].

7.3 CLASSIFICATION OF COMPUTATIONAL INTELLIGENCE MEDICAL DATA (CIMD)

Computational intelligence medical data (CIMD) is categorized into two methods: single method and hybrid method, which are further categorized into different types. A brief diagrammatic representation of CIMD classification is given in Figure 7.1 [11].

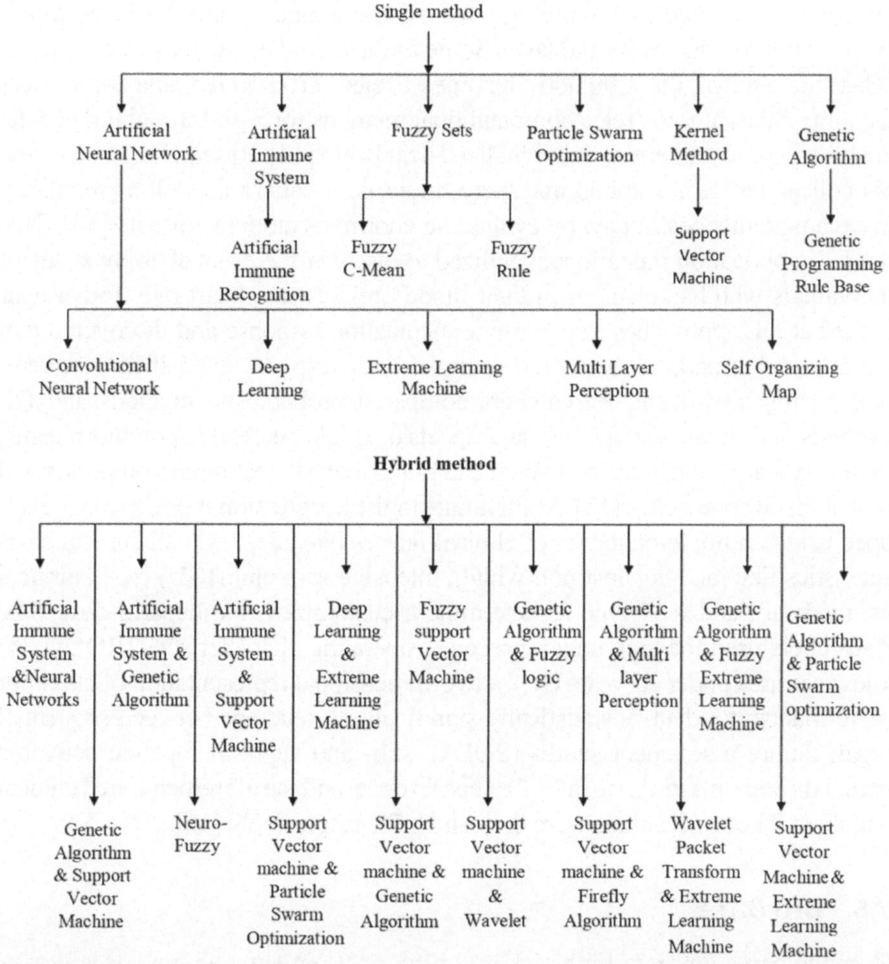

FIGURE 7.1 A schematic diagram depicting the classification of CIMD: Single and hybrid method.

Source: Reprinted with permission from Ref. [11]. Copyright 2022. Elsevier

7.4 COMPUTATIONAL APPROACHES TOWARD PERSONALIZED MEDICINE

While personalized medicine may not be a novel concept, the modern development of strong analysis techniques has expanded the market for predictive, preventative, participatory, and personalized treatment, sometimes referred to as P4 medicine [12]. The goal is to cut costs while enhancing care quality. Different areas of personalized medicine, including diagnosis, prognosis, and pharmacogenomics, have been examined by research groups using computational tools or by modifying or improving norms and laws. Some of these studies, such as Google Inc.'s "Baseline Study," the 1,00,000 Genomes Project (100 KGP), and the Cancer Genome Atlas, aim to create computational methods for high-throughput genetic analysis in order to deliver individualized healthcare [13]. Researcher *Forkan* and his colleagues demonstrated that there might be a pattern as well as regularity in each patient's health data by evaluating enormous amounts of data [14]. This model's application scenario was utilized to discover the exact aberrant status of individuals who had changes in their blood pressure and heart rate. Vidyasagar looked at DL approaches to determine medication response and discovered that there were biomarkers that could estimate drug response even if they weren't biologically significant. Researchers compared probabilistic methods and DL methods to estimate the operational impacts of single nucleotide polymorphisms. In their research, Krishnan and Westhead found that ML techniques outperformed probabilistic approaches [15]. Multivariate logistic regression models were developed using an implementation of clinical factors like age, sex, and clinical characteristics like race (against non-white), intensive care unit (ICU) type (surgical vs. medical), and ICU type to determine a customized first heparin dose. The researchers used the area under a receiver operating characteristics (ROC), also known as area under curve (AUC), a two-dimensional representation of classifier performance, to identify statistically significant correlations between sequential organ failure assessment scores (SOFA), sub- and supra-therapeutic activated partial thromboplastin time (aPTT), heparin dose, and the aforementioned clinical variables. The AUC values were 0.78 and 0.79, respectively [16].

7.5 BIG DATA

Humans can aggregate high-risk and high-cost patients, as well as low-risk and low-cost people, using big data and digitalization. Big data seems to be a vast collection of past records that can be used to forecast and estimate specific outcomes. Big data analytics may also be able to forecast the outcomes of people with numerous ailments or illnesses. Among the advantages of big data analytics in the medical sector are some of the following, which could also help us provide better treatment to patients:

1. **Operation of the Clinic:** Clinically identify and treat patients at a lower cost using effective research [17].
2. **Public Health:** Investigating illness patterns in order to track disease outbreaks and enhance public health promptly.

3. **Quick Development and More Precise Outcomes:** Public health: investigating illness patterns in order to track disease outbreaks and enhance public health in a timely manner. Quick development and more precise outcomes. An enormous quantity of data is used to detect requirements and provide better treatment to patients [18].
4. **Device/Remote Monitoring:** Collect and evaluate enormous volumes of data in real-time to monitor and forecast events.
5. **Medicine Based on Evidence:** Incorporate and examine numerous data structures, both organized and unstructured, for analytics and forecasting in the future.

   Predictive models for data analysis and a quicker decision-making process are being developed in research and development. Patients should be subjected to statistical tools and algorithms in order to enhance clinical tests and innovative treatment [19].

7.5.1 SOFTWARE USED FOR BIG DATA MANAGEMENT

There are various platforms for evaluating big datasets, as described in Figure 7.2. HDFS (Hadoop distributed file system) is among the most appropriate and effective tools for managing and processing huge amounts of data. Other technologies, such as the cloud and MongoDB, are excellent for handling large amounts of data. The techniques via which data is pre-processed until it is processed in analytics are known as data pre-processing. The empty field in the data is handled using a variety of approaches. The missing data can be completed manually or with the help of several approaches for filling in the missing data. Hot deck, mean filling, and nearest neighbor are three strategies for filling missing values. The missing data can be addressed in the following way [20]. An open-source data processing system called Hadoop can handle massive amounts of data by allocating chunks of datasets to servers, all of which solve different aspects of larger problems. The MapReduce implementation allows individuals to share the advantages of computing. Based on the development of enhanced efficiency, Hadoop splits a document into many blocks and stores them in different locations inside a group. Researchers explained how to use SAVANNA Hadoop to schedule big data applications using a data-aware methodology. Additionally, MongoDB and CouchDB are employed as database analytics applications and for new data aggregation [21]. MapReduce in big data is a reduction approach that combines sorting and mapping to create file indexing [22]. There are numerous data analysis methods available to govern and handle the examination of a vast amount of information in a dispersed computing system, such as data mining, the extract transforms load process, online analytical processing (OLAP), and querying [18]. Mishra et al. investigated cloud computing's basis, implications, and problems. It covers the most recent computer paradigms. It is crucial for the monitoring of complicated optimization problems as well as for virtualization, safety, and the distribution of resources. Even though analysis of data has enhanced understanding of many things, there remain some uncertainties. Cloud computing seems to be a computer-based computing system that is continuously scalable. In comparison to the previous version, it is a new solution to a conventional data analysis problem [23]. To shorten the makespan while maximizing cloud usage, Sarkhel and colleagues developed alternative task scheduling algorithms like 'minimum-level priority queue' (MLPQ), 'Mean-MIN-MAX' and 'Min-Median.' DDM, which is built on software applications, can be used to meet the needs of demanding data processing [24]. Based on storage and parallel computing capabilities, it may examine any extra data. In aspects of cloud computing platforms, this DDM redesigns the workflow process to better meet user demands, which can be neglected in place of concurrent job sequences [25]. Behera and colleagues investigated particle swarm optimization, which is mainly based on the metaheuristic evolutionary optimization method. It has a lot of appeal in the field of swarm intelligence due to its simple algorithm design [26].

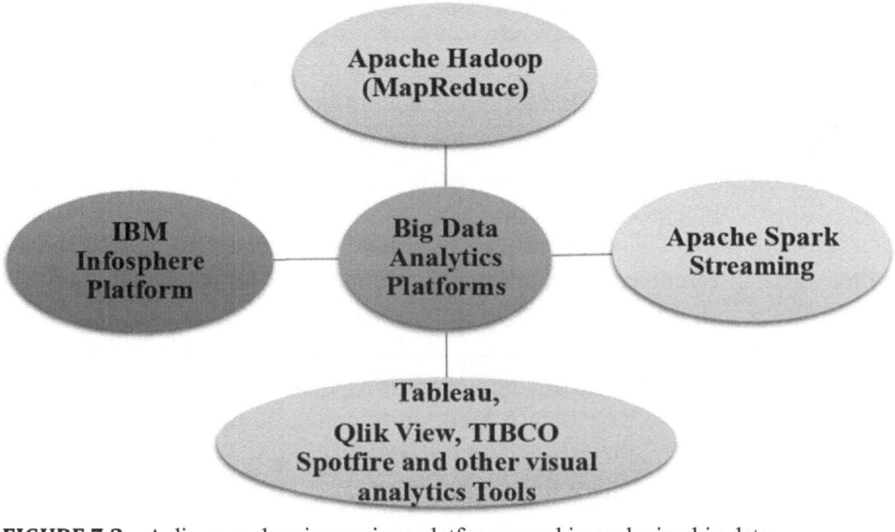

FIGURE 7.2 A diagram showing various platforms used in analyzing big data.

7.5.2 *STEPS INVOLVED IN PREDICTING BIG DATA*

The following steps were presented in a frame to analyze unprocessed or original data:

- Cleansing/ETL;
- Data joining;
- Feature extraction;
- Modeling and prediction (clustering, classification, etc.);
- Visualization of results;
- Analysis and reporting.

Steps for utilizing big data-driven predictive modeling for population health management are shown in Figure 7.3 [27].

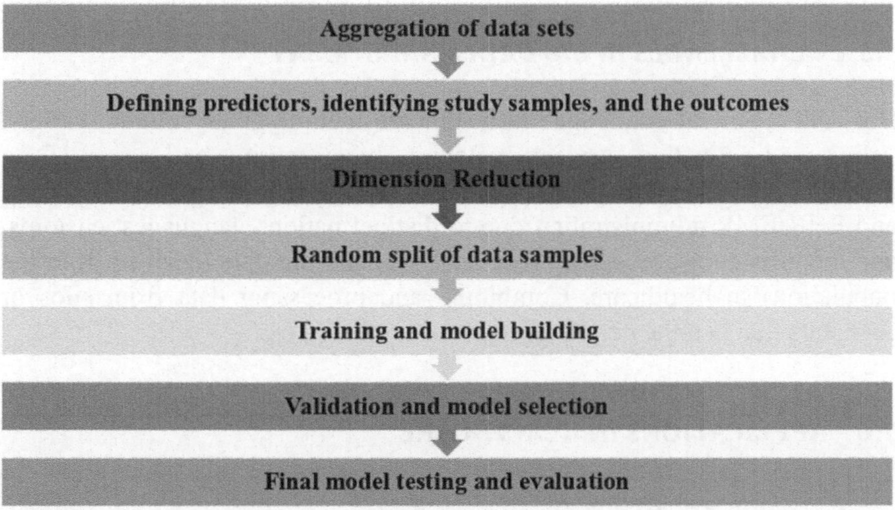

FIGURE 7.3 A flowchart depicting the steps involved in big data analysis.

- ➢ **Step 1:** Aggregation of Datasets: At the patient level, data from a variety of domains (e.g., laboratory results, claim statistics, genetic information, medical and prescription files as well as other EHR information) are combined into a single view.
- ➢ **Step 2:** Defining Predictors, Identifying Study Samples, and the Outcomes: For a specific study, observations and variables of interest are chosen.

- **Step 3:** Dimension Reduction: Data is dimensionally reduced using a procedure.
- **Step 4:** Random Split of Data Samples: At random, all data is split into the training session, verification, and testing data sets.
- **Step 5:** Training and Model Building: The training dataset is utilized to build the models during the training session.
- **Step 6:** Model Selection and Validation: After training, the validation dataset is utilized to assess each model's efficiency before selecting a final model.
- **Step 7:** Final Model Testing and Evaluation: The testing dataset assesses the final model's performance.

7.5.3 CHALLENGES IN BIG DATA MANAGEMENT

Big data's general challenges in healthcare include great volume, variety, validity, visualization, privacy, velocity, cybersecurity, and so on. Data mining from widely dispersed healthcare sources; transnational Medicare and EHR/EMR administration due to distinct nations, languages, customs, and inconsistency among big data analytics and big data (derived from the population) in healthcare. Combining and processing data from silos or segments that healthcare providers have created [27].

7.6 APPLICATIONS IN HEALTHCARE

1. **Public Health:** Avoid crises and give services to the general public, avert crises, target vaccinations, and identify at-risk individuals.
2. **Employ Genomic Analysis:** It will become the standard for medical records and the decision-making process in healthcare.
3. **Research and Development:** Develop clinical studies, obtain novel treatments to market faster, discover side effects before they hit the market, and minimize clinical trials and failures.
4. **Medicine is Based on Evidence:** Compile as well as interpreting a range of both structured and unstructured data to anticipate outcomes for at-risk patients.

5. **Patient Profile Analysis:** Identify those patients who would profit from lifestyle modifications and preventative medicines.

   Various applications of computational technology in healthcare are depicted in Table 7.1, while Table 7.2 shows the applications of big data in healthcare.

TABLE 7.1 The Applications of Different Techniques Used in Data Management Along with Their Impact and Characteristics

Technology	Intelligent Agent	Text Mining	Machine Learning
Impact	• Automatic management. • Efficient decision making. • Effective scheduling.	• Widen the scope of biomedical research.	• Robotic surgery system. • Diagnosis system/ prognosis method. • Strengthen medical signal. • Image processing system.
Main characteristics	• Autonomy flexibility. • Intelligent proactivity.	• Representation of information. • Recover from text.	• Learning from the facts which are known. • Predict the facts which are unknown fact.
Main applications	• In healthcare data management. • In decision support system. • In resource allocation. • In planning. • In action synchronization. • Prevalent healthcare.	• In biomedical research. • In knowledge management. • In discovery.	• Drug discovery and development. • In surgery. • In diagnosis. • In prognosis. • In signal processing. • Medical imaging.

7.7 PATIENT SELECTION

Since the enactment of the Health Information Technology for Economic and Clinical Health (HITECH) Act in 2009, there has been a rise in the accessibility of routinely collected E-health data, providing opportunities for more effective study among various groups. For instance, researchers are putting more emphasis on the development of pragmatic clinical trials (PCTs), which

TABLE 7.2 The Big Data Application in Healthcare Services

Sl. No.	Services in Healthcare	Big Data Application
1.	Public health	• Identify at-risk patients. • Targeted vaccines. • Prevent crises and assist populations.
2.	Research and development	• Find out about the side effects of a drug before it reaches the market. • Clinical trial design performance. • Reduce trials and failures. • Hasten the introduction of new treatments to the market. • Target medicines and devices.
3.	Evidence-based medicament.	• Predict the result of a patient who is at risk. • Compile and examine numerous sources of both organized and unorganized data.
4.	Genomic analytics	• Carrying out genetic analysis, which ought to frequently be a component of routine medical decision-making as well as medical user data.
5.	Patient profile analysis	• Identify patients benefiting from changes in lifestyle as well as preventive care.
6.	Device/remote monitors	• Collect enormous quantities of fast-moving information and evaluate them in real-time.

are relative efficacy studies carried out in reality and incorporated into normal clinical practice [28]. PCTs are intended to maximize the overall relevance and generalization of trial conclusions to practice through the use of a broad selection process, regular clinical sites and staff, minimal follow-up visits, as well as a basic design. The recruitment of underrepresented communities is difficult for both traditional and pragmatic research investigations. Since they frequently have superior accessibility to patients, clinical information, and research groups, university health centers, community hospitals, or other organizations focusing on patient care have historically handled several large observational investigations and clinical studies. Patients that do not meet the criteria are ignored in this procedure. Those patients who are not receiving clinical care but would profit from participating in research work are being neglected in this procedure. Active community involvement in medical trials may help increase enrollment in studies, particularly among underrepresented groups, shorten the project duration, and enhance the distribution and acceptance of research results in Populations. Figure 7.4 shows conventional studies and new strategies involved in patient selection [29].

7.7.1 RECRUITING TECHNIQUES

A thorough recruiting plan that is customized to the study issue should be created. There are a variety of recruitment techniques to choose from:

- All patients are enrolled at the same time, and the study begins at the same time.
- Patients are enrolled in the study in a "batch" method.
- Patients are continually recruited until the required sample size is reached.
- Patients are recruited until a specific deadline is met [30].

7.7.2 CONVENTIONAL STUDIES AND NEW STRATEGY

Our innovative approach searches the community as well as outside the medical environment for potential recruits. Selected participants give complete agreement for their complete inclusion and access to health records when preliminary data is obtained at the time of outreach. Participants are connected to a record at a healthcare location using IDs from the gathered data for eligibility confirmation and continuous collection of data via EHR inquiries. Patients can be followed up with immediate care, but researchers can also access EHR data for longitudinal information thanks to the connection to clinical records. This approach makes it easier to identify and attract people that are normally underrepresented [31].

Sensors are frequently employed in the collection of patient data. Various sensors can regularly gather personal health signs, including blood pressure, body temperature, breathing, and pulse rate, cardiac condition, and blood glucose level. Personalized e-Health and m-Health are made possible by MBANs and wearable biosensors, and the future era of E-health and M-health is expected to depend heavily on big data processing and the web of things.

Big data processing in healthcare is supported by such a distributed network built on clouds as well as other modern techniques like the internet of things (IoT). This infrastructure maintains large amounts of datasets, allows for the integration of health resources and legacy systems in hospitals, and ensures privacy and cyber-security. Through the creation of a trustful

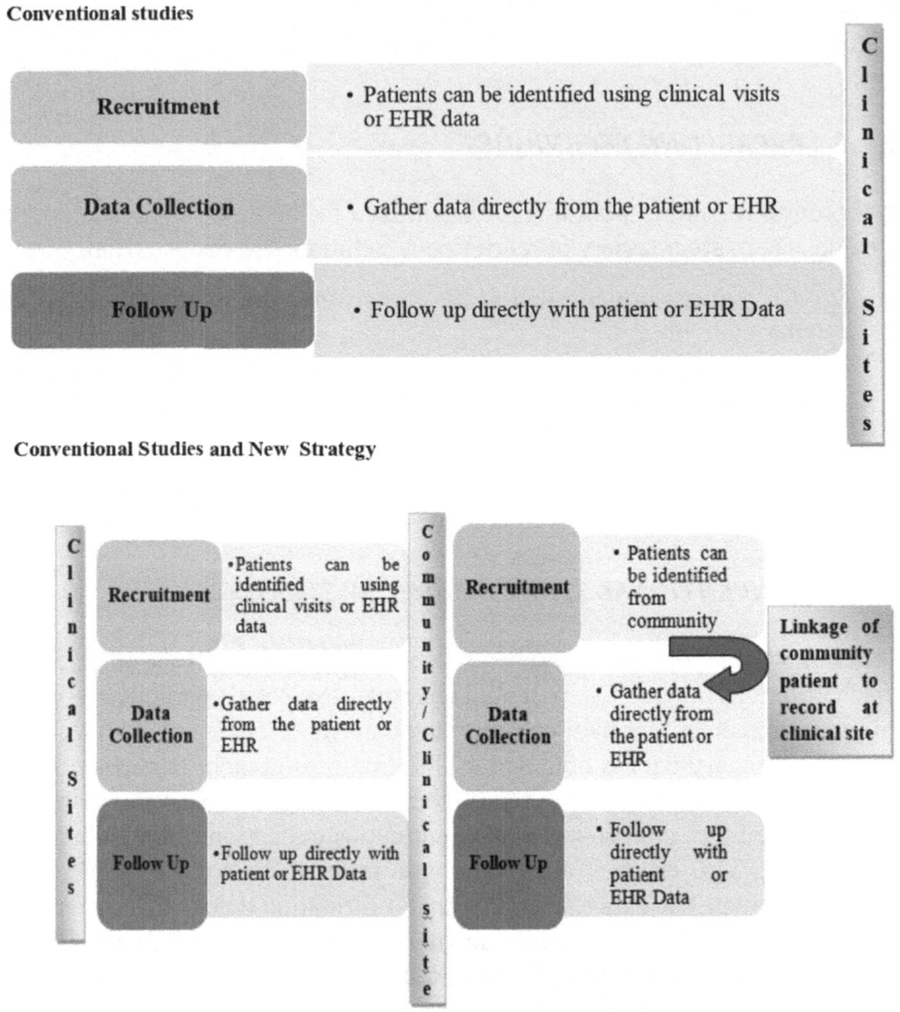

FIGURE 7.4 Diagrams showing the conventional studies and new strategies involved in patient selection.

cooperation environment with safe data exchange, blockchains assist in providing high-quality personal healthcare [27].

7.8 TREATMENT STRATEGY USING AI

Because ML and artificial intelligence (AI) researchers have been anxiously awaiting real-time data which is generated by the disease outbreak across the universe, the prompt transmission of COVID-19 individual information data, like physiologic traits and therapy outcomes, obtained from data processing for quick and easy access is critical, even though difficult. The workflow is depicted in Figure 7.5, but there are a few steps that now preclude the utilization of AI as well as ML to tackle COVID-19. A significant present hurdle is the lack of clinical datasets related to COVID-19 that can be processed and kept in easily available databases [32].

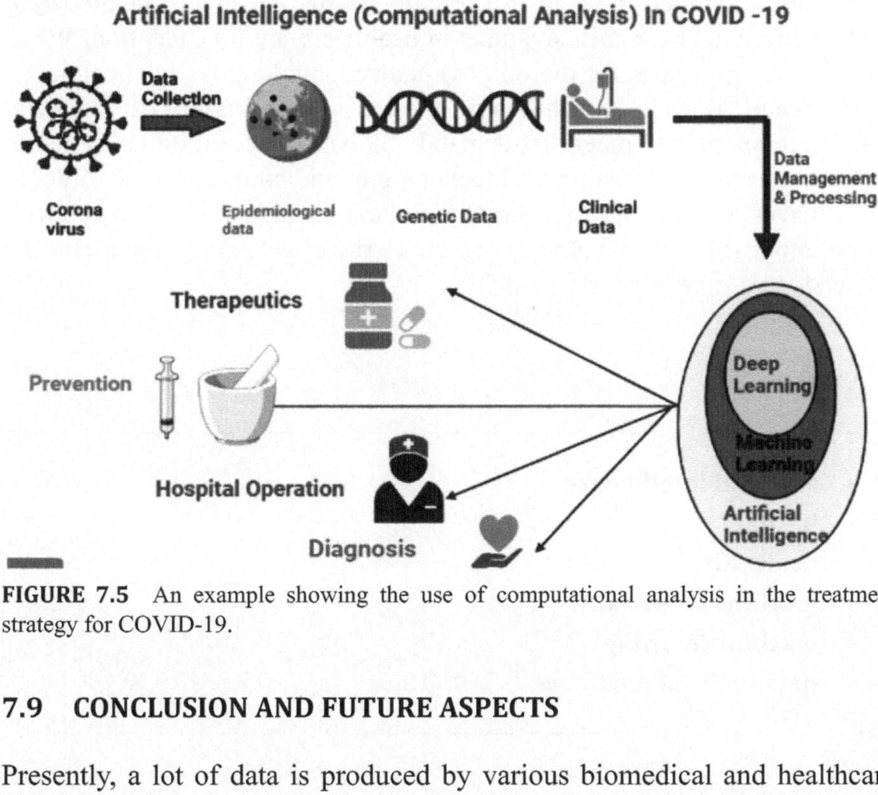

FIGURE 7.5 An example showing the use of computational analysis in the treatment strategy for COVID-19.

7.9 CONCLUSION AND FUTURE ASPECTS

Presently, a lot of data is produced by various biomedical and healthcare instruments like genomics, mobile biometric sensors, and smartphone applications. Therefore, we need to understand and evaluate what can be done with this data. For instance, such types of data analysis can provide a deeper understanding of many procedural, technical, medicinal, and other advancements in healthcare. The integration of computational systems for signal processing by both researchers and practicing physicians has grown. As a result, creating a detailed model of the human body by merging physiological data and "omics" approaches could be the next big goal. This revolutionary concept has the potential to improve our understanding of illnesses and aid in the creation of novel diagnostic tools. The constant increase in available genetic data, including intrinsic undetected mistakes from experiments and analytical procedures, necessitates additional attention. However, there are chances to implement systemic changes in healthcare research at every stage of this long process. Big data will benefit healthcare by predicting epidemics (concerning population health), offering early warnings of illness conditions, and assisting in the discovery of new biomarkers as well as intelligent future therapeutic techniques for improved quality of life. In conclusion, the world is changing quickly, and innovations in healthcare are no exception. While there is an urgent need for more individualized and long-lasting healthcare, both science, as well as technology, are providing a variety of beneficial novel technologies to meet that demand. Global collaboration is needed to support investments in both novel technologies and human assets in order to lead citizens into this new avenue of population health where data is developing into a substantial corporate asset, a critical economic input, and the cornerstone of new business models.

KEYWORDS

- **artificial intelligence**
- **big data**
- **healthcare**
- **machine analysis**
- **machine learning**
- **personalized medicine**

REFERENCES

1. Vayena, E., Dzenowagis, J., Brownstein, J. S., & Sheikh, A., (2018). Policy implications of big data in the health sector. *Bulletin of the World Health Organization., 96*(1), 66–68.
2. De Lusignan, S., Josephine, C. J., Poh, N., Michalakidis, G., Aaron, M. A., Desombre, T., & Krause, P., (2012). Conducting requirements analyses for research using routinely collected health data: A model driven approach. In: *Quality of Life Through Quality of Information* (Vol. 180, pp. 1105–1107). IOS Press.

3. Garapati, S. L., & Garapati, S., (2018). Application of big data analytics: An innovation in health care. *Comput Intell., 14*(1), 15–27.
4. Scheffler, R., Cometto, G., Tulenko, K., Bruckner, T., Liu, J., Keuffel, E., L., Preker, A., et al., (2016). *Health Workforce Requirements for Universal Health Coverage and the Sustainable Development Goals.* (Human resources for health observer, 17). World Health Organization: Geneva, Switzerland.
5. Lytra, M. D., Kwok, T. C., & Anna, V., (2019). Data analytics in smart healthcare: The recent developments and beyond. *Applied Sciences, 9*(14), 2812.
6. Frost, S., (2015). A Frost & Sullivan White Paper Drowning in Big Data? *Reducing Information Technology Complexities and Costs For Healthcare Organizations,* 12–14.
7. Paton, C., (2014). *Will Google Glass Become Standard Eyeware for Doctors*? Internet.
8. Elrazek, A., Mohamed, A., El-Hawary, B., Altaher, S., Akshaya, S. B., Alboraie, M., & Samy, S., (2017). Prediction of HCV vertical transmission: What factors should be optimized using data mining computational analysis. *Liver International, 37*(4), 529–533.
9. Cristianini, N., & Shawe-Taylor, J., (2000). *An Introduction to Support Vector Machines and Other Kernel-Based Learning Methods* (p. 23). Cambridge University Press.
10. Bellazzi, R., & Blaz, Z., (2008). Predictive data mining in clinical medicine: Current issues and guidelines. *International Journal of Medical Informatics, 77*(2), 81–97.
11. Ali, K., Amirrudin, K., Shahaboddin, S., Abdullah, G., Alinejad-Rokny, H., & Anthony, T. C., (2018). Computational intelligence approaches for classification of medical data: State-of-the-art, future challenges and research directions. *Neurocomputing, 276*(7), 2–22.
12. Hood, L., & Friend, S. H., (2011). Predictive, personalized, preventive, participatory (P4) cancer medicine. *Nature Reviews Clinical Oncology, 8*(3), 184–187.
13. Vicini, P., Fields, O., Eric, L., Litwack, E. D., Martin, A. M., Morgan, T. M., Pacanowski, M. A., et al., (2016). Precision medicine in the age of big data: The present and future role of large-scale unbiased sequencing in drug discovery and development. *Clinical Pharmacology & Therapeutics., 99*(2), 198–207.
14. Forkan, A. R. M., Khalil, I., Ibaida, A., & Tari, Z., (2015). BDCaM: Big data for context-aware monitoring—A personalized knowledge discovery framework for assisted healthcare. *IEEE Transactions on Cloud Computing, 5*(4), 628–641.
15. Krishnan, V. G., & Westhead, D. R., (2003). A comparative study of machine-learning methods to predict the effects of single nucleotide polymorphisms on protein function. *Bioinformatics, 19*(17), 2199–2209.
16. Soroushmehr, S. R. R., & Najarian, K., (2016). Transforming big data into computational models for personalized medicine and health care. *Dialogues in Clinical Neuroscience, 18*(3), 339–343.
17. Patel, H., & Gandhi, S., (2018). A review on big data analytics in healthcare using machine learning approaches. In: 2nd *International Conference on Trends in Electronics and Informatics (ICOEI)* (Vol. 11, pp. 84–90). IEEE.
18. Cichosz, S. L., Johansen, M. D., & Hejlesen, O., (2016). Toward big data analytics: Review of predictive models in management of diabetes and its complications. *Journal of Diabetes Science and Technology, 10*(1), 27–34.
19. Belle, A., Thiagarajan, R., Soroushmehr, S. M. R., Navidi, F., Beard, D. A., & Najarian, K., (2015). Big data analytics in healthcare. *BioMed Research International, 2015,* 1–16.

20. Sahu, S. N., Moharana, M., Martha, S. R., Bissoyi, A., Maharana, P. K., & Pattanayak, S. K., (2019). Computational biology approach in management of big data of healthcare sector. In: *Big Data Analytics for Intelligent Healthcare Management* (pp. 247–267). Academic Press.
21. Chen, C. L. P., & Zhang, C. Y., (2014). Data-intensive applications, challenges, techniques, and technologies: A survey on big data. *Information Sciences, 275*, 314–347.
22. Islam, N. S., Lu, X., Wasi-Ur-Rahman, M., Shankar, D., & Panda, D. K., (2015). Triple-H: A hybrid approach to accelerate HDFS on HPC clusters with heterogeneous storage architecture. In: *15th IEEE/ACM International Symposium on Cluster, Cloud and Grid Computing* (pp. 101–110). IEEE.
23. Das, H., Naik, B., & Behera, H. S., (2018). Classification of diabetes mellitus disease (DMD): A data mining (DM) approach. In: *Progress in Computing, Analytics, and Networking* (pp. 539–549). Springer, Singapore.
24. Mishra, B. S. P., Das, H., Dehuri, S., & Jagadev, A. K., (2018). *Cloud Computing for Optimization: Foundations, Applications, and Challenges* (p. 39). Springer International Publishing.
25. Sarkhel, P., Das, H., & Vashishtha, L. K., (2017). Task-scheduling algorithms in cloud environment. *Computational Intelligence in Data Mining* (Vol. 556, pp. 553–562). Springer, Singapore.
26. Tsoumakas, G., & Vlahavas, I., (2009). Distributed data mining. *Database Technologies: Concepts, Methodologies, Tools, and Applications* (pp. 157–164). IGI Global.
27. Wang, L., & Alexander, C. A., (2020). Big data analytics in medical engineering and healthcare: Methods, advances, and challenges. *Journal of Medical Engineering & Technology, 44*(6), 267–283.
28. Richesson, R. L., Green, B. B., Laws, R., Puro, J., Kahn, M. G., Bauck, A., Smerek, M., et al., (2017). Pragmatic (trial) informatics: A perspective from the NIH health care systems research Collaboratory. *Journal of the American Medical Informatics Association, 24*(5), 996–1001.
29. Holzer, J. K., Ellis, L., & Merritt, M. W., (2014). Why we need community engagement in medical research. *Journal of Investigative Medicine, 62*(6), 851–855.
30. Achilleas, T., Forough, F., Lesile, M., & Bhandari, M., (2010). Practical tips for surgical research: How to optimize patient recruitment. *Canadian Journal of Surgery, 53*(3), 205–210.
31. Zimmerman, L. P., Goel, S., Sathar, S., Gladfelter, C. E., Onate, A., Kane, L. L., Sital, S., et al., (2018). A novel patient recruitment strategy: Patient selection directly from the community through linkage to clinical data. *Applied Clinical Informatics, 9*(1), 114–121.
32. Alimadadi, A., Aryal, S., Manandhar, I., Munroe, P. B., Joe, B., & Cheng, X., (2020). Artificial intelligence and machine learning to fight COVID-19. *Physiological Genomics, 52*(4), 200–202.

CHAPTER 8

Artificial Intelligence in Healthcare to Improve the Quality of Life of Elderly

GAYATRI PRAJAPATI and KHWAIRAKPAM SHARMILA

Department of Human Development and Family Studies, School of Home Science, Babasaheb Bhimrao Ambedkar University, Lucknow, Uttar Pradesh, India

ABSTRACT

Artificial intelligence (AI) refers to a task that is primarily carried out by a computer with little to no human involvement. It's a computer program that can turn a machine into one with its own intelligence and behavior. AI should be capable of performing tasks that need human intelligence, including communication, decision-making, and visual perception, among others. By combining large volumes of data, it plays a critical role in diagnostic imaging. It has the potential to expand procedural guiding, intra-procedural analysis, robotics, healthcare, and clinical judgment capabilities. It can be challenging to recognize and diagnose a mental health illness in older individuals due to various reasons such as declining physical health conditions, impairments in cognitive or sensory function, or medication use. All these issues can make it difficult to identify and diagnose mental health issues in older people. Thus, this chapter aims to explore how AI can help in improving older person's quality of life. In older persons, the heterogeneity in the expression of mental health signs and symptoms and response to treatment has an impact on early and accurate diagnosis. A category of computer programs known as AI emphasizes the development and evaluation of different computer-based assistive technologies, which are solutions that preserve older people's independence and improve the safety and overall well-being of the elderly.

Creating Smart Healthcare with Blockchain and Advanced Digital Technology.
Rishabha Malviya and Sonali Sundram (Eds.)

8.1 INTRODUCTION

The ability of a computer or a robot that is controlled by a computer to carry out tasks that would typically be carried out by intelligent individuals is known as artificial intelligence (AI). The word is frequently used to refer to a project aimed at constructing systems that characterize human cognitive processes like reasoning, searching for meaning, generalizing, and learning from prior experience [1]. AI technologies have the potential to enhance the health and well-being of the elderly, but only if ageism is eliminated in their development, implementation, and use. The World Health Organization (WHO) has produced a new policy brief on AI for health that includes legal, non-legal, and technological methods that can be utilized to lower the danger of aging or aging through these technologies. These technologies are transforming several areas for the elderly, including public health and medicine, where they may assist in predicting health risks and events, enable medication research, and encourage the privatization of care management, among other things [2]. During a Dartmouth conference in 1956, American computer scientist John McCarthy et al. first used the term "artificial intelligence." Previously, Alan Turing proposed the Turing test as a measure of computer intelligence, and Dietrich Prinz wrote chess-playing software [3-5]. Most people agree that AI technologies will complement and increase human activity rather than taking the position of doctors and other healthcare professionals. AI is designed for the individual with a wide range of activities, including governmental workflows, clinical documentation, patient outreach, and more. It can also provide more specialized assistance, such as patient monitoring (PM), medical device automation, and image analysis. Divergent viewpoints exist regarding the best uses of AI in the healthcare industry. According to Forbes, the most crucial areas for advancement in 2018 will be administrative workflow, clinical decision assistance, robotic surgery, virtual assistants, and image analysis [6].

These similar themes were mentioned in the 2018 Accenture research, which emphasizes on the growth of AI in healthcare applications across 27 machines, dosing error reduction, and cybersecurity [7]. According to a 2019 McKinsey report, key topics include robotics-assisted surgery, electroceuticals, targeted and personalized treatment, and linked and cognitive devices [8]. AI is a rapidly expanding field that encompasses a wide range of technologies aimed at stimulating human cognition and intelligent behavior [9]. Using a user-centered approach, AI developers take into account a variety of older individuals as well as health-related quality of life to highlight the feasibility and appropriate purpose of such technology in target populations during design and evaluation [10]. In order to help with diagnosis and treatment delivery that is individualized for each patient's requirement, which includes long-term monitoring, care, management, and treatment, it may help with the proactive and impartial evaluation of mental health issues. Additionally, compared to younger adults, older persons display higher levels of comorbidity, chronicity, and complexity. Drug use, acute and chronic physical illnesses, and cognitive, sensory, or functional impairments can all make it more difficult to identify and diagnose mental health issues [11, 12]. For those with chronic conditions or who are severely ill, AI can help improve the quality of their treatment. The proposed treatment could also have a beneficial socioeconomic effect [13]. As part of the expanding trend in Fit Tech toward interactive personal training services, Avatar is an on-demand fitness software that was released on the App Store in May 2020. The centerpiece of 20 billion neurons' (TwentyBN) smartphone fitness software is personal trainer Avatar, an AI start-up financed by Microsoft's venture arm M12. Utilizing the machine vision and natural language processing capabilities of TwentyBn's AI platform, Virtual Coach communicates with users of the workout device in real-time. The Ally avatar develops a plan based on a user's fitness level and goals, leads them through an exercise, and offers verbal feedback on their form while encouraging them and making suggestions for improvement [14].

Healthcare is more readily available because of telemedicine and wearable technology. Additionally, they permit prompt responses that can keep patients out of hospitals while still providing them with continued, high-quality medical treatment [15]. AI has a lot of potential for improving the quality of life for persons who have temporary or permanent visual, hearing, mobility, cognition, and learning problems. People with disabilities have been shown to gain significantly from assistive devices driven by AI, particularly in terms of social interaction, day-to-day activities, and employment in the modern workplace. The inclusive design makes all of this feasible [16]. Today, as life expectancy rises, so do the numbers of the elderly and those in need of assistance. Most elderly people want to age, which means they want to remain in their surroundings as long as they can [17, 18]. However, any changes due to aging present challenges which are difficult to treat and overcome [19]. According to this viewpoint, research is concentrating on developing ICT (information and communication technology) based systems and, more recently, robotic systems to enable older persons to engage in both physical and mental activities (physical assist robots and socially assistive robots) [20, 21]. All the connected items will probably require integration with a larger system in order to produce the perfect home where individuals and robots will help the elderly with their health (i.e., a smart home) [19]. People with dementia can benefit from smart homes, and numerous research studies have looked at how to make dementia sufferers' lives easier. The Internet of Things (IoT) architectures' low-cost sensors might be a practical technique to identify unusual behavior in the home. To ensure safety, sensors have been put in a number of rooms of the house, such as the bedrooms, kitchens, and bathrooms. It is possible to install a sensor on the oven to track usage and alert the patient if the oven was not turned off after use. To notify the patient when the window is open when it is raining, a rain sensor can be attached near the window [22, 23].

Figure 8.1 describes AI programming focuses on three cognitive skills: learning, logical, and self-improvement. The Learning processes of AI programming focus on developing rules for receiving input and transforming it into useful information. Algorithms, or rules, provide computing equipment with step-by-step instructions for completing a task. The logic process of AI programming is focused on choosing the best algorithms to provide the desired results. AI programming's self-improvement procedures are designed to constantly fine-tune algorithms and ensure that they produce the most reliable outcomes possible [24].

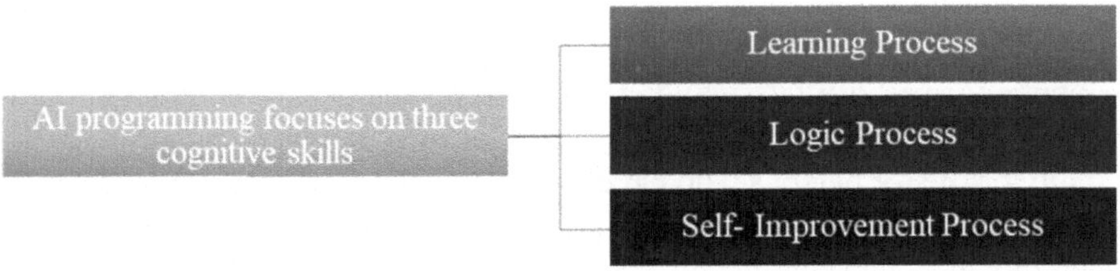

FIGURE 8.1 AI programming for cognitive skills.

It works mainly in three types: machine learning (ML), neural networks, and deep learning (DL) (Figure 8.2).

8.1.1 MACHINE LEARNING (ML)

This learning is a type of AI which employs statistical approaches in enabling computer programs to frame hypotheses and judgments based on previous data, allowing them to improve their performance over time. These optimization

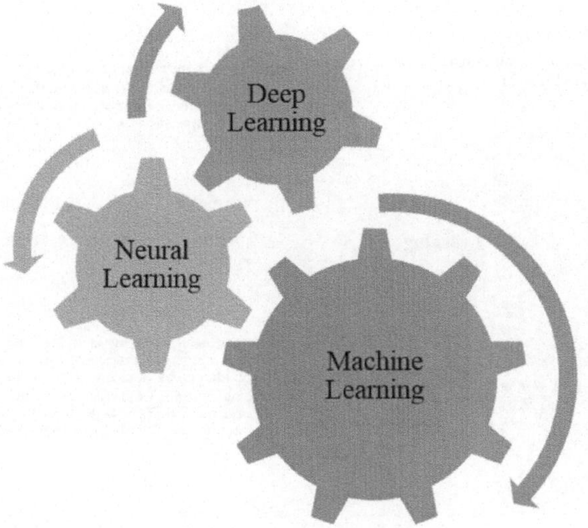

FIGURE 8.2 Subfield of artificial intelligence learning.

algorithms can gather and analyze broad volumes of data from several longitudinal observations, classify patterns, and apply predictive analysis to determine risk levels and offer behavioral or medical suggestions [25]. A statistical method known as ML is used to 'learn' by 'teaching' models with data and fitting them to the data. One of the most often used kinds of AI is ML. The most popular application of traditional ML in healthcare is Precision medicine, which determines which type of treatment and procedures are most likely to be effective on a patient based on several patient features and the context of the therapy [26]. Figure 8.3 described the three classic genres of ML.

8.1.2 NEURAL NETWORK

It is a piece of hardware or software that performs operations like those carried out by the neurons in the human brain [27]. An AI technique called a neural network instructs a computer to analyze data in a manner modeled after the human brain. Artificial neural networks so try to more accurately tackle complicated issues, such as summarizing documents or identifying faces [28]. A neural network which is also considered a kind of ML is composed of interconnected units (such as neurons) that process data by reacting to outside input and transmitting data between one another. To find the relationship and draw meaning from the undefined data, the procedure requires repeated runs over the data [29].

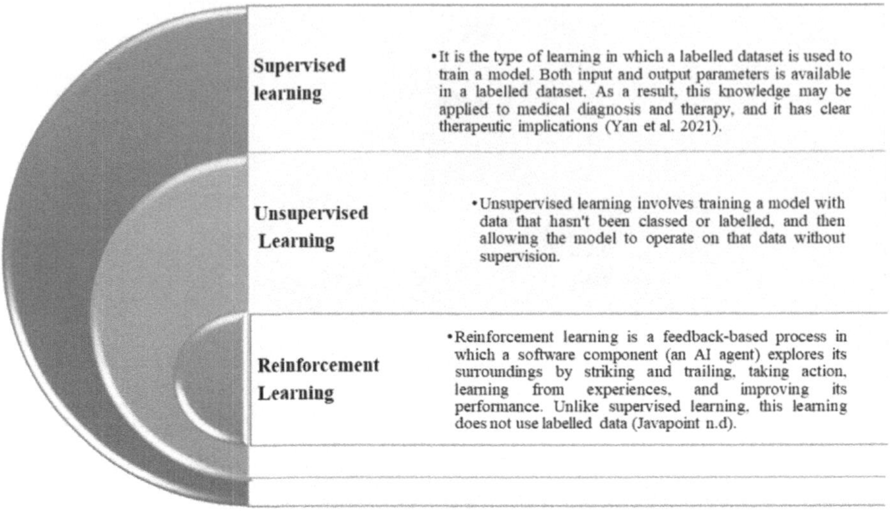

FIGURE 8.3 Types of machine learning.

8.1.3 DEEP LEARNING (DL)

Deep learning (DL) is a method of computer learning that employs interconnected neurons or nodes in a layered structure that is reminiscent of the human brain. Computers can use this to build an adaptive system that helps them learn from their errors and keep becoming better. It is a type of ML which employs massive neural networks with numerous layers of processing units to discover complicated patterns in enormous volumes of data. It takes advantage of increases in computing power and better training methodologies. Image and speech recognition are examples of common uses [29]. DL is considered the hardest form of ML. The quick processing architecture of today's graphics processing units and cloud has revealed thousands of elements that may have been concealed in such models. DL is frequently used in the healthcare industry to identify possibly malignant lesions using radiology pictures [26].

8.2 TYPES OF ARTIFICIAL INTELLIGENCE (AI)

There are several ways to categorize AI, but there are primarily two: classifications based on capabilities and those based on functional forms of AI. The many categories of AI are presented in Figure 8.4.

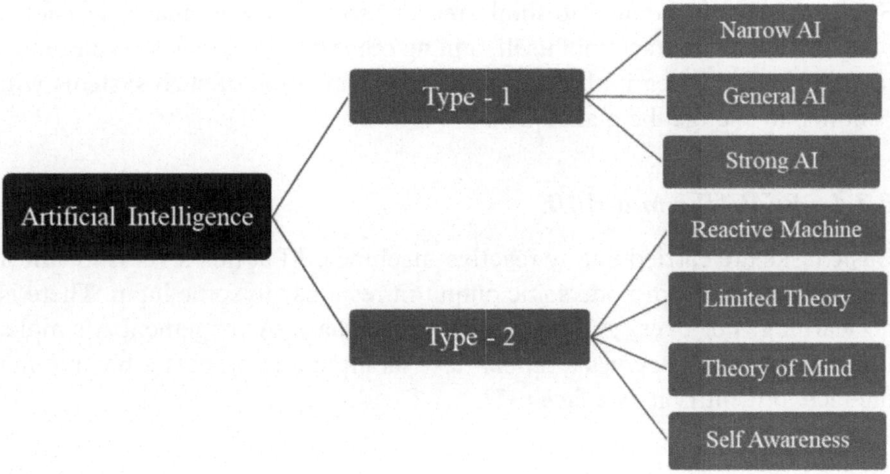

FIGURE 8.4 Types of artificial intelligence.

8.2.1 NARROW AI

A sort of AI known as narrow AI can intelligently carry out a certain task. The most prevalent and currently accessible type of AI is called narrow AI. Playing chess, e-commerce site purchasing recommendations, self-driving cars, speech recognition, and image identification are a few instances of limited AI [30].

8.2.2 GENERAL AI

The capacity of an AI agent to learn, comprehend, and act exactly like a human is known as artificial general intelligence. Massive reductions in training time will result from these systems' ability to independently develop numerous competences, discover linkages between different disciplines, and draw generalizations. Imitating multifaceted abilities, it will make AI systems similar to humans [31].

8.2.3 STRONG AI

Super AI is a level of system intelligence where machines are more intelligent than people and are capable of handling any task with cognitive abilities above and beyond those of humans. This is the outcome of typical AI.

Strong AI should be able to think, reason, solve puzzles, make decisions, plan, learn, and interact with itself, among other things. Super AI is currently just an idealized idea in the world of AI. The creation of such systems will continue to change the planet [30].

8.2.4 REACTIVE MACHINE

Basic tasks are carried out by reactive machines. AI at this level is the most basic. These kinds provide some output in response to some input. There is no learning. For every AI, this is the initial phase. Arrangement A simple, reactive machine receives a human face as input and outputs a box around the face to identify it as a face [32].

8.2.5 LIMITED MEMORY

Limited memory machines are those that can learn from past data other than having the reactive capabilities of purely reactive machines. This category of AI includes almost all applications that are currently known to exist. The vast majority of modern AI systems, including those that employ DL, are trained using training data, which is then stored in memory to create a reference model for future problem-solving.

Virtual assistants, chatbots, and self-driving cars are all examples of modern AI applications that use limited-memory AI [31].

8.2.6 THEORY OF MIND

This kind of AI should be able to interact socially and comprehend people's feelings, ideas, thoughts, and expectations [33]. Theory of mind represents a sophisticated class of AI technology, even though there have been many advancements in this area and only exists as an idea. The development of this form of AI is still ongoing. Kismet is one application of the theory of mind AI. A researcher at the Massachusetts Institute of Technology created Kismet, a robot head, in the late 1990s. Kismet can simulate and identify human emotions. Although Kismet can track gazes and express attention to people, these two capabilities are still major advances in the theory of mind AI. Another use of the theory of mind AI is Sophia from Hanson Robotics. Sophia can see because of cameras that are built into her eyes and computer algorithms. She can maintain eye contact, identify people, and follow faces [34].

8.2.7 SELF-AWARENESS

Self-awareness AI hypothetically can understand its internal conditions, traits, and states as well as perceive human emotions. This kind of AI would enable machines to not only comprehend and evoke the emotions of individuals with whom they interact, but also to have emotions, beliefs, and desires [35].

8.3 ARTIFICIAL INTELLIGENCE (AI)

Artificial intelligence (AI) is used in many fields like healthcare, education tools, retail, manufacturing, transportation, etc.

8.3.1 EDUCATION TOOLS

AI can assist professors and students improve papers and research using tools like plagiarism checkers and citation finders. In the blink of an eye, AI systems can comprehend spoken language and use their databases to do extensive study. This helps them to double-check the spelling, punctuation, and other aspects of literary work [36].

8.3.2 RETAIL

AI refers to a set of technologies, in order to predict, forecast, inform, and help merchants make data-driven business decisions, ML and predictive analytics that can gather, process, and analyze vast amounts of data are needed. In addition to learning important information about various market demographics and enhancing various customer care touch points, AI in retail has provided businesses with high-end data and analytics to help them run their stores more efficiently and capitalize on new business prospects [37].

8.3.3 MANUFACTURING

Improved integration of the IoT and sensors increased data availability and developments in robotics. Automation is propelling manufacturing into a time of significant innovation and transformation [38]. AI applications aid in the identification of some particular man-made issues for which AI technology can provide answers, resulting in major improvements in productivity, quality, efficiency, safety, and cost [39].

8.3.4 TRANSPORTATION

All modes of transportation are becoming safer, cleaner, smarter, and more comfortable as a result of AI. Vehicles, infrastructure, drivers, and transportation users may all benefit from AI in case of delivering transportation services. AI aids in the detection of market trends, risk identification, traffic congestion reduction, greenhouse gas and air pollution emissions reduction, transportation design and management, and travel demand and pedestrian behavior analysis [40].

8.3.5 HEALTHCARE TECHNOLOGY

AI is becoming more prevalent in healthcare technology as new tools are used to diagnose, create medications, and monitor patients. The approach may be learnt and improved as it is used, as learn more about the patient or the substance, and adjust to get better and better [36].

The recent effective uses of AI in healthcare have been enabled by the increasing availability of data on healthcare and the quick development of large data analysis methodologies. Strong AI algorithms can uncover therapeutically important facts buried in massive volumes of data when guided by appropriate clinical questions, which can help clinical decision-making [41]. A person may have at least one chronic condition, like hypertension, diabetes, or arthritis, with increasing age. Along with chronic diseases, frailty is a prevalent problem among older adults [42]. From a scientific and psychological standpoint, the area of aging mental health is concerned with both healthy and pathological aging, including physical illness, neurodegeneration, psychological, and cognitive changes, and mental issues in people of 65 years and older people. Clinical applications and care delivery for such disorders are the main areas of interest in geriatric mental health research. Technology improvements like the widespread availability of smartphones, other wearable sensors, and embedded sensors have changed the clinical care and research environment in inclusion to the introduction of huge datasets (such as electronic health records (EHRs)). Such complex data can be dynamically interpreted using AI techniques and generate astonishing insights, which could improve diagnostic methods and outcomes. By learning and implementing such tailored predictors to assist decision-making in medicine. AI has the potential to improve mental health treatment and research on aging [11]. AI systems that are able to be applied in the field of medicine must first be "trained" utilizing data produced by clinical procedures like screening, diagnosis, and treatment assignment, among others. Learn the relationship between the subject's features and the consequences of interest so that they can be employed by similar groupings of topics. These clinical data may be in the form of demographic information, medical notes, electronic records from medical equipment, or physical examination, among other things, but are not restricted to those [41]. Because they are portable, accurate, and simple to use, healthcare wearables have special benefits for both doctors and patients. They generally use weak or limited AI, which is the kind of AI that they exploit. These features, however, are more than sufficient for wearables to improve lifestyle and handle emergencies. For instance, after a patient leaves the hospital, wearables with AI capabilities may make their lives easier. Wi-Fi armbands with essential recorders, prescription reminders, and live doctor chat are all part of the technology. Additionally useful for remote heart monitoring, and wearables devices. With the help of ML algorithms built into heart monitors and smartphone apps; doctors can remotely monitor the health of the heart. This enables them to spot murmurs that would be difficult for the human ear to pick up on and are early indicators of structural heart disease [15].

8.4 APPLICATION OF AI TO MEDICAL FIELDS

The introduction of AI in medicine correlates with the modern era's introduction of AI. Since the early 1950s, when physicians attempted to improve their diagnosis using computer-assisted programs, AI has been used in medicine. Gunn's 1976 investigation into the potential use of computer analysis to diagnose sudden abdominal discomfort was the first successful attempt to apply AI techniques in the area of surgery [43]. The following are common patterns in artificially intelligent healthcare systems. This type of system begins with a sizable amount of data, applies ML algorithms to it to extract information, and then uses that information to generate useful outputs to address a specific issue in the medical system. Patient diagnosis, medication development, and other applications of AI in medical science include matching patient symptoms with relevant clinicians [5, 44]. AI research in medicine, which was once limited to certain disciplines, such as oncology, dermatology, radiology, neurology, and cardiology, is now encompassing all aspects of healthcare, including surgical robots [43].

8.4.1 ARTIFICIAL INTELLIGENCE (AI) IN DERMATOLOGY

Digitalization, telehealth, and informatics are increasingly interwoven in the field of dermatology. Consequently, applications of AI in dermatology are also possible. Acne, lichen planus, pityriasis lichenoides, dermatomyositis, and seborrheic dermatitis are further dermatological disorders where AI has found a function. AI in psoriasis primarily focuses on enhancing image recognition-based psoriasis categorization algorithms [45, 46]. Massive skin image databases are incredibly valuable since they allow AI in the field of dermatology and provide essential foundational information for the technology. Important challenges for the advancement of skin imaging are how to perform supplemental diagnoses of diseases using AI and how this enormous skin imaging data will be used to give basic resources for dermatological AI [47]. In 2011, dermatologists and researchers launched SkinVision. Every subject is allowed to learn about their skin health through this health prevention tool. Early skin cancer detection is now achievable gratitude to SkinVision, which also enables early treatment to cut down on costs. An AI remote diagnostic and treatment tool for skin tumors in the elderly has been released, and it is developed based on the dermoscopy graphic data of the Chinese Skin Image Database (CSID) and the underlying technical foundation. The "handheld dermoscopy + mobile application" approach used by this AI technology is portable. The first broad platform in China for AI-assisted skin patient diagnosis and therapy is called AIDERMA. AIDERMA primarily consists of three functional sections:

- Doctor consultation;
- Assisted diagnosis and therapy; and
- Ongoing learning [48].

Dermatology, at all facets of the national level, including people development, financial support for scientific research, technology development, and market capital, has given AI attention never before seen. The field of dermatology still has a lot of potential for AI. Future dermatologists will benefit from more expert, precise, and individualized auxiliary diagnosis and treatment. However, the advancement of AI theory and technology enables the development and quality improvement of database resources and multidisciplinary and cross-disciplinary collaboration. The ultimate objective is to improve how AI benefits both patients and doctors [49].

8.4.2 ARTIFICIAL INTELLIGENCE (AI) IN RADIOLOGY

Since its inception, radiology has seen two significant technological advances. First, the ability to detect pathology with ultrasonography, MRI, and CT is fundamentally better than with X-rays. Picture archive and computer systems (PACS) subsequently markedly increased the productivity and diagnostic precision of radiologists. AI is poised to bring about yet another dramatic technical development in the field of radiology (AI). Radiology practice could be drastically changed by AI. AI cannot only interpret radiologic studies more quickly and accurately than human radiologists but also extract additional information from them that radiologists would not have seen (radiomics) [50]. Computer vision techniques highlight obtrusive things in the image by distilling radiologist-defined criteria into a pattern-recognition issue [51]. These algorithms do not, however, generalize across diseases and imaging modalities and are frequently task-specific. In radiography, qualified medical professionals visually evaluate medical scanning and findings of the report to locate, describe, and track diseases. Such evaluation is mostly based on experience and education and is occasionally subject to interpretation. Radiologists periodically change the viewing planes, window width, and level settings as they visually look through stacks of images. Radiologists are taught to recognize abnormalities based on changes in imaging intensity or the emergence of aberrant patterns using their training, experience, and comprehension of the healthy radiograph [52]. These imaging data continue to grow faster than the number of skilled readers that are readily available. These findings have sparked an investigation into the clinical utility of AI-generated biomarkers [53]. AI is quite good at spotting difficulty patterns in image data, and it can automatically generate a quantitative assessment. When AI is included as a tool to support clinicians in their workflow, radiological assessments that are more precise and reproducible may then be made [54].

8.4.3 ARTIFICIAL INTELLIGENCE (AI) IN OPHTHALMOLOGY

In ophthalmology, cataract and glaucoma are both highly prevalent conditions. It is not unexpected that there aren't many stories about using ML to treat anterior segment illnesses. The most common cause of blindness in the world is cataracts, which is a clouding of the lens. A primary effect of glaucoma is optic nerve damage, which can result in permanent blindness. Even though glaucoma cannot be cured, appropriate care can decrease the disease's progression. Therefore, it is crucial to find glaucoma early. Examination of the optic nerve, visual field, retinal nerve fiber thickness, and intraocular pressure are the primary factors in glaucoma diagnosis [55]. Retina experts had little experience with digital healthcare, which can involve telemedicine, and AI. Although possible, interactions with AI in the retina were thought to be best saved for later deployment. AI may be a tool doctors can employ to track patients for illness progression, as retina specialists and their patients have learnt [56]. By extending and expanding the usage of digital ophthalmology, AI and its applications in ophthalmology have the potential to increase the availability, productivity, and accessibility of current resources and boost the overall effectiveness of eye care services [57]. Traditional feature-based ML methods served as the foundation for the first applications of AI in ophthalmology. These ML techniques, commonly referred to as "supervised learning," required skilled ophthalmologists to categorize certain clinical traits and severity in images to construct the AI solutions. DL, commonly referred to as "unsupervised learning," is a new AI technique that is educated without the use of expert feature labeling. Instead, DL uses full images that have been clinically diagnosed (or rated for severity) by specialists, allowing the AI to "learn" the predictive features for classification of diagnosis or grading, with error rates that are better than those previously accepted [58].

8.4.4 ARTIFICIAL INTELLIGENCE (AI) IN CARDIOLOGY

According to Mayo Clinic, integrating AI tools and technology into clinical practice can help both those who already have heart disease and those who are at higher risk for developing it. The AI cardiovascular team at the clinic is utilizing these new methods to diagnose and predict early risk factors for major and complex heart issues. In order to improve treatment outcomes, AI is being utilized to program computers to interpret data swiftly and consistently. Uses include improving diagnostic imaging capabilities and speeding up the treatment of strokes and heart problems. Over the past 20 years, interventional cardiology has made major advancements in the treatment of cardiovascular disease. Heart failure, coronary artery disease (CAD), valvular heart disease, cardiac arrhythmias, pericardial disease, myocardial disease, congenital heart disease, and pericardial disease can all be treated in the catheterization lab, even though percutaneous coronary intervention (PCI) is its main focus [59]. AI imaging technologies are showcasing their ability to do image interpretation, quality control, diagnostics, and workflow improvements [60]. AI and ML can assist in the discovery of novel variations or phenotypes within large cardiovascular imaging data sets, which can enhance our understanding and result in fresh therapeutic approaches for CAD [61]. They can also facilitate catheter-based interventions through the robotic application, enhance clinical decision-making, organize workflow in the catheterization laboratory, and forecast appropriate placement to lessen or prevent paravalvular leakage [62]. Cardiovascular single-photon emission imaging (for the classification of the three layers of the coronary artery) and MRI are additional applications of AI in cardiac imaging analysis. Intravascular ultrasound (for detecting the extent of lumen and media-adventitia), optical coherence tomography (for the classification of the three layers of the coronary artery), and cardiac single-photon emission imaging (for the classification of the three layers of the coronary artery) are also included. One of the most crucial factors in the diagnosis of CVD is cardiovascular imaging. DL will improve the accuracy, simplicity, and speed of imaging diagnostics in the future [63].

8.4.5 ARTIFICIAL INTELLIGENCE (AI) IN NEUROLOGY

Neurodegenerative diseases like Parkinson's, Alzheimer's, and amyotrophic lateral sclerosis have all benefited from artificial intelligence (ALS) [9]. AI has been used to analyze speech recordings, cognitive test results, and, most frequently, neuroimaging since it offers a variety of AI-based picture analysis choices. The rate of brain atrophy and other biomarkers of Alzheimer's disease can be measured automatically by AI systems [64]. DL algorithms have the potential to automate the triage procedure by correctly identifying head-related CT scan abnormalities that need rapid treatment. When radiologists' work is incorporated into ML, neuroimaging could be replaced as a source of digitized image data since these algorithms will soon be more accurate than the trained human eye [65]. The use of AI in neuroscience contributes to a better understanding of how the organic brain functions intelligently. A paradigm change in healthcare is being caused by the expanding availability of healthcare data and the quick development of analytical methodologies [66].

8.4.6 ARTIFICIAL INTELLIGENCE (AI) IN PATHOLOGY

The field of pathology focuses on illness diagnosis primarily through the examination of tissue, cell, and bodily fluid samples. The Pathology AI System is a computer application that offers automated pathology or helps pathologists in their work. Pathology AI systems' main function is to analyze digital slide pictures using ML and image analysis. A task, such as providing a diagnostic or score, or a subtask, such as sorting cells into several cell kinds, can be taught from the data using ML [67]. The huge amount of data generated during the patient care lifecycle has the potential to be handled by AI systems in order to improve disease diagnosis, classification, prediction, and prognosis. Using whole-slide scanners, the process of scanning histopathology, immunohistochemistry, or cytology slides is referred to as "digital pathology." Computational methods are also used to interpret, organize, and analyze these digitized whole-slide images [68]. It is natural to introduce algorithmic intelligence in the pathology area, at least in the phylogenetic features of cells and tissues, in order to create a consistent and maybe more precise diagnosis. Morphology-based automated disease diagnosis is now a reality in a variety of digital pathology tools, from micro-cameras to complete slide imaging scanners [69]. Although the advantages of digital pathology are extensively characterized in terms of the quality, effectiveness, and flexibility it gives to services, the adoption of this technology is still in its infancy. AI image analysis can be used as a system to prioritize cases, select those that are most likely to be benign, or alert pathologists to instances that could be fatal. In a busy department, this enables simplification and better workload prioritizing. Clinical applications for prostate cancer, basal cell carcinoma, and breast cancer lymph node metastasis training in a DL full slide image analysis system have been observed [70].

8.4.7 ARTIFICIAL INTELLIGENCE (AI) IN ONCOLOGY

Oncology has benefited greatly from advances in AI because cancer is a disease of the genome [71]. A cancer diagnosis is the starting point for developing clinical management and traditionally relevant therapy methods, and its AI-based refinement is a significant accomplishment. Additionally, it suggests that drug discovery, therapy administration, and follow-up plans should all be considered in the development of AI as it moves forward. The development of genuine AI must follow a broad and multidisciplinary pattern in order to show a clear improvement in managing cancer patients. The three particular cancer kinds that are now benefiting more from AI-based techniques in clinical practice are Breast cancer, prostate cancer, and lung cancer [72]. Predicting clinical outcomes, enhancing cancer imaging diagnostics with treatment response evaluation, and accelerating drug development and translational oncology are all areas where AI has shown potential at the moment [73]. Using more aggressive treatment modalities will not only conserve healthcare resources but also reduce negative side effects. Lesions that are malignant or pre-cancerous should be accurately diagnosed to help limit overtreatment. Predicting pre-cancerous lesions in cervical cancer screening has proven to be highly accurate when using AI algorithms that support the examination of colposcopy pictures. At the time of diagnosis, AI-based correct cancer classification lessens the need for intrusive interventions and pointless surgery [71].

8.4.8 ARTIFICIAL INTELLIGENCE (AI) IN ROBOTICS

Through the use of AI, systems may learn, solve issues, and make decisions on their own without the assistance of carefully written instructions [74]. According to AI in Robotics (2019), AI provides robots with a computer vision to navigate, sense their environment, and determine how to react. ML, which is a component of computer programming and AI, robots learn how to carry out their tasks from humans. Robots that are artificially intelligent combine robotics with AI. Robots operated by AI use various AI methods, including reinforcement learning, computer vision, and ML. AI algorithms are required to enable the robot to carry out more difficult jobs [75]. Robots with AI are more productive because they can learn to detect new items on their own. However, robotics is being employed for industrial purposes and in many other disciplines to accomplish a variety of tasks with desired accuracy and high efficiency and is superior to humans in certain situations [76]. Assistive robotics, such as human-computer interaction (HCI) technologies, in specific, seek to develop intelligent robots, artificial limbs, rehabilitation robots, robotic systems, and companion-type robots that engage in physical and mental activities to preserve healthy lifestyles in older people by enticing their users to create training programs in these areas [77, 78]. A few examples are robots used for medical procedures such as endoscopic operations, robotic assistants for patient aid and rehabilitation, robots integrated into implants and prostheses, and robots that assist doctors and other healthcare workers with their jobs. Some of these tools were created by several companies expressly to enhance the interaction between people and machines while dealing with patients and from the perspective of care. The majority of robots now under development use some type of AI technology to perform better in terms of classification, language recognition, image processing, and other areas [23].

8.5 NURTURING ARTIFICIAL INTELLIGENCE (AI) TECHNOLOGY IN CARE, BUILDING RELATIONSHIPS, AND HEALTH OUTCOMES FOR ELDERLY

Older people want to age in place and have relationships. Therefore, AI health monitoring systems may have an impact on older persons' emotional, psychological, and relational dimensions in addition to clinical health outcomes [79]. Even with the aid of AI technology, health monitoring and care management are conducted within and via interactions between dependent individuals and those who provide for them [80]. Therefore, in order to advance older individuals' autonomy and efficient health monitoring, it is important to have a reflective grasp of the multiple factors that frame how older adults and potential carers receive, offer, and use AI health monitoring. Driving real health outcomes requires an understanding of the elderly or patients' health as a whole, including the factors that shape their behavior. More support will be needed to help consumers interpret health data and make their decisions, as well as to develop systems and skills that can change their unhealthy behaviors [81]. Another study described the kind of AI-assisted care-facilitating gadgets, such as assistance with dressing, hand washing, and fall detection. As developers of AI health monitoring systems continue to expand their solutions, the moment has come to integrate ethical concerns while designing and implementation of such emerging technologies [25, 82]. Social robots that incorporate sensors may increase elders' self-assurance and comfort with being alone [83]. In order to lessen mental and emotional suffering, isolation, and separation, minimize social isolation, foster independent living and mental health, and encourage a healthy lifestyle, psychological and emotional assistance is required. End-user education and training can greatly assist in achieving this goal by encouraging a sense of assurance about managing a specific health condition and progressively enhancing general psychological well-being [84]. Fall prediction and prevention AI techniques are currently being developed. This can encourage elders with illnesses like Parkinson's disease to leave the house instead of keeping them there out of fear of falling. AI's advantages for healthcare could someday have demonstrable effects on clinical systems. AI can assist elders in greater self-care and longer home stays [83]. According to a report from the Institution of Engineering and Technology (2022), Fitness enthusiasts may now measure their vital signs using many types of applications, sensors, and wearable gadgets. In order to increase performance, the gadgets analyze data from exercise routines like yoga and gym workouts using algorithms. For people trying to lose weight, diet applications offer the caloric content of foods, and smart scales can keep body measurements in the cloud so that trends can be shown over time. These tools provide people with the capacity to enhance their health and well-being by accurately describing the impact of nutrition and exercise on the body [14].

8.6 IMPROVE AGE-RELATED COGNITIVE DECLINE THROUGH AI

Approximately 80% of older persons and 77% of them have multiple chronic diseases, according to the National Council on Aging (NCOA). These trends also apply to areas other than physical health: According to the NCOA, one in four senior citizens have a mental condition, such as depression, anxiety disorders, or dementia. Organizations are starting to use cutting-edge tools, such as AI and data analysis techniques, to better understand the requirements of older people in order to meet the challenges brought on by an aging population. Clinical staff can gain insights from patient data using AI and data analytics tools to better understand specific illnesses and how they manifest differently in diverse patient populations [85]. Dementia research has frequently used AI. One of the most advanced ML techniques, deep neural network, is frequently employed with genetic and neuroimaging data because it can make predictions by identifying generalizable nonlinear latent patterns and identify the early stages of dementia [16].

In reality, attempts to combat age-related cognitive loss without drugs have been made, and the outcomes are encouraging. Exercise, animal therapy, cognitive training between the therapist and patient, and human-robot interaction (HRI) are some of these intervention techniques. HRI has the advantage of enhancing patient relationships, mood, and emotional expressiveness in those with dementia [86–88]. Additionally, unheard-of advances in AI have recently returned to the scientific and popular consciousness. These advancements in robotics, cognitive psychology, and AI have shown to be at least somewhat effective in postponing the symptoms of various degrees of age-related cognitive decline [89]. According to Duckworth [90], social isolation increases depressive symptoms and reduces cognitive attention. Anxiety can also limit the ability to think abstractly [90–92]. Despite being intended for use in aged care, some technologies could not be in line with people's values or satisfy their need for social connection. People with dementia might find joy and peace from the robot "Paro" [93]. New features including sensor data (digital), handwriting data (text), and speech data (audio) present special chances to spot new signs of cognitive deterioration. There are home-based motion sensors for detecting cognitive impairments, computerized handwriting analysis, tasks that record people washing their hands, multi-modal wearable activity monitors, and speech recordings. These data (in particular from wearable sensors and the environment) have the potential to provide continuous, long-term monitoring of cognitive development [94]. Another helpful robot that has received a lot of attention is the MARIO project, which aims to manage active and healthy aging with the aid of caring service robots. The research intends to address the issues of dementia, loneliness, and isolation, which are frequently observed in elderly individuals. The MARIO Kompa companion robot was created to foster contact with end users, support physicians and caregivers in completing dementia diagnostic tests, and improve acceptance by dementia patients through the provision of real feelings and emotions [23].

8.7 ASSISTIVE DEVICES WITH AI

Assistive technologies are computer-based solutions that preserve older people's independence and improve safety. Third, telehealth or telemedicine solutions include video systems that let patients communicate with carers and passive monitoring devices, remote data transmission between patients and caregivers, and healthcare professionals. The use of assistive technologies such as sensors and warning systems that notify carers of any changes in the care recipient's location or behavior is one example of behavior monitoring [95, 96]. AI has the potential to improve "inclusion, participation, and independence for people with disabilities," according to the United Nations Conference on the Rights of Persons with Disabilities, which was held in June 2019. Applications of AI in assistive technology are already being developed by numerous companies to improve accessibility [16]. AI has a great deal of potential for improving the quality of life for persons who have temporary or permanent problems with their vision, hearing, mobility, cognition, or learning. People with disabilities have been shown to gain a lot from AI-powered assistive devices, particularly in terms of social interaction, modern-day living, and work. This is all made feasible via inclusive design [16]. According to the Global Disability Innovation Hub [97], assistive technology (such as hearing aids, wheelchairs, communication aids, glasses, prostheses, and memory aides) can enable people to live healthy, fulfilling lives that are independent and respectable, as well as fully engage in society [97]. New forms of AT may become possible as a result of AI technology (like Microsoft's Seeing AI project, which employs intelligent cameras to assist the blind and partially sighted). Additionally, it might make ATs more accessible. AI will also enable blind or low-vision individuals to take advantage of various types of assistive technologies, such as Braille, computer amplification software, mechanical magnifiers, and expanded letter keyboards [98]. Robots that resembled people and were used as service or socially assistive robots (SARs). An artificial agent with traits or qualities resembling either human or animal behavior is known as a SAR [99, 100]. These robots are employed to help the elderly with activities of independent life. After it was understood that elderly people needed assistance and help, advanced technological healthcare was used in a domestic setting to ensure that their well-being, security, and safety were maintained. People can stay in their comfortable homes while yet having access to urgent therapy to improve their health appreciation to remote health monitoring (RHM) in smart homes. As inhabitants live in a community of retirees, smart homes offer care combined with activities to keep residents mentally and physically engaged and healthy. Different home design concepts featured various features, such as health-checking devices that were monitored by a centralized medical center for readings of blood pressure, electrocardiogram (ECG), oximetry, and glucose levels. In addition, the home has emergency preparedness and handicap accessibility elements that are integrally linked to the global emergency medical aid system to deliver telemedicine in a home [101]. Not all medical disorders or chronic diseases that necessitate the constant presence of medical personnel or technology for life-critical screening are acceptable for home telecare, even though this notion of home is intended to assist the elderly [102]. Smart home assisted living for the elderly (SHALE) is a domiciliary service that offers healthcare and wellness management tools in a home and is supported by technological innovations such as wearable medical devices, advanced sensor technologies, and wireless communications [103]. It is intended to promote senior citizens' independence and quality of life, lessen the burden on caregivers, facilitate everyday activities in the home, and keep an eye on seniors who are taking medicine [104–106]. The adoption of new technology is strongly influenced by the cohort's demographics and the innovation's perceived relative benefits in terms of cost and benefit. Health innovations are more likely to be quickly adopted if they efficiently solve problems, make activities easier, incorporate user support, encourage participation, and are generally fun to use [107]. According to the Pew Research Center [108], 11% of persons over 50 use mobile devices to measure health indicators including blood pressure, physical activity level, or blood sugar [108]. Between the ages of 65 and 69, older persons use online e-health resources at their highest rate. The availability and capacity of healthcare for older persons are rising thanks to digital health tools. These technologies offer strategies to enhance clinical outcomes for older persons and their caregivers, as well as ways to improve the quality of life for older adults and their caregivers, from enabling remote monitoring to promoting independence [107]. Technology also makes it more likely that family members and friends will continue to provide social support, which is possible with the potential of providing care remotely. However, older adults may get more comfortable and accepting of certain devices over time, they frequently worry about keeping their freedom out of anxiety that they won't become overly reliant on them [109]. The use of assistive devices by elderly persons who live at home helps with mobility, fosters social interaction, lessens depression, and reduces hospitalization. It was shown that using assistive technology, including ICT, robotics, telemedicine, sensor technology, medication management software, and video games, efficiently helped elderly persons live independently safely and actively [110, 111].

8.8 CONCLUSION

Machines can learn from experience, adapt to new inputs, and carry out human-like activities owing to AI. Computers may be taught to perform particular jobs using these technologies by processing large volumes of data and identifying patterns in the data. AI is anticipated to be used in the areas of clinical care, drug development, risk prediction, diagnosis, and therapy in the medical field. The use of AI in medicine is expanding quickly. ML, cognitive computing, and big data analytics are the core components of these technologies. Clinicians who use it can diagnose illnesses and improve therapeutic procedures. AI can decrease the rate of misdiagnosis and increase the effectiveness of diagnostics when used in conjunction with conventional medical techniques. These tools could help caregivers be more organized and supported in their work. A type of AI assistance tool for caregiving, like those to help with dressing or hand washing or fall detection.

Monitoring activity and foreseeing serious diseases before they manifest are two excellent uses of portable and wearable technology. For various reasons, including boosting their drive for healthy living, they find them helpful in enhancing their physical and emotional health. With the number of older people increasing, the rapid innovation of assistive devices is becoming more familiar in the day-to-day lives of the elderly. The literature review also reveals that appropriately designed assistive devices with the help of AI can have many benefits for the elderly in improving their quality of life.

ACKNOWLEDGMENT

The authors profoundly appreciated all the respondents who participated in this study. The author also acknowledges and is grateful for the immense help received from the scholars whose articles are cited and included in references in this chapter.

CONFLICT OF INTEREST

The authors declared that there is no conflict of interest regarding the publication of the chapter.

FUNDING

The authors received no specific funding for this work.

KEYWORDS

- **artificial intelligence**
- **assistive devices**
- **deep learning**
- **healthcare**
- **machine learning**
- **quality of life**

REFERENCES

1. Copeland, B. J., (2022). *Artificial Intelligence.* In: Encyclopedia Britannica.
2. *Ensuring Artificial Intelligence (AI) Technologies for Health Benefit Older People [Internet].* Who.int. Available from: http://who.int/news/item/09-02-2022-ensuring-artificial-intelligence-(ai)-technologies-for-health-benefit-older-people (accessed on 4 December 2023).
3. McCarthy, J., Minsky, M. L., Rochester, N., & Shannon, C. E., (2006). A proposal for the Dartmouth summer research project on artificial intelligence. *AI Mag.* [Internet], *27*(4), 12–14. Available from: https://ojs.aaai.org//index.php/aimagazine/article/view/1904 (accessed on 4 December 2023).
4. Turing, A. M., (2021). Computing machinery and intelligence 1950. In: *Ideas That Created the Future* (pp. 147–164). The MIT Press.
5. Basu, K., Sinha, R., Ong, A., & Basu, T., (2020). Artificial intelligence: How is it changing medical sciences and its future? *Indian J. Dermatol. [Internet], 65*(5), 365–370. Available from: http://dx.doi.org/10.4103/ijd.IJD_421_20.
6. Marr, B., (2018). *How is AI Used in Healthcare – 5 Powerful Real-World Examples That Show the LATEST ADVances [Internet].* Forbes. vailable from: https://www.forbes.com/sites/bernardmarr/2018/07/27/how-is-ai-used-in-healthcare-5-powerful-real-world-examples-that-show-the-latest-advances/?sh=225ce51a5dfb (accessed on 4 December 2023).
7. Kalis, B., Collier, M., & Fu, R., (2018). 10 promising AI applications in health care. *Harvard Business Review [Internet].* Available from: https://hbr.org/2018/05/10-promising-ai-applications-in-health-care (accessed on 4 December 2023).
8. Singhal, S., & Carlton, S., (2019). *The Era of Exponential Improvement in Healthcare?* [Internet]. Mckinsey.com. McKinsey & Company; Available from: https://www.mckinsey.com/industries/healthcare-systems-and-services/our-insights/the-era-of-exponential-improvement-in-healthcare (accessed on 4 December 2023).
9. Belić, M., Bobić, V., Badža, M., Šolaja, N., Đurić-Jovičić, M., & Kostić, V. S., (2019). Artificial intelligence for assisting diagnostics and assessment of Parkinson's disease: A review. Clin. Neurol. *Neurosurg. [Internet], 184*(105442), 105442. Available from: http://dx.doi.org/10.1016/j.clineuro.2019.105442.
10. Kolovson, S., Pratap, A., Duffy, J., Allred, R., Munson, S. A., & Areán, P. A., (2020). Understanding participant needs for engagement and attitudes towards passive sensing in remote digital health studies. *Int. Conf. Pervasive Comput. Technol. Healthc. [Internet], 2020*, 347–362. Available from: http://dx.doi.org/10.1145/3421937.3422025.
11. Renn, B. N., Schurr, M., Zaslavsky, O., & Pratap, A., (2021). Artificial intelligence: An interprofessional perspective on implications for geriatric mental health research and care. *Front Psychiatry [Internet], 12,* 734909. Available from: http://dx.doi.org/10.3389/fpsyt.2021.734909.
12. Gallo, J. J., Rabins, P. V., & Anthony, J. C., (1999). Sadness in older persons: 13-year follow-up of a community sample in Baltimore, Maryland. *Psychol. Med. [Internet], 29*(2), 341–350. Available from: http://dx.doi.org/10.1017/s0033291798008083.
13. Faculty of Engineering, Physical Sciences. *Artificial Intelligence to Improve Quality of Life for Elderly People Who Are Chronically Ill [Internet].* University of Leeds. Available from: https://eps.leeds.ac.uk/computing/news/article/5533/

artificial-intelligence-to-improve-quality-of-life-for-elderly-people-who-are-chronically-ill (accessed on 4 December 2023).

14. Bannister, P., Fiet, C., & Nag, R. (2022). *Artificial Intelligence and Ageing [Internet].* The Institution of Engineering and technology.theiet.org. Available from: https://www.theiet.org/media/9629/artificial-intelligence-and-ageing.pdf (accessed on 4 December 2023).
15. Karp, R., (2021). *Integrating Wearable Sensors and AI in MedTech [Internet].* Fluffy Spider. Fluffy Spider Technologies. Available from: https://fluffyspider.com/blog/integrating-wearable-sensors-and-ai-in-medtech/ (accessed on 4 December 2023).
16. EdTech, M., (2019). *How AI is Making Assistive Technologies More Powerful [Internet].* MagicBox. Available from: https://medium.com/magicbox/how-ai-is-making-assistive-technologies-more-powerful-670aa043bfcf (accessed on 4 December 2023).
17. European Commission, (2017). Directorate-General for Economic and Financial Affairs and Economic Policy Committee of the European Communities. *The 2018 Ageing Report: Underlying Assumptions and Projection Methodologies*. Luxembourg: Publications Office of the European Union.
18. Marek, K. D., & Rantz, M. J., (2000). Aging in place: A new model for long term care. *Nurs. Adm. Q [Internet], 24*(3), 1–11. Spring. Available from: http://dx.doi.org/10.1097/00006216-200004000-00003.
19. Beer, J. M., & Owens, O. L., (2018). *Social Agents for Aging-in-Place* (pp. 237–259). In: Aging, Technology and Health [Internet]. Elsevier. Available from: http://dx.doi.org/10.1016/b978-0-12-811272-4.00010-5.
20. Consilium Research & Consultancy, (2020). *Scoping Study on the Emerging Use of Artificial Intelligence (AI) and Robotics in Social Care.* Technical Report, Skills for Care.
21. Cortellessa, G., De Benedictis, R., Fracasso, F., Orlandini, A., Umbrico, A., & Cesta, A., (2021). AI and robotics to help older adults: Revisiting projects in search of lessons learned. *Paladyn [Internet], 12*(1), 356–378. Available from: http://dx.doi.org/10.1515/pjbr-2021-0025.
22. Demir, E., Köseoğlu, E., Sokullu, R., & Şeker, B., (2017). Smart home assistant for ambient assisted living of elderly people with dementia. *Procedia Comput. Sci. [Internet], 113*, 609–614. Available from: http://dx.doi.org/10.1016/j.procs.2017.08.302.
23. Bohr, A., & Memarzadeh, K., (2020). The rise of artificial intelligence in healthcare applications. In: *Artificial Intelligence in Healthcare [Internet]* (pp. 25–60). Elsevier. Available from: http://dx.doi.org/10.1016/b978-0-12-818438-7.00002-2.
24. Burns, E., Laskowski, N., & Tucci, L., (2022). *What Is Artificial Intelligence (AI)?* Definition, benefits and use cases [Internet]. SearchEnterpriseAI. TechTarget. Available from: https://www.techtarget.com/searchenterpriseai/definition/AI-Artificial-Intelligence (accessed on 4 December 2023).
25. Ho, A., (2020). Are we ready for artificial intelligence health monitoring in elder care? *BMC Geriatr. [Internet], 20*(1), 358. Available from: http://dx.doi.org/10.1186/s12877-020-01764-9.
26. Davenport, T., & Kalakota, R., (2019). The potential for artificial intelligence in healthcare. *Future Healthc. J. [Internet], 6*(2), 94–98. Available from: http://dx.doi.org/10.7861/futurehosp.6-2-94.

27. Vaishnavi, P., (2022). *AI Neural Network [Internet]*. Mindmajix. Available from: https://mindmajix.com/neural-network-in-artificial-intelligence (accessed on 4 December 2023).
28. AWS, (2020). *What Is a Neural Network [Internet]*. Available from: https://aws.amazon.com/what-is/neural-network/#:~:text=A%20neural%20network%20is%20a,that%20resembles%20the%20human%20brain (accessed on 4 December 2023).
29. *Artificial Intelligence: What it is and Why it Matters [Internet]*. Sas.com. Available from: https://www.sas.com/en_in/insights/analytics/what-is-artificial-intelligence.html (accessed on 4 December 2023).
30. *Types of Artificial Intelligence* – javatpoint [Internet]. www.javatpoint.com. Available from: https://www.javatpoint.com/types-of-artificial-intelligence (accessed on 4 December 2023).
31. Joshi, N., (2019). *7 Types of Artificial Intelligence [Internet]*. Forbes. Available from: https://www.forbes.com/sites/cognitiveworld/2019/06/19/7-types-of-artificial-intelligence/?sh=30ea174c233e (accessed on 4 December 2023).
32. Johnson, J. *4 Types of Artificial Intelligence [Internet]*. BMC Blogs. Available from: https://www.bmc.com/blogs/artificial-intelligence-types/ (accessed on 4 December 2023).
33. Gn, C. K., (2018). *Artificial Intelligence: Definition, Types, Examples, Technologies [Internet]*. Medium. Available from: https://chethankumargn.medium.com/artificial-intelligence-definition-types-examples-technologies-962ea75c7b9b (accessed on 4 December 2023).
34. Biswal, A., (2020). *7 Types of Artificial Intelligence that you Should Know in 2022 [Internet]*. Simplilearn.com. Simplilearn. Available from: https://www.simplilearn.com/tutorials/artificial-intelligence-tutorial/types-of-artificial-intelligence (accessed on 4 December 2023).
35. *Types of Artificial Intelligence – AI Types & Techniques* (2022). [Internet]. Intellipaat Blog. Intellipaat. Available from: https://intellipaat.com/blog/types-of-artificial-intelligence/ (accessed on 4 December 2023).
36. *What Is AI Technology and How is it Used? [Internet]* (2020). Western Governors University. [cited 2022 May 11]. Available from: http://wgu.edu/blog/what-ai-technology-how-used2003.html (accessed on 4 December 2023).
37. Marotta, D., (2020). *Artificial Intelligence: How AI is Changing Retail [Internet]*. Hitachi Solutions. Available from: https://global.hitachi-solutions.com/blog/ai-in-retail/ (accessed on 4 December 2023).
38. Monostori, L., Kádár, B., Bauernhansl, T., Kondoh, S., Kumara, S., Reinhart, G., et al., (2016). Cyber-physical systems in manufacturing. *CIRP Ann. Manuf. Technol. [Internet], 65*(2), 621–641. Available from: http://dx.doi.org/10.1016/j.cirp.2016.06.005.
39. Arinez, J. F., Chang, Q., Gao, R. X., Xu, C., & Zhang, J., (2020). Artificial intelligence in advanced manufacturing: Current status and future outlook. *J. Manuf. Sci. Eng. [Internet], 142*(11), 1–53. Available from: http://dx.doi.org/10.1115/1.4047855.
40. Niestadt, M., Debyser, A., Scordamaglia, D., & Pape, M. (2019). Europa.eu. Available from: https://www.europarl.europa.eu/RegData/etudes/BRIE/2019/635609/EPRS_BRI(2019)635609_EN.pdf (accessed on 4 December 2023).
41. Jiang, F., Jiang, Y., Zhi, H., Dong, Y., Li, H., Ma, S., et al., (2017). Artificial intelligence in healthcare: Past, present, and future. *Stroke Vasc. Neurol. [Internet], 2*(4), 230–243. Available from: http://dx.doi.org/10.1136/svn-2017-000101.

42. Yu, K. H., Beam, A. L., & Kohane, I. S., (2018). Artificial intelligence in healthcare. *Nat. Biomed. Eng. [Internet], 2*(10), 719–731. Available from: http://dx.doi.org/10.1038/s41551-018-0305-z.
43. Pai, V. V., & Pai, R. B., (2021). Artificial intelligence in dermatology and healthcare: An overview. *Indian J. Dermatol. Venereol. Leprol. [Internet], 87*(4), 457–467. Available from: http://dx.doi.org/10.25259/IJDVL_518_19.
44. Güneş, E. D., Yaman, H., Çekyay, B., & Verter, V., (2014). Matching patient and physician preferences in designing a primary care facility network. *J. Oper. Res. Soc. [Internet], 65*(4), 483–496. Available from: http://dx.doi.org/10.1057/jors.2012.71.
45. Jafari, M. H., Nasr-Esfahani, E., Karimi, N., Soroushmehr, S. M. R., Samavi, S., & Najarian, K., (2017). Extraction of skin lesions from non-dermoscopic images for surgical excision of melanoma. *Int. J. Comput. Assist. Radiol. Surg. [Internet], 12*(6), 1021–1030. Available from: http://dx.doi.org/10.1007/s11548-017-1567-8.
46. Abraham, A., Sobhanakumari, K., & Mohan, A., (2021). Artificial intelligence in dermatology. *Journal of Skin and Sexually Transmitted Diseases [Internet], 3*(99), 99–102. Available from: http://dx.doi.org/10.25259/jsstd_49_2020.
47. Chang, J., (2018). The value of internet platform in skin image ecology. *Dermatology Bulletin, 35*, 242–246.
48. Haenssle, H. A., Fink, C., Schneiderbauer, R., Toberer, F., Buhl, T., Blum, A., et al., (2018). Man against machine: Diagnostic performance of a deep learning convolutional neural network for dermoscopic melanoma recognition in comparison to 58 dermatologists. *Ann. Oncol. [Internet], 29*(8), 1836–1842. Available from: http://dx.doi.org/10.1093/annonc/mdy166.
49. Li, C. X., Shen, C. B., Xue, K., Shen, X., Jing, Y., Wang, Z. Y., et al., (2019). Artificial intelligence in dermatology: Past, present, and future. *Chin. Med. J. (Engl) [Internet], 132*(17), 2017–2020. Available from: http://dx.doi.org/10.1097/CM9.0000000000000372.
50. Deyer, T., & Doshi, A., (2019). Application of artificial intelligence to radiology. *Ann. Transl. Med. [Internet], 7*(11), 230. Available from: http://dx.doi.org/10.21037/atm.2019.05.79.
51. Nagaraj, S., Rao, G. N., & Koteswararao, K., (2010). The role of pattern recognition in computer-aided diagnosis and computer-aided detection in medical imaging: A clinical validation. *Int. J. Comput. Appl. [Internet], 8*(5), 18–22. Available from: http://dx.doi.org/10.5120/1207-1729.
52. Castellino, R. A., (2005). Computer aided detection (CAD): An overview. *Cancer Imaging [Internet], 5*(1), 17–19. Available from: http://dx.doi.org/10.1102/1470-7330.2005.0018.
53. Boland, G. W. L., Guimaraes, A. S., & Mueller, P. R., (2009). The radiologist's conundrum: Benefits and costs of increasing CT capacity and utilization. *Eur. Radiol. [Internet], 19*(1), 9–11. discussion 12. Available from: http://dx.doi.org/10.1007/s00330-008-1159-7.
54. Hosny, A., Parmar, C., Quackenbush, J., Schwartz, L. H., & Aerts, H. J. W. L., (2018). Artificial intelligence in radiology. *Nat. Rev. Cancer [Internet], 18*(8), 500–510. Available from: http://dx.doi.org/10.1038/s41568-018-0016-5.
55. Du, X. L., Li, W. B., & Hu, B. J., (2018). Application of artificial intelligence in ophthalmology. *Int. J. Ophthalmol. [Internet], 11*(9), 1555–1561. Available from: http://dx.doi.org/10.18240/ijo.2018.09.21.

56. Joshua, M., (2022). *The Offerings and Limitations of Digital Health Care in Ophthalmology [Internet].* Ophthalmology Times. Available from: https://www.ophthalmologytimes.com/view/the-offerings-and-limitations-of-digital-health-care-in-ophthalmology (accessed on 4 December 2023).
57. Ting, D. S. W., Pasquale, L. R., Peng, L., Campbell, J. P., Lee, A. Y., Raman, R., et al., (2019). Artificial intelligence and deep learning in ophthalmology. *Br. J. Ophthalmol. [Internet], 103*(2), 167–175. Available from: http://dx.doi.org/10.1136/bjophthalmol-2018-313173.
58. Gunasekeran, D. V., & Wong, T. Y., (2020). Artificial intelligence in ophthalmology in 2020: A technology on the cusp for translation and implementation: A technology on the cusp for translation and implementation. *Asia Pac. J. Ophthalmol. (Phila) [Internet], 9*(2), 61–66. Available from: http://dx.doi.org/10.1097/01.APO.0000656984.56467.2c.
59. Narula, S., Shameer, K., Salem, O. A. M., Dudley, J. T., & Sengupta, P. P., (2016). Machine-learning algorithms to automate morphological and functional assessments in 2D echocardiography. *J. Am. Coll Cardiol [Internet]., 68*(21), 2287–2295. Available from: http://dx.doi.org/10.1016/j.jacc.2016.08.062.
60. Dey, D., Slomka, P. J., Leeson, P., Comaniciu, D., Shrestha, S., Sengupta, P. P., et al., (2019). Artificial intelligence in cardiovascular imaging: JACC state-of-the-art review. *J. Am. Coll. Cardiol. [Internet], 73*(11), 1317–1335. Available from: http://dx.doi.org/10.1016/j.jacc.2018.12.054.
61. Seetharam, K., Raina, S., & Sengupta, P. P., (2020). The role of artificial intelligence in echocardiography. *Curr. Cardiol. Rep. [Internet], 22*(9), 99. Available from: http://dx.doi.org/10.1007/s11886-020-01329-7.
62. Seetharam, K., Shrestha, S., & Sengupta, P. P., (2021). Cardiovascular imaging and intervention through the lens of artificial intelligence. *Interv. Cardiol. [Internet], 16*, e31. Available from: http://dx.doi.org/10.15420/icr.2020.04.
63. Yan, Y., Zhang, J. W., Zang, G. Y., & Pu, J., (2019). The primary use of artificial intelligence in cardiovascular diseases: What kind of potential role does artificial intelligence play in future medicine? *J. Geriatr. Cardiol. [Internet], 16*(8), 585–591. Available from: http://dx.doi.org/10.11909/j.issn.1671-5411.2019.08.010.
64. Six, O., (2020). *Artificial Intelligence in Neurology: Promising Research and Proven Applications [Internet].* Quantib.com. Available from: https://www.quantib.com/blog/artificial-intelligence-neurology-promising-research-and-proven-application (accessed on 4 December 2023).
65. Vishnu, V. Y., & Vinny, P. W., (2019). The neurologist and artificial intelligence: Titans at crossroads. *Ann. Indian Acad. Neurol. [Internet], 22*(3), 264–266. Available from: http://dx.doi.org/10.4103/aian.AIAN_493_18.
66. Ganapathy, K., Abdul, S. S., & Nursetyo, A. A., (2018). Artificial intelligence in neurosciences: A clinician's perspective. *Neurol. India [Internet], 66*(4), 934–939. Available from: http://dx.doi.org/10.4103/0028-3886.236971.
67. Lange, H., Luengo, C., & Biosciences, F. (2020). *Pathology AI (Artificial Intelligence) Reference Guide [Internet].* Digitalpathologyassociation.org. Available from: https://digitalpathologyassociation.org/_data/cms_files/files/PathologyAI_ReferencGuide.pdf (accessed on 4 December 2023).
68. Cui, M., & Zhang, D. Y., (2021). Artificial intelligence and computational pathology. *Lab Invest. [Internet], 101*(4), 412–422. Available from: http://dx.doi.org/10.1038/s41374-020-00514-0.

69. Chang, H. Y., Jung, C. K., Woo, J. I., Lee, S., Cho, J., Kim, S. W., et al., (2019). Artificial intelligence in pathology. *J. Pathol. Transl. Med. [Internet], 53*(1), 1–12. Available from: http://dx.doi.org/10.4132/jptm.2018.12.16.
70. Moxley-Wyles, B., Colling, R., & Verrill, C., (2020). Artificial intelligence in pathology: An overview. *Diagn. Histopathol. (Oxf.) [Internet], 26*(11), 513–520. Available from: http://dx.doi.org/10.1016/j.mpdhp.2020.08.004.
71. Farina, E., Nabhen, J. J., Dacoregio, M. I., Batalini, F., & Moraes, F. Y., (2022). An overview of artificial intelligence in oncology. *Future Sci. OA [Internet], 8*(4), FSO787. Available from: http://dx.doi.org/10.2144/fsoa-2021-0074.
72. Luchini, C., Pea, A., & Scarpa, A., (2022). Artificial intelligence in oncology: Current applications and future perspectives. *Br. J. Cancer [Internet], 126*(1), 4–9. Available from: http://dx.doi.org/10.1038/s41416-021-01633-1.
73. Kann, B. H., Thompson, R., Thomas, C. R. Jr., Dicker, A., & Aneja, S., (2019). Artificial intelligence in oncology: Current applications and future directions. *Oncology (Williston Park), 33*(2), 46–53.
74. Martin, A., (2021). *Robotics and Artificial Intelligence: The Role of AI in Robots [Internet].* Available from: https://aibusiness.com/verticals/robotics-and-artificial-intelligence-the-role-of-ai-in-robots (accessed on 4 December 2023).
75. Javaprint. *Robotics and Artificial Intelligence [Internet].* Available from: https://www.javatpoint.com/robotics-and-artificial-intelligence (accessed on 4 December 2023).
76. Bisen, V. S., (2020). *AI in Robotics: Use of Artificial Intelligence in Robotics [Internet].* VSINGHBISEN. Available from: https://medium.com/vsinghbisen/ai-in-robotics-use-of-artificial-intelligence-in-robotics-726a4e9ade18 (accessed on 4 December 2023).
77. Pérez, P. J., Garcia-Zapirain, B., & Mendez-Zorrilla, A., (2015). Caregiver and social assistant robot for rehabilitation and coaching for the elderly. *Technol. Health Care [Internet], 23*(3), 351–357. Available from: http://dx.doi.org/10.3233/THC-150896.
78. Penteridis, L., D'Onofrio, G., Sancarlo, D., Giuliani, F., Ricciardi, F., Cavallo, F., et al., (2017). Robotic and sensor technologies for mobility in older people. *Rejuvenation Res. [Internet], 20*(5), 401–410. Available from: http://dx.doi.org/10.1089/rej.2017.1965.
79. Ienca, M., Wangmo, T., Jotterand, F., Kressig, R. W., & Elger, B., (2018). Ethical design of intelligent assistive technologies for dementia: A descriptive review. *Sci. Eng. Ethics [Internet], 24*(4), 1035–1055. Available from: http://dx.doi.org/10.1007/s11948-017-9976-1
80. Kittay, E. F., (2013). *Love's Labor: Essays on Women, Equality, and Dependency [Internet]* (1st edn.). London, England: Routledge. Available from: https://www.taylorfrancis.com/books/mono/10.4324/9781315021218/love-labor-eva-feder-kittay (accessed on 4 December 2023).
81. Szwartz, G., & Godby, S. (2020). *Understanding Human Behavior in Designing a Future of Health [Internet].* Deloitte Insights. Available from: https://www2.deloitte.com/us/en/insights/industry/health-care/health-behavior-change-technology.html (accessed on 4 December 2023).
82. Xie, B., Tao, C., Li, J., Hilsabeck, R. C., & Aguirre, A., (2020). Artificial intelligence for caregivers of persons with Alzheimer's disease and related dementias: Systematic literature review. *JMIR Med. Inform [Internet], 8*(8), e18189. Available from: http://dx.doi.org/10.2196/18189.
83. Greulich-Smith, T., (2018). *Can Artificial Intelligence Care for the Elderly?* [Internet]. GovInsider. Available from: https://govinsider.asia/innovation/artBeeDHaenssleificial-intelligence-ageing-population/ (accessed on 4 December 2023).

84. Kouroubali, A., Kondylakis, H., Logothetidis, F., & Katehakis, D. G., (2022). Developing an AI-enabled integrated care platform for frailty. *Healthcare (Basel) [Internet], 10*(3), 443. Available from: http://dx.doi.org/10.3390/healthcare10030443.
85. Kent, J., (2020). *Using AI, Data Analytics to Enhance Person-Centered Care for Seniors [Internet].* Healthitanalytics.com. Available from: https://healthitanalytics.com/features/using-ai-data-analytics-to-enhance-person-centered-care-for-seniors (accessed on 4 December 2023).
86. Gross, H. M., Schroeter, C., Mueller, S., Volkhardt, M., Einhorn, E., Bley, A., Langner, T., et al., (2011). 'I'll keep an eye on you: Home robot companion for elderly people with cognitive impairment. In: *IEEE International Conference on System, Man Cybernatics (SMC)* (pp. 2481–2488).
87. Martín, F., Agüero, C., Cañas, J. M., Abella, G., Benítez, R., Rivero, S., Valenti, M., & Martínez-Martín, P., (2013). Robots in therapy for dementia patients. *Journal of Physical Agents, 7*(1), 48–55.
88. Sabanovic, S., Bennett, C. C., Chang, W. L., & Huber, L., (2013). PARO robot affects diverse interaction modalities in group sensory therapy for older adults with dementia. In: *Proc IEEE 13th International Conference of Rehabilitation Robotics (ICORR)* (pp. 1–16).
89. Nouchi, R., & Kawashima, R., (2014). Improving cognitive function from children to old age: A systematic review of recent Smart Ageing intervention studies. *Adv. Neurosci. (Hindawi) [Internet], 2014*, 1–15. Available from: http://dx.doi.org/10.1155/2014/235479
90. Duckworth, A., (2016). *Grit: Passion, Perseverance, and the Science of Success*. New York, NY, USA: Scribbner.
91. D. G. Emotional Intelligence, (2005). New York, NY: Bantam Dell Publishing Group.
92. Vogan, A. A., Alnajjar, F., Gochoo, M., & Khalid, S., (2020). Robots, AI, and cognitive training in an era of mass age-related cognitive decline: A systematic review. *IEEE Access [Internet], 8*, 18284–18304. Available from: http://dx.doi.org/10.1109/access.2020.2966819.
93. Waycott, J., Zhao, W., Kelly, R. M., & Robertson, E., (2022). Technology-mediated enrichment in aged care: Survey and interview study. *JMIR Aging [Internet], 5*(2), e31162. Available from: http://dx.doi.org/10.2196/31162.
94. Graham, S. A., Lee, E. E., Jeste, D. V., Van, P. R., Twamley, E. W., Nebeker, C., et al., (2020). Artificial intelligence approaches to predicting and detecting cognitive decline in older adults: A conceptual review. *Psychiatry Res. [Internet], 284*, 1–7. Available from: http://dx.doi.org/10.1016/j.psychres.2019.112732.
95. Khosravi, P., & Ghapanchi, A. H., (2016). Investigating the effectiveness of technologies applied to assist seniors: A systematic literature review. *Int. J. Med. Inform. [Internet], 85*(1), 17–26. Available from: http://dx.doi.org/10.1016/j.ijmedinf.2015.05.014.
96. Pilotto, A., Boi, R., & Petermans, J., (2018). Technology in geriatrics. *Age Ageing [Internet], 47*(6), 771–774. Available from: http://dx.doi.org/10.1093/ageing/afy026.
97. Hub GDI, (2022). *Powering Inclusion: AI and Assistive Technology*. Call for evidence [Internet]. Global Disability Innovation Hub. Available from: https://www.disabilityinnovation.com/news/ai-and-assistive-technology (accessed on 4 December 2023).
98. Ribeiro, J., (2021). *How A.I. Can Empower Assistive Technology and Reduce Inequality [Internet].* Towards Data Science. Available from: https://towardsdatascience.com/how-a-i-can-empower-assistive-technology-and-raise-inclusiveness-abf616e78377 (accessed on 4 December 2023).

99. Broekens, J., Heerink, M., & Rosendal, H., (2009). Assistive social robots in elderly care: A review. *Gerontechnology [Internet], 8*(2). Available from: http://dx.doi.org/10.4017/gt.2009.08.02.002.00.
100. Hegel, F., Muhl, C., Wrede, B., Hielscher-Fastabend, M., & Sagerer, G., (2009). Understanding social robots. In: *The 2nd International Conference of Advance Computer-Human Interaction*. Cancun, Mexico.
101. The use and effects of telemedicine on complementary, alternative, and integrative medicine practices: a scoping review. *BMC Complement Med Ther.* 2023 Aug 2;23(1):275. doi: 10.1186/s12906-023-04100-x. PMID: 37533042; PMCID: PMC10394941.
102. Botsis, T., Demiris, G., Pedersen, S., & Hartvigsen, G., (2008). Home telecare technologies for the elderly. *J. Telemed. Telecare [Internet], 14*(7), 333–337. Available from: http://dx.doi.org/10.1258/jtt.2008.007002.
103. Demiris, G., & Hensel, B. K., (2008). Technologies for an aging society, a systematic review of —Smart home applications. *Yearbook of Medical Informatics.*
104. Cavallo, F., Aquilano, M., & Arvati, M., (2015). An ambient assisted living approach in designing domiciliary services combined with innovative technologies for patients with Alzheimer's disease: A case study. *Am. J. Alzheimers Dis. Other Demen. [Internet], 30*(1), 69–77. Available from: http://dx.doi.org/10.1177/1533317514539724.
105. Zhang, D., Hariz, M., & Mokhtari, M., (2008). Assisting elders with mild dementia staying at home in pervasive computing and communications. In: *Sixth Annual IEEE International Conference* (pp. 692–697).
106. Basarudin, N. A., Yeon, A. L., Yusoff, Z. M., Dahlan, N. H. M., & Mahdzir, N., (2018). Smart home assisted living for elderly: The needs for regulations. *J. Soc. Sci. Res. [Internet],* (6), 7–13. Available from: http://dx.doi.org/10.32861/jssr.spi6.7.13.
107. Reynolds, A., & Osborne, T. F., (2017). Promoting technology adoption and engagement in aging. In: *Using Technology to Improve Care of Older Adults*. New York, NY: Springer Publishing Company.
108. Smith, A., (2014). *Older Adults and Technology Use [Internet].* Pew Research Center: Internet, Science & Tech. Available from: https://www.pewresearch.org/internet/2014/04/03/older-adults-and-technology-use/ (accessed on 4 December 2023).
109. Prajapati, G., & Sharmila, K., (2021). A pilot study on assistive device usage and mental wellbeing of elderly. *Annals of the Romanian Society for Cell Biology, 25*(6), 13144–13154.
110. Prajapati, G., & Sharmila, K., (2020). Role of assistive devices in wellbeing of elderly: A review. *Indian Journal of Gerontology, 34*(3), 394–402.
111. Joshi, A., Mishra, S., Jain, D., Ludhiani, S., & Rajput, A., (2022). *Bioinformatics Tools and Big Data Analytics for Patient Care* (Vol. 1, p. 240). Routledge Taylor & Francis Group.

CHAPTER 9

Affordable Healthcare: The Promise of Blockchain

ABHITAV TIWARI,[1] MALLIKA TAMMINANA,[2] SHALINI PERADA,[3] B. SRIVIDYA,[3] SHIVLAL YADAV,[4,5] ANKITA MOHARANA,[6] and DHANALEKSHMI U. MEENAKSHI[7]

[1]*Guru Ghasidas Vishwavidalaya, Bilaspur, Chhattisgarh, India*

[2]*Bharat School of Pharmacy, Hyderabad, Telangana, India*

[3]*RITEE College of Pharmacy, Raipur, Chhattisgarh, India*

[4]*Birla Institute of Technology, Mesra, Ranchi, Jharkhand, India*

[5]*Department of Pharmacy, Central University of Rajasthan, Bandrashindri Kishangarh, Ajmer, Rajasthan, India*

[6]*Arka Jain University, Tata, Jamshedpur, Jharkhand, India*

[7]*College of Pharmacy, National University of Science and Technology, Muscat, Oman*

ABSTRACT

Blockchain technology might revolutionize the healthcare business. MPI, AAI, and Interoperability are the most common examples of this technology. MPIs provide patients with a unique identity that can follow them across settings, enabling more seamless and scalable care delivery. Blockchain technology would eliminate third parties and streamline operations. Smart contracts would be implemented between parties to automatically adjudicate disputes. Improving how healthcare claims are assessed may reduce widespread claim fraud. This reduction in fraud would benefit providers and payers. Blockchain might increase interoperability between systems and organizations. This is

Creating Smart Healthcare with Blockchain and Advanced Digital Technology.
Rishabha Malviya and Sonali Sundram (Eds.)

crucial for advancement in our present health ecosystem, which comprises several IT legacy systems that don't interact properly. Our present health environment is inefficient because of this. Patients may select who can access their data (and how much), protecting their privacy (either private or public). Blockchain technology would enhance the healthcare supply system overall. Smart contracts allow fewer intermediaries, which streamlines transactions and increases efficiency. All stakeholders would have a more complete image of the patient's record, improving transparency. The use of blockchain technology in the supply chain would assist pharmaceutical enterprises and manufacturers, as well as clinical trials and patient-centered longitudinal health research. We explore how blockchain and associated information technologies might improve healthcare and make it inexpensive for patients.

9.1 AN INTRODUCTION TO HEALTHCARE BLOCKCHAIN

The Blockchain system is widely regarded as one of the most influential technological developments of the 21st century. It increases the efficiency of operational and regulatory verification by making supply chains more visible and traceable across a wide range of businesses. Distributed ledger technology (DLT) is better known by its "blockchain" appellation, which has garnered the interest and investment of the banking and finance sectors [1]. A blockchain is a distributed, continuously growing list of documents, or "blocks," that are linked in a chain via a procedure called "mining." Pending transactions provide a mathematical challenge. In order to ensure that each block is secure, miners use computers to construct a hash, which is a unique string of letters and numbers. Each block contains a timestamp, the data connected with the transactions, and the cryptographic hash of the previous block. It records data from all previous blocks and transactions to build a network or chain. Changes to even a single block may have a domino effect, potentially stopping the whole blockchain in its tracks. When the blockchain processes the data and simultaneously locks in all computers on the network, an immutable digital record is formed which can't add new blocks to the chain [2]. One of the distinctive features of blockchain is the increased transparency and security that comes from sharing information and transactions through an irreversible P2P network. Blockchain technology has found widespread use in the worlds of cryptocurrency and financial transactions. The benefits of blockchain technology are being used by a wide range of industries, from the entertainment industry to the industrial sector and even the healthcare sector. Blockchain technology has the potential to improve healthcare interoperability, which would ultimately benefit patients. Security, privacy, and interoperability are all enhanced, and patients may become the ecosystem's focal point. Therefore, blockchain technology may be utilized to enhance patient privacy and control over their medical information while simultaneously simplifying the usage of mobile applications and remote monitoring. Blockchain technology has the potential to solve many problems and alleviate many worries in the healthcare industry. In Figure 9.1, we can see how blockchain can be used as a potential roadmap for the healthcare system, and it was started as a small project to reduce duplicity and result in patients controlling access rights to their data [3]. The healthcare business is now experiencing two major challenges: data security and data ownership. Data breaches with far-reaching consequences have occurred because of insufficient safeguards around the storage and transmission of sensitive medical information. The Office of Civil Rights (OCR) of the Department of Health and Human Services reports that in 2018, 13 million healthcare records were compromised across several data breaches. Furthermore, the average cost of a data breach was $7.91 million, with healthcare having the highest per capita cost of any sector [4]. This was according to a survey by IBM Security's Ponemon Institute. As the popularity of personalized medicine and wearables rises, so does the risk that individuals may lose full authority over their health records. There are serious ethical considerations associated with each of these cases. Numerous applications of blockchain technology are now being explored in the healthcare industry.

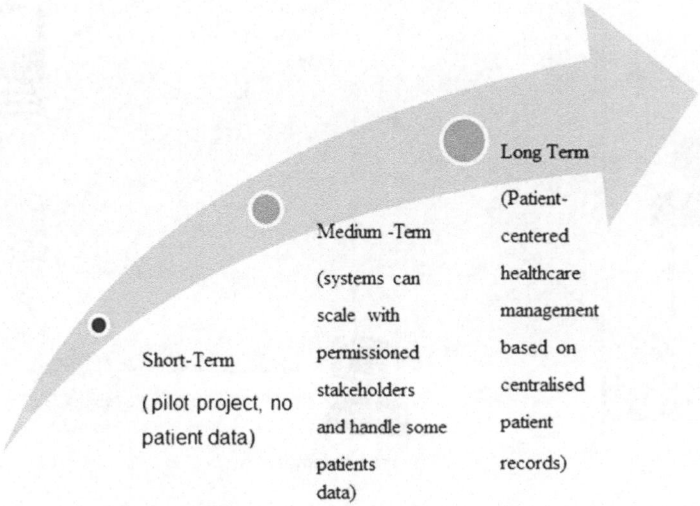

FIGURE 9.1 Potential roadmap of blockchain for the healthcare system.

The use of blockchain technology and virtual currency is now being hailed as the "solution" to a number of issues that exist across a broad variety of industries. It would seem that the general public is split in its attitude towards this technology, with some individuals applauding its powers and implementation while others argue that it is all hype and no substance. It is possible, as of the middle of 2018, to locate blockchain technology anywhere on the Gartner hype cycle between the "peak of exaggerated expectations" and the "trough of disappointment," depending on your perspective. "The core ideas of blockchain technology sound enticing for health data," as stated by the healthcare industry, due to blockchain's "decentralized and encrypted ways of sharing, exchanging, and storing information." However, the paradigm shifts in information dissemination made possible by blockchain technology introduce new challenges in terms of privacy and security [5]. Blockchain technology could change how we share clinical data by making it safer for patient and provider identities and credentials, streamlining the management of the health supply chain, facilitating data sharing and consent for research and clinical trials (including data monetization), processing insurance and claims, and detecting and reducing fraud. In Figure 9.2, we can see how

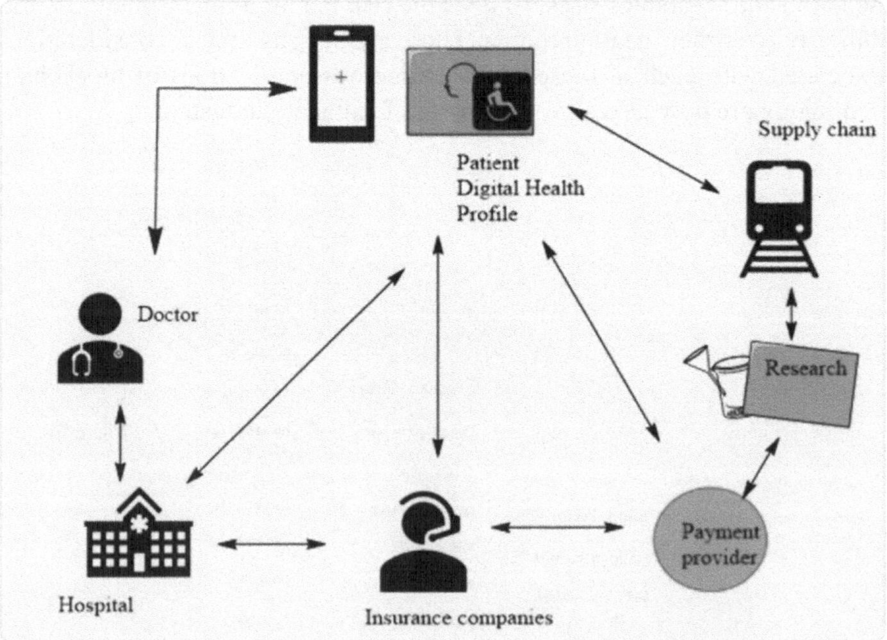

FIGURE 9.2 Interrelation between patient and providers in process of blockchain technology.

blockchain technology works in the healthcare system and have all inter-relation between the patients and providers. Keeping track of a patient's information when it's been spread out in several locations is challenging, as is dealing with the flood of new clinical data and the forking of blockchains that result from consensus changes. Hybrid approaches are used to keep track of rules and references to data stored in a centrally protected system or on a private blockchain. Since this is so close to centralized ownership, some may argue that it undermines the goal of decentralization.

9.2 KEY CHARACTERISTICS OF BLOCKCHAIN TECHNOLOGY

9.2.1 DECENTRALIZATION

Modern healthcare facilities and organizations are often designed around centralized processes, making it easy for one entity to be overwhelmed. The healthcare system as a whole might be negatively affected by the centralized approach owing to issues like a single point of failure in the event of a natural catastrophe or malevolent intent. Blockchain's decentralized nature makes it a secure, efficient, and democratic tool. The blockchain's decentralized nature might help improve patient data access and security, opening the door to new systems in which patients have the ultimate knowledge of their information [6].

9.2.2 TRANSPARENCY

The immutability of blockchain is a fascinating feature. Health data openness paves the way for a definitive and auditable accounting of all patient interactions. Current healthcare data management solutions are unable to deliver privacy, security, and openness simultaneously. Blockchain not only preserves privacy and provides for authorized access to healthcare data, but it also offers increased openness.

All health-related transactions may be easily looked up and tracked thanks to the public blockchain. Because of the immutability of the blockchain, healthcare organizations may more easily track a drug's origins, history of production, and distribution chain, among other details. More transparency in healthcare will boost service quality and efficiency. The blockchain's openness is achieved via the use of cryptography and access control methods [7–9].

9.2.3 IMMUTABILITY

Current centrally managed healthcare systems are very susceptible to hacking and data theft, hence the immutability of healthcare data is a major concern [10]. As a further distinguishing feature, blockchain technology cannot be altered once it has been created. It's a word for how unchangeable the information in a blockchain ledger is. This unique quality could make auditing a more time- and cost-efficient process. Furthermore, it has the potential to build trust in and guarantee the accuracy of health data sent between hospitals. The blockchain guarantees its immutability through the use of cryptographic hashing. Each digital block that makes up a blockchain is used to calculate a hash based on the data in the preceding block and the data added to the current block [11].

9.2.4 DATA PROVENANCE

Healthcare providers should be able to provide detailed accounts of data generation, access, and transfer to earn patients' confidence. Using blockchain technology, you can trace the evolution of your data from its creation to the current day. Blockchain technology may be used to store and verify health records, making them more reliable and auditable. Blockchain technology offers the possibility of securing the provenance of health data, which in turn protects healthcare systems from being hacked or changed. The use of this technology also improves the healthcare industry's traceability. By computing hash values of the provenance record and transmitting them to the consensus nodes, consensus nodes maintain a consistent ledger of all authorized transactions [12].

9.2.5 DISTRIBUTED LEDGER AND CONSENSUS

By bringing together two essential components of technology, the distributed ledger and consensus methods, blockchain has the potential to provide a number of advantages. Reduced inefficiencies in operations mean lower overhead costs and DLT may help achieve this. All patient records are replicated throughout the network's blockchain nodes, making them verifiable and available to all users. Blockchains are designed to update themselves at regular intervals, guaranteeing that all data is always accurate and in sync with other files. Conversely, consensus algorithms validate blockchain transactions.

They make it possible for all parties engaged in healthcare systems to accept a common reality. Additionally, they aid in guaranteeing the veracity of blockchain transactions [13].

9.2.6 ANONYMITY AND PROGRAMMABILITY

Public blockchains have several advantages over private ones, including anonymity and programmability. Anonymity protects the privacy of all parties involved in a transaction, whether they are the sender or the recipient. As a result of their programmability, smart contracts may be used to automate previously manual processes, such as those involving financial transactions. Codes in the smart contracts may be automatically executed depending on the terms agreed upon by the parties involved in a transaction. These codes aid in the regulation of auditable and finalized transactions. They make it possible for anonymous parties to carry out dependable transactions and agreements without the need for a third party or an extrajudicial enforcement mechanism [14, 15].

9.2.7 HEALTH SUPPLY CHAIN MANAGEMENT (SCM)

While supply chain management (SCM) is essential in any business where resources and commodities are being transported, it is of critical importance in the pharmaceutical industry for monitoring raw materials, production, and distribution. Substandard or fake drug delivery may have devastating consequences for the individuals who are supposed to benefit from these medicines. There was "up to $200 billion in annual revenue" from the "global market for fake, substandard, counterfeit, and gray market medications" in 2016. The safety and well-being of patients are directly tied to the reliability of their medicine supply. Low-income markets and developing nations frequently have higher concentrations of substandard, falsified, and counterfeit pharmaceuticals [16]. The volume of imported pharmaceuticals also affects the reliability of product authenticity claims, particularly in the presence of a deficient or nonexistent SCM infrastructure. The United States, however, has also been the target of counterfeit pharmaceuticals. While the management and integrity of the pharmaceutical supply chain are crucial, blockchain technology also has the potential to enhance the security of medical equipment and supplies. Implanted medical technology, such as cardiac pacemakers and drug infusion pumps, is vulnerable to hacking and manipulation. The US Food and Drug Administration (FDA) and the European Union (EU) require that all medical devices have a unique device identifier, which can be stored and managed using blockchain technology, along with the tracking and distribution of firmware updates, which can be handled employing smart contracts. Medical device tracking via the use of blockchain technology is being spearheaded by a collaboration between Edinburgh Napier University, NHS (National Health Service) Scotland, and Spiritus Development. Tracking medical devices might lead to faster recalls and more effective notifications, boosting device safety and efficiency.

The immutability of a blockchain-based medical device monitoring system may be put to use in the fight against device loss, theft, and tampering of any kind. "By lowering or eliminating fraud and mistakes, decreasing delays from paperwork, enhancing inventory management, recognizing problems more swiftly, minimizing courier costs, and strengthening customer and partner confidence," blockchain technology may significantly enhance SCM [17].

9.3 HOW CAN BLOCKCHAIN TECHNOLOGY BE MADE AFFORDABLE FOR CUSTOMERS?

There are a number of different ways in which blockchain technology has the potential to revolutionize the healthcare industry. There are many examples of this, some of which include the master patient identifier (MPI), autonomous automated adjudication, and interoperability. MPIs provide a single-person identity that can follow the patient into multiple settings; this makes it possible for more streamlined and scalable delivery of healthcare across a variety of healthcare providers (and perhaps beyond healthcare, where data is equally relevant). The preparation of claims and other healthcare transactions between parties would be significantly streamlined if autonomous automated adjudication were used. This streamlining would be significant. Blockchain technology could, in essence, do away with the requirement of a third party, which would result in a more streamlined process. In this method, smart contracts would be used between the various parties in order to facilitate automated claims adjudication. Improving the way claims are processed in the healthcare industry has the potential benefit of lowering the incidence of widespread claim fraud [18]. A reduction in fraudulent activity would be to everyone in the healthcare industry's advantage, from patients to providers to payers. As a matter of policy, state Medicaid programs are increasingly addressing the identification and prevention of fraud in an increasing number of cases. According to estimates provided by the Government Accountability Office (GAO) of the United States, fraud in the Medicaid program exceeds $14 billion annually, which corresponds to approximately 4% of total program expenditures. This percentage is likely to increase as total program expenditures continue to rise. According to the results of another study, Medicaid fraud may be directly responsible for between 15% and 22% of all spending because services are billed for more than they are worth. These findings indicate that the implementation of a blockchain application that makes use of a smart contract and maintains a verifiable record of all service and payment operations may be able to eradicate the widespread fraud and overpayment that occurs within the Medicaid system. Interoperability between systems and organizations could potentially improve thanks to blockchain technology. This is necessary in order for us to make progress in our current health ecosystem, which is made up of a wide variety of disparate IT legacy systems that have accumulated over time and do not efficiently interact with one another. If blockchain technology were implemented, it would be possible to replace all of these separate systems with a unified and interoperable solution. Through the use of smart contracts and a completely auditable history, Blockchain would make it possible for participants to conduct peer-to-peer (P2P) transactions with one another.

The transactions that take place on a blockchain would be cryptographically secure and irreversible, and they would enable participants to maintain their anonymity. In addition, interoperability would be possible, blockchain applications in the healthcare industry. Using keys that users would have access to, patients would be able to determine who could access their data and to what extent. This would give patients more control over their personal information (whether private or public). Smart contracts make it possible to cut down on the number of intermediaries traditionally involved in transactions, which leads to improved transactional efficiency [19]. These transactions would promote transparency by providing all interested parties with a more complete picture of the patient's medical record. In addition to transactions based on contracts, clinical transactions that are based on electronic health records (EHRs) could also take place on the blockchain. Because of this, medical professionals would be able to have access to the data about numerous aspects of the patient throughout the patient's lifetime, which would result in more openness (this access would be restricted so that providers had access to the data only when necessary). Improvements to the supply chain that are powered by blockchain technology would be extended to include pharmaceutical companies and manufacturers, in addition to pharma clinical trials and patient longitudinal health research. The development of blockchain technology might result in financial benefits for the federal government by simplifying the processes involved in supply chain transactions. For instance, one of the challenges that people who receive Medicaid must deal with is a high turnover, which is brought on by shifting economic criteria. When a receiver moves easily between several government platforms, keeping their identity may be easier with the use of blockchain technology. This would be of especially great benefit if account-based plans from the private sector were made accessible to those enrolled in Medicaid (with the hope of a reduction in costs and better outcomes). Other government programs, such as commercial prescription insurance, might also gain from a simpler method of providing medical care that involves all parties in the supply chain. There has been an increase in the number of industries that are implementing various applications of blockchain technology. According to Deloitte, 35% of organizations in the health and life sciences are interested in using blockchain technology, and 28% of respondents want to spend 5 million dollars or more (10% expect to invest 10 million dollars or more) [20]. It is expected that the reduction in the number of intermediaries (and delayed payment networks) would result in savings in the banking industry of $15–20 billion by the year 2022. Blockchain technology is being used by a growing number of companies, with the real estate and supply chain industries leading the charge. Several companies are operating in the healthcare industry. Blockchain technology has been put to use in a wide number of application domains by Ramzi Abujamra and David Randall. These domains include Gem (in cooperation with Philips Healthcare Blockchain Lab), Pokit Dok, Healthcoin, Hashed-Health, and many more. The Hyperledger Healthcare Working Organization is a group that is working toward the goal of accelerating the commercial adoption of blockchain technology via the open-source collaboration of healthcare member companies. The application cases for blockchain technology are many, and it can bring about a revolutionary change in the health information systems that are now in place.

Many researchers are concentrating on public health information technology (IT) not just because of the influence it has on the healthcare system in the United States but also due to the challenges connected with integrating and deploying this technology also, the use of blockchain technology has the potential to not only make the creation and maintenance of applications easier but also to lead to cost reductions in comparison to the existing IT infrastructure. Figure 9.3 presents the many facets and applications of Blockchain technology that may be found in the healthcare sector [21].

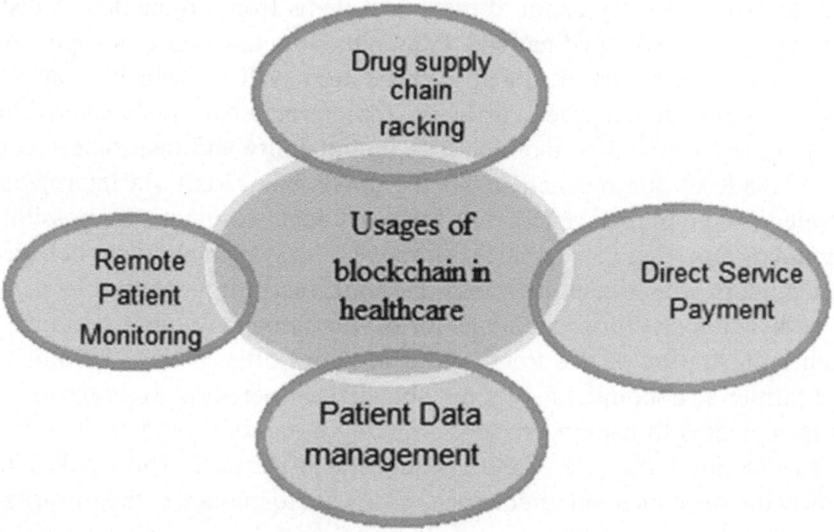

FIGURE 9.3 Application of blockchain in healthcare.

9.4 BLOCKCHAIN TECHNOLOGY AND ITS GLOBAL USES

People in low-income situations, those who have just fled their homes, and the homeless may not be able to break the loop of receiving public and private aid because they lack "transaction identity," a notion that helps explain why they are repeatedly denied access to these resources. The term "transaction identity" refers to the sum of one's life experiences and the interactions that shape one's reputation and place in society. The DLT at the heart of the blockchain is already being put to use throughout the world to address the problem of transaction identification in developing nations. These initiatives depend on humanitarian DLT projects from across the world. This version differs from others in that it uses DLT or blockchain without tying it in any way to virtual currencies such as bitcoin. Helping refugees in the Middle East, poor farmers in South America and HIV patients in Africa establish transaction identities, connect records, and actively participate in global economic and social systems has been made easier through the DLT platform, which is mobile-friendly, inexpensive, and effective. These global examples of blockchain technology's use to address humanitarian use cases

[22]. This is because these use cases avoid putting vulnerable populations at risk from cryptocurrency volatility and data-hacking risks. With the help of a major pharmaceutical corporation, blockchain technology is being used to track the whole supply chain of medicinal items from production to distribution in underdeveloped nations. Example: Drug assistance is supplied to people who aren't part of global identification systems, which creates the possibility of theft and poses a difficulty for international supply chains since the drugs are difficult to monitor. The immutability and distributed ledger entries made by the blockchain for the goods being sent via intermediate suppliers in the global system and final recipients eliminate the possibility of fraud or reporting inaccuracies. Moreover, the system monitors deliveries to customers whose identities may be confirmed through the blockchain network. Microenterprise solutions for paying farmers in Latin America are another illustration of this trend; these solutions often include establishing each farmer's economic identity on a blockchain network. Most farmers do not have access to banking services, forcing them to depend on intermediaries to facilitate the sale of their products and get paid. The result is that farmers are dependent on middlemen, who want to maximize their profits by negotiating low prices for the goods they source.

Blockchain technology improves farmers' economic conditions and integrates them into the global economy by eliminating the need for intermediaries and helping to create an economic identity for these farmers, who can now sell their produce directly to buyers and get paid directly through mobile payments [23]. What's intriguing about these international examples is that they may allow disenfranchised community members in resource-poor contexts to build and take ownership of their identity without the need for a middleman, such as a mobile phone or internet access. In addition, under their identities, they can integrate their many forms of economic and social information through blockchain technology into a single, incorruptible, and the independently verifiable global database. Healthcare, education, government aid, and microloans are only a few areas where similar information and data-sharing challenges exist, but the aforementioned cases may be applied everywhere. That the same DLT platform may be used to link social and health data for Austin's homeless population is not a huge leap of the imagination [24].

9.5 INSIGHTS ON BLOCKCHAIN'S PROSPECTS

Cost, quality, and patient experience indicators are now widely spread but may be gathered using blockchain and novel data privacy measures. Because of this, important issues concerning the genuine worth of medical therapies may be asked and addressed. Clinical pathway systems that need complete data recall for contract reconciliation are a perfect match for blockchain because of the distributed ledger architecture and verified transaction block characteristics. To leave an auditable trail, all patient-level data from various sources may be captured in a safe and private setting, evaluated to ensure it relates to the proper unique person, and then permanently stamped in the ledger with a unique cryptographic signature. Future VBCs (Vietnam Blockchain Corporation), especially in customized medical applications, will have many more data pieces available to quantify the numerous aspects of value, making scalability a crucial feature. Because of the data's intrinsic mobility in this data flow architecture, VBCs may have as many participants as needed. It also provides an abundance of real-world evidence for examination. As a result, the chronic data blockage syndrome will be largely eliminated in a blockchain-enabled VBC future, and the world as we know it now would be drastically altered. With the elimination of HIEs, pharmaceutical firms, health insurers, and healthcare providers may more freely implement VBCs. All parties to a contract would have access to the distributed ledger of data without needing to worry about data security or juggling different B2B agreements, thereby eliminating the need for middlemen. The data would be almost real-time and suitable for CQI, which is key to a VBC's overarching aim of establishing a learning health system [25]. Because there would no longer be a "tollgate" B2B agreement required for the sake of data interchange, the conventional data suppliers of today would need to adjust to a future where the prices of data collection would decrease drastically. The current disjointed and data-hoarding environment would no longer force VBCs to deal with crippling overhead expenses and a lack of data. In the future, contracts might be written with clear, mutually agreed-upon guidelines for who has access to what parts of a patient's medical record.

The adoption of EHRs and evaluation of quality indicators and outcomes would form a perfect virtuous loop. Between now and then, we have to keep working on making PHI interoperable and safe, develop the capacity to aggregate and standardize data, and use big data methods to provide meaningful information that can be used to improve clinical or performance outcomes. Digital-clinical technologies in the patient interaction arena complement artificial intelligence (AI) in managing data streams to determine appropriate courses of action for individual patients [26]. Ultimately, we can leverage innovations for health improvement and monitor quality and outcomes for continuous improvement if we get patients, providers, and communities involved. Once barriers are removed, key data sets necessary for successful VBCs, including clinical data, claims data, and sociodemographic data will be able to integrate to offer a holistic and longitudinal perspective of the impact of pharmacotherapy on a patient and patients in a community. This would aid VBCs and the FDA in their post-marketing monitoring efforts by providing a deeper insight into the effects of individual treatments on individual patients. Using blockchain, which is a great tool for provenance and security, only the necessary data will be accessible, with little risk, and with the patient's agreement (as opposed to permission-less blockchain networks, such as Bitcoin). Possibilities expand in a setting where the price of sharing information is effectively nothing. By working together, public and private healthcare payers may more readily exchange and compare data, strengthening their collective potential to influence health policy and practice [27]. According to the HIPAA Omnibus Rule, a clinical data owner has the responsibility of providing the patient with their data in the format, manner, and form requested by the patient. When patients agree to the safe and confidential exchange of their personal health information (PHI), HIPAA is transformed into a dynamic data-flow regulation. The difficulty arises in establishing the identity of a patient requesting access to, or the exchange of, their protected health information. Internet fraud and identity theft continue to be major problems despite efforts to address these issues outside of the blockchain. A HIPAA-driven data aggregation rule might be quite effective in any case. It has the potential to bridge the gap between current but insufficient patient data, complete but out-of-date plan data, and provider data that is both current and comprehensive but outdated. Consumer Data on sociodemographic determinants of health, which is not currently linked directly to any system, might be imported if the patient consents to its full use [28].

9.5.1 RECORDS MANAGEMENT

The adoption of electronic records systems by healthcare providers at large has been considered the "holy grail" of health IT. The utilization of EHRs was required under the 2009 law that has enabled much of the industry's development, but recent sector and government studies suggest that execution of these standards is lagging, with quite diverse adoption rates among providers. The adoption of EHRs received a massive financial boost as a result of this. Throughout the process of implementation, several milestones have been established, both by the enabling legislation and by CMS guidelines and regulations.

Meaningful Use Stage 1, which was intended to streamline data collection and sharing, was completed in 2012. Stages 2 and 3 followed. Step 2 of a program to improve clinical practices for all eligible healthcare providers and institutions, with a report to CMS due by the end of 2014. The plan called for blockchain technology to be used extensively in the healthcare sector during the third and final phase of the effort. Originally scheduled for widespread implementation by 2016, the use of EHRs by providers has been postponed until 2017 [29] in the pursuit of improved clinical outcomes. Results from this and other research show that hospitals and provider professionals have had varying degrees of success at various points in the adoption process. Adoption rates and progress toward Stage 3 EHR standards are of tremendous interest to physicians and lawmakers. Inconsistent adoption amongst professional providers and institutions has been noted in recent statistics, even though the usage of EHRs has increased from 20% of providers embracing the technology in 2002 to over 60% presently. The adoption rate is lower among physicians aged 55 and above and in rural hospitals than in urban hospitals. These lower-than-anticipated adoption rates raise serious questions about the feasibility of achieving Stage 3 attestation and meaningful use standards by the vast majority of professional providers, especially given the fact that many health IT firms have struggled to achieve CMS guidelines with their clients and many small providers has struggled to implement Stage 2 standards. Special challenges arise for federal agencies throughout the process of implementing EHR standards. EHR technology integration and improving interoperability have proven difficult for both the Department of Defense and the Veterans Administration. Potential answers to the aforementioned issues may be found in adopting a blockchain system for government records management and EHRs in particular. Interoperability and data security are only two of the issues that may be ameliorated via the use of application programming interfaces [30].

9.5.2 MEDICAID MANAGEMENT INFORMATION SYSTEMS

The Affordable Care Act (ACA) gave the Department of Health and Human Services (HHS) and the Centers for Medicare and Medicaid Services (CMS) the power to build health IT systems. This was done to make it easier to run the programs created by the law. The ACA must coordinate multiple programmatic uses of outdated IT to verify eligibility, enroll participants, and provide ongoing programmatic support (including Medicaid and numerous social programs). Fundamental to the actual carrying out Authors: Ramzi Abujamra and David Randall State-by-State policy changes have made ACA programs more complicated than originally anticipated. Before the passage of the Patient Protection and ACA, the CMS established a regulatory and financial framework designed to provide states with the resources to make rapid and extensive investments in healthcare IT. In order to help states improve their enrollment and eligibility processes, the federal government offers funding via a variety of mechanisms.

The implementation relies heavily on the creation of an IT infrastructure for Medicaid (MITA). The Medicaid Information Technology Architecture (MITA) is a countrywide framework for improving healthcare administration and technology development throughout the Medicaid system [31]. Among MITA's numerous goals is the establishment of standardized, interoperable frameworks for the development of comprehensive, bidirectional communication systems. The Medicaid MITS Architecture guidelines are crucial for states to integrate the different Medicaid MITS components. The MMIS is a unified collection of processes and computer processing activities (subsystems) that are created at the general design level to accomplish its key aims. "Mechanized claims processing and information retrieval systems" and "systems mechanization" are defined in 42 CFR 433.111 and Section 1903(a)(3) of the Act, respectively, for use under Title XIX. To better serve claimants, providers, and those asking about benefits; to speed claims processing through electronic methods; to increase management's access to important data for strategic decision making, and to control and decrease administrative expenses for the Title XIX program. Blockchain, the DLT, may solve these issues at a cheaper cost than traditional hardware and software infrastructure. In light of the inevitable evolution of both the MMIS program and blockchain technology, we argue that the two should be integrated into one another.

9.5.3 BENEFITS ADMINISTRATION

Blockchain technology might significantly improve efficiency and reduce the cost of managing employee benefits. Given the rate of change in areas like benefits design, enrollment, beneficiary engagement, and provider payment systems, it is reasonable to anticipate difficulties with interoperability. A fundamental challenge in health IT is the lack of compatibility across various systems. It is suggested that using blockchain applications, which provide potentially infinite flexibility and assist the efficient functioning of different systems, help solve these problems. The administration of benefits makes use of a wide variety of different systems, each of which was developed to gather and analyze data from a specific set of sources. This is especially true of government-funded healthcare programs like Medicaid and Medicare, as well as federal and state-level health insurance marketplaces. It has been shown that the intricacy of these systems' integration is one of their defining characteristics. The complex nature of the healthcare system is only one of the numerous barriers to widespread blockchain use. Data privacy and the availability of sensitive patient-specific information is one of the major roadblocks in the creation of a healthcare blockchain application. It has been suggested that developing systems using the Proxy pattern to facilitate data flow is an efficient solution to address the challenge of user authentication [34]. When it is considered that blockchain technology may be used in a variety of ways and addresses important issues like data privacy and interoperability, it's simple to understand the promise of blockchain applications. There are a variety of procedures and systems that may be able to meet the needs and hurdles with the new technology, including wellness programs, enrollment, and eligibility systems, and the records management systems outlined above concerning EHR deployment. There are some significant flaws in the distribution of benefits that may be traced back to the existing centralized structure of health IT. Furthermore, it is suggested that the present national health IT infrastructure is inflexible, making it difficult and costly to adapt to new technology through programmed means. For example, the current approaches used to ascertain enrollment eligibility are hampered by irrational, rigid logic rules that frequently hinder them from recognizing the requirements of a specific situation. This is in part due to the concentration and rigidity of many contemporary networks. Centralized benefit administration creates data silos to keep people out and data secure, which is commendable in today's cyber security atmosphere but impedes personalization of benefits and inhibits timely coordination among many stakeholders. It is proposed that the need for safe and easily available data is at the root of such well-known issues as data input redundancy, fraud, and excessive service use. Because of the centralized nature of current systems, there is a limited understanding of what data should be exchanged with whom and who should store it. It is believed that by deploying decentralized apps in a blockchain ecosystem through smart contracts, many of the issues and limitations of centralized technology may be alleviated. There may be far-reaching advantages for the healthcare system if benefits and treatment are managed in a decentralized fashion. Our proposed use of smart contracts would result in ramifications like automatic qualification for and acceptance of benefits. A blockchain application might likely open the way for personalized treatment by enabling smart care contracts that do not disrupt administrative or clinical processes [35]. The convergence of clinical and administrative systems that are modifiable through blockchain smart contracts is expected to lead to the removal of duplicate procedures typical of centralized data silo systems. An obvious alternative would be portals that allow for communication between the many systems needed for blockchain deployment. In the context of the records management use case, the need for interoperability was emphasized. Blockchain applications that collaborate using smart contract design in the vein of the Ethereum model can facilitate the development of a so-called "smart benefit" design system by allowing providers to modify patients' data via specific permissions, as required by the Health Insurance Portability and Accountability Act (HIPAA). It is further anticipated substantial savings in IT system integration and continuing maintenance and changes as a consequence of the flexibility of the applications propose are made possible by the blockchain's superiority over current health IT systems [36].

9.6 RECENT CASE STUDIES

9.6.1 ESTONIAN E-HEALTH SYSTEM

Healthcare in Estonia has been revolutionized by the widespread use of cutting-edge IT and associated e-solutions. E-health records (including prescriptions, patient questions, and billing data) for 95–90% of Estonian patients are monitored and accessible in a secure manner through e-patient portals. A patient's medical records (such as test results and X-rays) may be accessed in one central place through the e-portal by the treating physician. The Estonian government started a blockchain-based effort in 2016 to safeguard the health records and system access logs of the country's 1.3 million citizens. The project's end purpose is to store the log files that record the data processing activities related to the health records. The healthcare business is particularly vulnerable to data breaches owing to malicious hacking or fraudulent insider behavior; however, the numerous benefits of blockchain technology may help mitigate this threat. Access to patient medical records was timestamped and documented in an encrypted digital ledger. All patient information is stored permanently in a database using cryptographic hash methods. The project may achieve its goal of providing administrators with continuous, real-time awareness of the integrity of stored patient data, enabling them to identify breaches and take remedial action before any permanent damage is done. In addition, it aims to improve the Estonian healthcare system in terms of decentralization, security, transparency, tamper-proofness, immutability, and suitability without adding to the budget [37].

9.6.2 BLOCKCHAIN FOR HEALTHCARE AND PHARMA DATA IN THE UAE

The primary objectives of the system are to increase the safety of data and the capacity for storing it across national healthcare networks. The blockchain-based system is designed to make it easier to find doctors, hospitals, pharmacies, and other medical facilities via MoHAP's (Ministry of Health and Prevention) software. This blockchain-based software is expected to deliver the most precise and unchangeable drug data, including manufacturing, authorized agent, active component, and cost. A registration of healthcare professionals and facilities might be kept in the MoHAP system, making verification for regulatory agencies easier. It also helps ensure the data is accurate and consistent, which is crucial to fostering trust and openness in the healthcare sector. Due to the immutability of the data, all healthcare professionals will have the same level of access to reliable information that can guide efficient decision-making. The MOHAP system has the potential to automate workflow processes, improve sustainability, and boost operational efficiency [38].

9.6.3 PERMISSIONED BLOCKCHAIN FOR MEDICAL DEVICE TRACKING IN SWISS HOSPITALS

Swiss hospitals have been at the center of several implant and false controversy cases in recent years. To combat these issues, Swiss hospitals have created a blockchain-based system for reliable and efficient monitoring of medical equipment. Following a consensus among healthcare facilities, all transactions are recorded on a blockchain, making them unchangeable and readily traceable. This system is built on top of Hyperledger, a private blockchain. The GS1 standard ensures uniformity in all kinds of transactional messaging (Switzerland: GS1 FG BIG Switzerland Ideal Message Healthcare, EDI 3.1 XML). This infrastructure is preferable to more traditional approaches since it eliminates the need for a middleman to get necessities like medical supplies. Every supply chain transaction is recorded on the blockchain network. Blockchain technology might be used to keep track of the whereabouts of individual medical devices, therefore enhancing patient security. As the blockchain-based platform can be integrated with all participants (including the manufacturer, smart logistics, and the patient file) in the supply chain [39], it may be possible to construct a secure and traceable platform for medical equipment in Swiss hospitals.

9.6.4 PATIENTORY DAPP SOLUTION

Many medical facilities would benefit from sharing patient records, but there is currently no reliable method for doing so. This is complicated by the fact that most hospitals now use incompatible versions of EHRs. In order to provide patients flexible, interoperable, and secure access to their electronic medical information, Patientory has developed a DApp solution that employs a private permissioned blockchain. Blockchain's unique qualities make it possible to keep patients' medical records in a distributed and secure way across several nodes. It also ensures that all transaction records are immutable and cannot be altered. The Patientory DApp system removes the requirement for a central repository or controller of EHRs, allowing for their safe, easy, and rapid transfer across institutions. Recent poll results suggest that, despite the DApp's beta status, the vast majority of users see it as a useful healthcare solution and an excellent tool for tracking exercise and diet. By enabling improved medical record-keeping and access, putting a stop to counterfeit medications, and providing for traceability of clinical trials, pharmaceuticals, and medical credentials, blockchain technology has enormous potential to disrupt and change the present healthcare industries [40]. We believe that most of the current healthcare data management systems are centralized, and as a consequence, they often fail to provide trustworthy data provenance, transparency, audit, secure, and tamper-proof data storage, dependability, trust, and traceability. Fortunately, there may be a way to mitigate some of the damage caused by these issues with the use of blockchain technology [41].

9.7 OPEN RESEARCH CHALLENGES

9.7.1 SCALABILITY

Numerous benefits exist for the healthcare sector when it is used as public blockchains; however, mainstream adoption may be hampered by scalability concerns. The capacity of traditional transaction networks to handle thousands of transactions per second is well established. For instance, the number of Visa transactions that may be processed per second ranges from 1,770 to 2,000. Alternatively, Ethereum blockchains are very slow in this sense, able to execute just around 20 transactions per second [42]. When it comes to private blockchains, scalability is not a huge worry since the nodes that do the actual processing are supervised by reliable third parties. The issue of scalability may be addressed in several ways. An option that aims to add a second layer to the primary blockchain network and enable rapid transactions is the Lightning Network. Another method involves dividing a blockchain into smaller sections, or "shards," and distributing the task of processing transactions among the nodes. Since each node doesn't have to download and store the whole blockchain's data, transaction rates may be increased through parallelization. It is possible that switching to a proof-of-stake (PoS) consensus mechanism rather than sharding would facilitate the app's scalability. Directed acyclic graphs (DAGs) are an alternative strategy that requires chaining together a set of related transactions. DAG can swiftly validate a high number of transactions [43].

9.7.2 NAVIGATE REGULATION AND UNCERTAINTY

Another challenge is figuring out how to make blockchain technology comply with various national privacy laws and regulations (such as HIPAA and GDPR). Moreover, many companies are reluctant to use this technology due to the lack of clear guidelines for what constitutes compliance. Blockchain-related legislation and regulation are in their early stages of development. These rules and regulations are expected to be comprehensive, so firms should monitor the regulatory climate as it develops. Establishing and maintaining open lines of communication with regulators, who may be contacted by healthcare providers for queries or guidance, is crucial. Blockchain is governed in various ways, depending on the country. Governments in places like Singapore and Switzerland are creating regulatory tokens to make it easier for their citizens to use blockchain technology. Unlike other countries, the United States delegated regulatory authority to individual states. In the EU, public blockchain technology is struggling to gain popularity due to strict privacy restrictions. China supports initiatives that would open the door for the mass use of blockchain technology, despite the country's ban on cryptocurrencies. Healthcare providers and government agencies should work together to standardize blockchain legislation and processes in order to fully exploit the blockchain's promise in the healthcare sector [44].

9.7.3 INTEROPERABILITY

If blockchain technology is to fulfill its potential in healthcare, interoperability difficulties must be tackled. Interoperability across different blockchain networks is essential for facilitating cross-chain communication. However, although developers may like the absence of blockchain standards, the resulting interoperability issues cause serious communication challenges. There is a huge hurdle to interoperability caused by the existence of several blockchain networks, each with its consensus process, transaction mechanism, and smart contract capabilities. One solution to this issue is to make use of current blockchain network standards. To guarantee interoperability in their blockchain-based supply chain operations, companies like IBM and Microsoft use data standards produced by the Global Standards Organization (GS1). A further alternative is to establish new standards. A standardized Ethereum blockchain has been constructed, for instance, by the Enterprise Ethereum Alliance (EEA) [45].

9.8 BLOCKCHAIN IMPLEMENTATION

In its simplest form, a blockchain is just a series of blocks that are encrypted to prevent tampering. One of its primary selling qualities in a number of industries is that it is unchangeable. A reliable and trustworthy record of transactions may be built on the basis of a consensus, thanks to the immutability of information stored in a blockchain. ProvChain, a blockchain-based architecture that offers chain-of-custody for data objects in the cloud, demonstrates this immutability, suggesting that blockchain is particularly well-suited to tasks in which data integrity is of paramount importance. Inconsistencies in consensus methods are one place where blockchain implementations deviate from one another. Bitcoin's proof-of-work (PoW) algorithm, HashCash, is designed to be expensive to use in order to prevent denial-of-service attacks. Every Bitcoin miner participates in the PoW process to validate the blockchain and distribute Bitcoins, which is also a vote towards the consensus on the blockchain. The Ethereum Yellow Paper states that Ethereum uses a Dagger-Hashimoto-inspired PoW algorithm called Ethash. However, the PoS Casper algorithm is being considered for adoption by Ethereum. Considering that the combined electricity consumption of Ethereum and Bitcoin is higher than that of the entire country of Ireland, this is done to address the protocol's extremely high energy requirements due to PoW. Ethereum also differentiates itself from Bitcoin by allowing the use of smart contracts. Every machine in the system executes a set of instructions encoded in a set of rules called "smart contracts" [46]. These contracts are executed automatically, binding all parties involved on the blockchain to the terms stipulated in the contract. They lay out the benefits, obligations, and penalties associated with the contract in the same way that a standard contract would. Contracts and laws written in this format may be utilized in place of traditional paper versions. Confidence in the community as a whole is another popular trust model in a blockchain setting. The new Coco framework from Microsoft allows for the creation of consortiums that are neutral with regard to blockchain technology. In the healthcare sector, this might comprise a group of affiliated institutions such as hospitals or, in the United Kingdom, the NHS trusts, as well as suppliers of necessary tools and supplies. Without the need for miners, smart contracts are executed exclusively on the hardware of the trusted partner. This improvement allows a blockchain instance based on Coco to process 1,600 transactions per second, bringing blockchain very close to the performance of the top payment processors. Coco is also suitable for use in many trusted execution contexts, such as those offered by Intel Software Guard Extensions, Microsoft Virtual Secure Mode, and Arm's Trust Zone [47].

9.9 CLINICAL TRIALS

Using blockchain technology in clinical trials and the management of trial subject consent has the potential to dramatically increase transparency, auditability, and accountability among medical professionals and researchers [48–50]. The maintenance of an inalterable record of patient permission is one method by which clinical trials may guarantee compliance with the informed consent regulations of the nation in question. Since one of the most common kinds of healthcare fraud involves forged informed consent documents, this is of the utmost importance. Forging patient consent and altering data are only two examples of why authenticating study participants is important. Benchoufi, Porcher, and Ravaud proposed improving the system by implementing a smart contract system that prevents doctors from using patient data until a key is granted at the end of an auditable smart contract method demanding authorization at each phase of the research. Refusal of consent is possible at any time throughout this process. Participants in clinical studies may be able to maintain their data under their control if consent forms are recorded in a blockchain, which would also provide an audit trail for scientists, doctors, and regulators [51, 52].

9.10 FUTURE PROSPECTS AND CONCLUSIONS

It is predicted that blockchain's broad adoption would disrupt global economic and social systems just as much as the introduction of the internet did. Recent price gains in Bitcoin just hint at how the market sees its potential in the future [53, 54]. The real value of Bitcoin and other cryptocurrencies lies in the underlying blockchain technology, which is a distributed ledger (DLT). Blockchain technology has many additional technical explanations, but the clearest layman explains that it is a DLT that provides each participant with their own encrypted and immutable copy of the transaction [55, 56]. The potential of information sharing for a value-based healthcare future may be expressed in more comfortable business lingo for individuals who are willing to experiment and take risks. For what purpose are we working, is one that must be asked again and again by healthcare practitioners, insurance companies, and pharmaceutical firms. Do we believe that lower per-transaction costs and more precise and timely data may get us there? As a consequence of the proliferation of information across the world, the answer to the question "What business are we in?"—may also evolve. The competitive environment for healthcare payers, providers, and pharmaceutical companies may shift as a result. The result might change depending on who we ask. Finally, synergies across companies, departments, industries, and even regions may result from this massive transformation in health IT. On the contrary, this information is very beneficial to the patient. Even though the aforementioned elements may result in some creative destruction of enterprises operating under the current data ownership hierarchy, the overall benefits of embracing blockchain and related technologies are clear. With a strong commitment to giving each person the best care possible and the use of new tools and technologies like blockchain, we can create a data-driven and value-based healthcare system [57].

ACKNOWLEDGMENTS

I would like to thank my co-authors for contributing their time, support, and knowledge to the completion of the work.

CONFLICTS OF INTEREST

The authors declare no conflict of interest.

KEYWORDS

- **blockchain technology**
- **e-health system**
- **healthcare system**
- **interoperability**
- **master patient identifier**
- **medical device tracking**
- **supply chain management**

REFERENCES

1. Rauchs, M., Glidden, A., Gordon, B., Pieters, G. C., Recanatini, M., Rostand, F., & Zhang, B. Z., (2018). *Distributed Ledger Technology Systems: A Conceptual Framework*. Available at SSRN 3230013.
2. Ponemon Institute, (2018). *Cost of Data Breach Study: Impact of Business Continuity Management*. https://www.continuitycentral.com/index.php/news/business-continuity-news/3366-the-2018-cost-of-data-breach-study-impact-of-business-continuity-management/(accessed on 23 June 2023)
3. Ertz, M., & Boily, É., (2019). The rise of the digital economy: Thoughts on blockchain technology and cryptocurrencies for the collaborative economy. *International Journal of Innovation Studies*, *3*(4), 84–93.
4. Till, B. M., Peters, A. W., Afshar, S., & Meara, J. G., (2017). From blockchain technology to global health equity: Can cryptocurrencies finance universal health coverage? *BMJ Global Health*, *2*(4), e000570.
5. Sadiku, M. N., Akhare, Y. P., & Musa, S. M., (2019). Emerging technologies in healthcare: A tutorial. *Int. J. Adv. Sci. Res. Eng. (IJASRE)*, *5*, 199–204.
6. Kumar, T., Ramani, V., Ahmad, I., Braeken, A., Harjula, E., & Ylianttila, M., (2018). Blockchain utilization in healthcare: Key requirements and challenges. In: *2018 IEEE 20th International Conference on e-Health Networking, Applications, and Services (Healthcom)* (pp. 1–7). IEEE.
7. Schneider, A., (2003). Decentralization: Conceptualization and measurement. *Studies in Comparative International Development*, *38*(3), 32–56.
8. Meijer, A., (2014). Transparency. In: *The Oxford Handbook of Public Accountability*.

9. Meijer, A., (2009). Understanding modern transparency. *International Review of Administrative Sciences*, *75*(2), 255–269.
10. Potanin, A., Östlund, J., Zibin, Y., & Ernst, M. D., (2013). Immutability. In: *Aliasing in Object-Oriented Programming – Types, Analysis, and Verification* (pp. 233–269). Springer, Berlin, Heidelberg.
11. Pechtchanski, I., & Sarkar, V., (2005). Immutability specification and its applications. *Concurrency and Computation: Practice and Experience*, *17*(5, 6), 639–662.
12. Glavic, B., Dittrich, K. R., Kemper, A., Schöning, H., Rose, T., Jarke, M., & Brochhaus, C., (2007). Data provenance: A categorization of existing approaches. *BTW'07: Datenbanksysteme in Buisness, Technologie und Web*, (103), 227–241.
13. Glavic, B., (2021). Data provenance. *Foundations and Trends® in Databases*, *9*(3, 4), 209–441.
14. Shahaab, A., Lidgey, B., Hewage, C., & Khan, I., (2019). Applicability and appropriateness of distributed ledgers consensus protocols in public and private sectors: A systematic review. *IEEE Access*, *7*, 43622–43636.
15. Xinyi, Y., Yi, Z., & He, Y., (2018). Technical characteristics and model of blockchain. In: *2018 10th International Conference on Communication Software and Networks (ICCSN)* (pp. 562–566). IEEE.
16. Clauson, K. A., Breeden, E. A., Davidson, C., & Mackey, T. K., (2018). *Leveraging Blockchain Technology to Enhance Supply Chain Management in Healthcare: An Exploration of Challenges and Opportunities in the Health Supply Chain.* Blockchain in healthcare today.
17. George, G., Haas, M. R., & Pentland, A., (2014). Big data and management. *Academy of Management Journal*, *57*(2), 321–326.
18. Hussien, H. M., Yasin, S. M., Udzir, S. N. I., Zaidan, A. A., & Zaidan, B. B., (2019). A systematic review for enabling of develop a blockchain technology in healthcare application: Taxonomy, substantially analysis, motivations, challenges, recommendations, and future direction. *Journal of Medical Systems*, *43*(10), 1–35.
19. Marian, O., (2018). Blockchain havens and the need for their internationally-coordinated regulation. *NCJL & Tech.*, *20*, 529.
20. Tiik, M., (2010). Rules and access rights of the Estonian integrated e-Health system. In: *Medical and Care Compunetics 6* (pp. 245–256). IOS Press.
21. Wiley, D. C., & Cory, A. C. (2013). Health insurance portability and accountability act. In *Encyclopedia of School Health.*ß SAGE Publications, Inc. 295–295.
22. Koteska, B., Karafiloski, E., & Mishev, A., (2017). Blockchain implementation quality challenges: A literature. In: *SQAMIA 2017: 6th Workshop of Software Quality, Analysis, Monitoring, Improvement, and Applications* (Vol. 1938, pp. 5–8).
23. Wu, J., & Tran, N. K., (2018). Application of blockchain technology in sustainable energy systems: An overview. *Sustainability*, *10*(9), 3067.
24. Khatoon, A., (2020). A blockchain-based smart contract system for healthcare management. *Electronics*, *9*(1), 94.
25. Bates, D. W., (2000). Using information technology to reduce rates of medication errors in hospitals. *BMJ*, *320*(7237), 788–791.
26. Ilgen, J. S., Eva, K. W., De Bruin, A., Cook, D. A., & Regehr, G., (2019). Comfort with uncertainty: Reframing our conceptions of how clinicians navigate complex clinical situations. *Advances in Health Sciences Education*, *24*(4), 797–809.

27. Yaga, D., Mell, P., Roby, N., & Scarfone, K., (2019). *Blockchain Technology Overview.* arXiv preprint arXiv:1906.11078.
28. Drossman, D. A., & Ruddy, J., (2020). Improving patient-provider relationships to improve health care. *Clinical Gastroenterology and Hepatology*, *18*(7), 1417–1426.
29. Brookman, J., Rouge, P., Alva, A., & Yeung, C., (2017). Cross-device tracking: Measurement and disclosures. *Proc. Priv. Enhancing Technol.*, *2017*(2), 133–148.
30. Foth, M., (2017). The promise of blockchain technology for interaction design. In: *Proceedings of the 29th Australian Conference on Computer-Human Interaction* (pp. 513–517).
31. Alla, S., Soltanisehat, L., Tatar, U., & Keskin, O., (2018). Blockchain technology in electronic healthcare systems. In: *IIE Annual Conference. Proceedings* (pp. 901–906). Institute of Industrial and Systems Engineers (IISE).
32. Abdellatif, A. A., Al-Marridi, A. Z., Mohamed, A., Erbad, A., Chiasserini, C. F., & Refaey, A., (2020). ssHealth: Toward secure, blockchain-enabled healthcare systems. *IEEE Network*, *34*(4), 312–319.
33. Soltanisehat, L., Alizadeh, R., Hao, H., & Choo, K. K. R., (2020). Technical, temporal, and spatial research challenges and opportunities in blockchain-based healthcare: A systematic literature review. *IEEE Transactions on Engineering Management.*
34. Ratta, P., Kaur, A., Sharma, S., Shabaz, M., & Dhiman, G., (2021). Application of blockchain and internet of things in healthcare and medical sector: Applications, challenges, and future perspectives. *Journal of Food Quality*, *2021.*
35. Jabarulla, M. Y., & Lee, H. N., (2021). A blockchain and artificial intelligence-based, patient-centric healthcare system for combating the COVID-19 pandemic: Opportunities and applications. In: *Healthcare* (Vol. 9, No. 8, p. 1019). MDPI.
36. Chen, M., Malook, T., Rehman, A. U., Muhammad, Y., Alshehri, M. D., Akbar, A., & Khan, M. A., (2021). Blockchain-enabled healthcare system for detection of diabetes. *Journal of Information Security and Applications*, *58*, 102771.
37. Ali, A., Almaiah, M. A., Hajjej, F., Pasha, M. F., Fang, O. H., Khan, R., & Zakarya, M., (2022). An industrial IoT-based blockchain-enabled secure searchable encryption approach for healthcare systems using neural network. *Sensors*, *22*(2), 572.
38. Arul, R., Alroobaea, R., Tariq, U., Almulihi, A. H., Alharithi, F. S., & Shoaib, U., (2021). IoT-enabled healthcare systems using blockchain-dependent adaptable services. *Personal and Ubiquitous Computing*, 1–15.
39. Sharma, P., Moparthi, N. R., Namasudra, S., Shanmuganathan, V., & Hsu, C. H., (2021). Blockchain-based IoT architecture to secure healthcare system using identity-based encryption. *Expert Systems*, e12915.
40. Attaran, M., (2022). Blockchain technology in healthcare: Challenges and opportunities. *International Journal of Healthcare Management*, *15*(1), 70–83.
41. Pablo, R. G. J., Roberto, D. P., Victor, S. U., Isabel, G. R., Paul, C., & Elizabeth, O. R., (2022). Big data in the healthcare system: A synergy with artificial intelligence and blockchain technology. *Journal of Integrative Bioinformatics*, *19*(1).
42. Namasudra, S., Sharma, P., Crespo, R. G., & Shanmuganathan, V., (2022). *Blockchain-Based Medical Certificate Generation and Verification for IoT-Based Healthcare Systems*. IEEE Consumer Electronics Magazine.
43. Azbeg, K., Ouchetto, O., & Andaloussi, S. J., (2022). BlockMedCare: A healthcare system based on IoT, blockchain and IPFS for data management security. *Egyptian Informatics Journal.*

44. Mustafa, M., Alshare, M., Bhargava, D., Neware, R., Singh, B., & Ngulube, P., (2022). Perceived security risk based on moderating factors for blockchain technology applications in cloud storage to achieve secure healthcare systems. *Computational and Mathematical Methods in Medicine, 2022.*
45. Chelladurai, U., & Pandian, S., (2022). A novel blockchain-based electronic health record automation system for healthcare. *Journal of Ambient Intelligence and Humanized Computing, 13*(1), 693–703.
46. Ghosh, T., Roy, A., & Misra, S., (2022). B2H: Enabling delay-tolerant blockchain network in healthcare for society 5.0. *Computer Networks, 210*, 108860.
47. Luong, D. A., & Park, J. H., (2022). Privacy-preserving blockchain-based healthcare system for IoT devices using zk-SNARK. *IEEE Access.*
48. Wang, S., Wang, J., Wang, X., Qiu, T., Yuan, Y., Ouyang, L., & Wang, F. Y., (2018). Blockchain-powered parallel healthcare systems based on the ACP approach. *IEEE Transactions on Computational Social Systems, 5*(4), 942–950.
49. Saha, A., Amin, R., Kunal, S., Vollala, S., & Dwivedi, S. K., (2019). Review on "Blockchain technology based medical healthcare system with privacy issues." *Security and Privacy, 2*(5), e83.
50. Banotra, A., Sharma, J. S., Gupta, S., Gupta, S. K., & Rashid, M., (2021). Use of blockchain and internet of things for securing data in healthcare systems. In: *Multimedia Security* (pp. 255–267). Springer, Singapore.
51. Tariq, N., Qamar, A., Asim, M., & Khan, F. A., (2020). Blockchain and smart healthcare security: A survey. *Procedia Computer Science, 175*, 615–620.
52. Dimitrov, D. V., (2019). Blockchain applications for healthcare data management. *Healthcare Informatics Research, 25*(1), 51–56.
53. Gökalp, E., Gökalp, M. O., Çoban, S., & Eren, P. E., (2018). Analyzing opportunities and challenges of integrated blockchain technologies in healthcare. *Eurosymposium on Systems Analysis and Design*, 174–183.
54. Shukla, R. G., Agarwal, A., & Shukla, S., (2020). Blockchain-powered smart healthcare system. In: *Handbook of Research on Blockchain Technology* (pp. 245–270). Academic Press.
55. Abu-Elezz, I., Hassan, A., Nazeemudeen, A., Househ, M., & Abd-Alrazaq, A., (2020). The benefits and threats of blockchain technology in healthcare: A scoping review. *International Journal of Medical Informatics, 142*, 104246.
56. Zaabar, B., Cheikhrouhou, O., Jamil, F., Ammi, M., & Abid, M., (2021). HealthBlock: A secure blockchain-based healthcare data management system. *Computer Networks, 200*, 108500.
57. Malviya, R., Ghinea, G., Dhanaraj, R. K., Balusamy, B., & Sundram, S., (2022). *Deep Learning for Targeted Treatment* (p. 436). Scrivener Publishing.

CHAPTER 10

Smart Contracts: Medical Insurance Contract for Patient

KAMLESH KUMAR RAGHUVANSHI,[1] SUBODH KUMAR,[1] SUSHIL KUMAR,[2] and SUNIL KUMAR[3]

[1]Department of Computer Science, Ramanujan College, University of Delhi, Delhi, India

[2]Department of Computer Science, Shyam Lal College(M), University of Delhi, North Campus, Delhi, India

[3]Department of Instrumentation, Shaheed Rajguru College of Applied Sciences for Women, University of Delhi, Delhi, India

ABSTRACT

Smart contract is an automated process which follows the protocols decided by the concerned authorities. The concerned parties use terms and conditions and make decisions based on a set of conditions and make it a rulebook at the time of implementation. The rulebook contains the code that is stored and processed using blockchain technology over the distributed ledger. Any changes are also reflected in the recorded distributed ledger. The medical insurance contract is also part of the smart contract where a patient claims the reimbursement from the working organization or third party. Medical insurance with smart contracts for patients forms the backbone of modern insurance technology. Blockchain-based tools have been used by different authorities in formalizing relationships to achieve their objectives. Although, medical insurance with smart contracts guarantees the performance of an outcome. Various developments have taken place during its implementation. One party may not be desirous to pursue the smart contract, others may

Creating Smart Healthcare with Blockchain and Advanced Digital Technology.
Rishabha Malviya and Sonali Sundram (Eds.)

disagree on the rulebook and also some parties may delay performance obligations. It may exhibit the outcome of a smart contract as magnificent. Smart contracts and blockchains are growing rapidly as intelligent systems for a wide range of applications that require information exchange and sharing across heterogeneous networks. In this chapter, blockchain-based technology has been discussed that allows customers and healthcare companies to agree with the execution of medical insurance smart contracts. Smart contracts and individual clients' data have been expressed using health standards and semantic webs. A smart data access policy has been used to evaluate smart contracts. Machine learning (ML), artificial intelligence (AI) and blockchain technology play an important role to enhance security and preventing various attacks on smart contract's medical insurance.

10.1 INTRODUCTION

It was estimated that general insurance, i.e., non-life premium collected in the fiscal year 2020 amounted to INR 1,893 billion, while the healthcare or medical insurance industry in India brought in amounts of 516 billion Indian rupees. It is to be noted that the premium or amount collected in the Fiscal year 2020 was 27% of all. When it comes to the total amount of premiums contributed to the insurance industry in India, the medical insurance market is only next to the vehicle insurance policy segment. Furthermore, amidst the consistent rise over the last 10 years, it is anticipated that only around 10% of India's population is protected by private medical insurance. This does not include the population that is covered by government-sponsored medical insurance programs. Multiple key stakeholders make up the Indian health insurance ecosystem, including insurance firms, stakeholders, supplier health centers, intermediaries, intermediary administrators, financial institutions, insurance industry technology, ventures, examination, dispensary, additional features or economic value service providers, regulatory agencies, and the executive as a potential buyer of public welfare insurance course of action. These stakeholders communicate with one another via an intricate web of procedures that are interconnected and heavily reliant on paper and data. However, there is a fragmentary flow of information, which makes the interaction between the many stakeholders difficult. It is vital to establish a trustworthy blockchain network in order to enhance the interaction process. This would allow for the execution of processes to be improved via many nodes in a decentralized way, while also providing accuracy and consistency, transparency, and data integrity. It's possible that using blockchain technology and functions and state or smart contracts might be a better approach to keep data and carry out agreements while ensuring that everyone involved is held responsible for their actions. In a way that is visible, immutable, and non-disputable, blockchain technology may automatically gather data for harmony like terms for the policy, agreements on charges and pertinent data, and the implementation with the help of smart contracts which depend on the agreed rules and services.

Concerns about data security and privacy will be adequately handled even though the information will be easily available to everyone. Additionally, the records cannot be altered in any way. Adoption of blockchain technology may go a long way toward assuring confidence, enhancing the consumer experience, and thereby assisting in the supplementary expansion of the medical insurance market share. The use of blockchain technology as an emulsion for the administration of medical information and the interchange of healthcare information has gained favor worldwide. The deployment of electronic records of health information based on blockchain technology in Estonia is a case in point because it protects the integrity of data, lessens the risk of internal data vulnerabilities, and makes it possible for organizations in both the public and private sectors to communicate and share information without any friction. At the commencement of a blockchain cycle, the quality of the data, standard protocols, procedures, and dependability are all very important, and they need to continue to get better for the blockchain to be effective.

10.2 ECOSYSTEM FOR MEDICAL INSURANCE IN INDIA AND PROSPECTS

The ecosystem of medical insurance in India is made up of a number of important players. The contact between all of these different parties is often complex and requires a substantial amount of data to be exchanged. The use of blockchain technology has the potential to enhance this contact process between a number of different parties. The following groups of people are considered to be stakeholders in India's medical insurance ecosystem.

These many stakeholders communicate with one another via a convoluted web of procedures that are heavily reliant upon one another and require extensive use of paper and data. Many of the participants in the medical insurance ecological systems are using automation for combined causes; nonetheless, the method has not so far become completely frictionless.

Figure 10.1 shows the healthcare architecture which contains insurance companies, diagnostics, pharmacies, beneficiaries, hospital providers, value-added service providers, third-party administrators (TPAs), reinsurers, government regulators, etc. Even though technology has been of assistance to India's healthcare assurance ecological system and the coordination between various collaborators to improve the efficiency of complicated operations. As a direct consequence of this, the whole ecosystem moved away from the use of manual methods and toward digital ones to collect and process data such as underwriting data, claiming records, and health records. However, there is a fragmentary exchange of information, which makes the interaction between the many stakeholders difficult. The distributed ledger technology (DLT) (blockchain) has the potential to facilitate the smooth sharing of information and increase trust amongst all parties involved via a participatory approach.

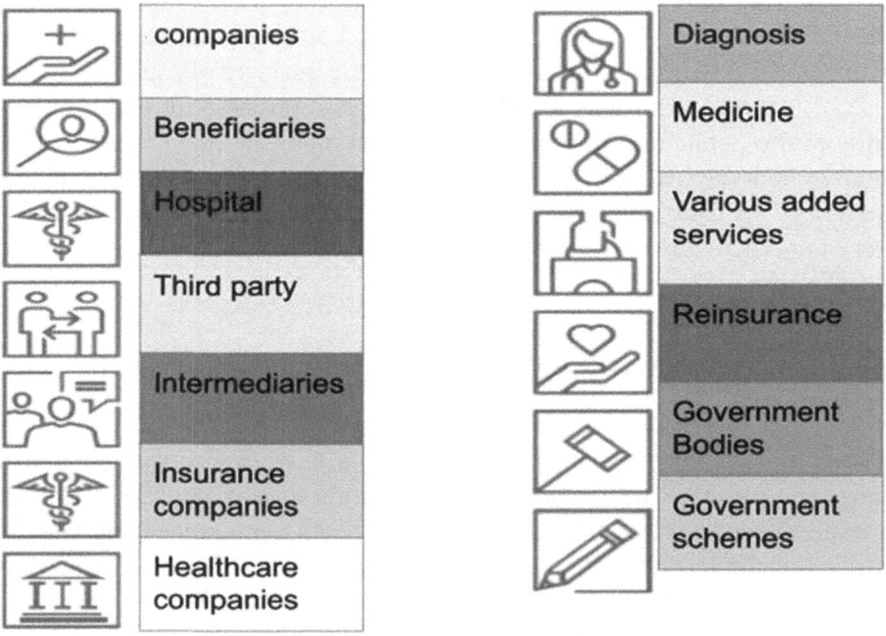

FIGURE 10.1 Complete healthcare architecture.

The requirement for fine-grained access control, transparency, and intrusion proof makes the establishment of a trustworthy network an absolute necessity. Blockchain technology and smart contracts implemented within a decentralized and distributed ledger may revolutionize the way health insurance ecosystems transparently manage records and carry out operations using a participatory method in which relevant stakeholders act as nodes. The capacity of blockchain technology and smart contracts to successfully perform complicated processes in a transparent and participatory manner will be the most important factor determining their level of commercial success. This would rely on the subsequent cost advantages to insurers, which would come about as a consequence of operational efficiency, lower administrative expenses, and the avoidance of excessive claiming reimbursement as well as enhanced customer service.

10.3 MEDICAL INSURANCE AND ITS FUTURE PERSPECTIVES IN THE INDIAN SUBCONTINENT

Medical insurance has become the next highest contributor category to the common assurance market in India as of fiscal year 20 (FY20), behind only the vehicle insurance segment in terms of size. In India's general insurance business, the value of the medical insurance and motor insurance markets combined accounts for more than two-thirds of the total value. It is projected that the health insurance sector's contribution to the most common assurance organization's gross written premium will rise from approximately 10% in the Fiscal Year 2005 to approximately 27% in Fiscal Year 2020. This represents a significant increase from the prior year's figure of approximately 10%. About 40% of the Indian population is covered by various plans like Ayushman Bharat schemes, and Jan Aarogya Yojna which was introduced in September of 2018. In India, the private sector and the government are working together to spread awareness about the benefits of purchasing health insurance, with the ultimate goal of steadily expanding the number of people who are covered by health insurance throughout the country. The connection between the many stakeholders must take place in a way that is both effective and transparent electronically, in a way that is both irreversible and visible, and that it addresses all issues connected to the information's confidentiality.

10.4 WHAT EXACTLY IS A BLOCKCHAIN, AND WHO IS IN CHARGE OF IT?

The blockchain is a solitary, decentralized, unchangeable, barely record of arrangement, which is upgraded when various, independent actors gain agreement on the legitimacy of newcomers by stakeholders. This ledger is immutable because it cannot be altered once it has been written into. Blockchain can be used as a concept and a decentralized distributed digital ledger. All the transactions are logged on a variety of nodes around the network. Users reach an agreement on what constitutes acceptable records of occurrences and then accept such records. Once the information has been input, it is not possible to change it or remove it, which makes the information immutable. Because the health insurance industry contains several stakeholders that regularly communicate data, modify, and validate data, and are reliant on the drift of information and limited for fruitful project management, blockchain is a good fit for this sector.

10.5 CONTROLLER OF BLOCKCHAIN TECHNOLOGY?

10.5.1 PUBLIC BLOCKCHAIN

Fully decentralized, meaning that anybody may join the network, perform transactions, and take part in the validation process of other users' transactions.

10.5.2 PERMISSIONED BLOCKCHAIN

A decentralized system in which some players are granted unique privileges inside the system. There are several restrictions on who may add data to a database.

10.5.3 PRIVATE BLOCKCHAIN

Only a small group of people are eligible to become nodes in the network. Everyone who takes part will be familiar with one another and will have rights according to the roles they play.

10.5.4 BLOCKCHAIN TECHNOLOGY SELECTION

Figure 10.2 shows the blockchain technology (BCT) process. First, the number of data sources has been selected. Data sources either maybe single or multiple. It depends upon the requirements. If there is a single data source, then it may be noted that the centralized data source contains all the information to be used. If there are multiple data sources, then it is further bifurcated based on the access to data. It may be open to all or restricted to some authorized person. If the access is restricted, then all unauthorized persons or clients are blocked automatically. Whereas in the case of open access data centers, first person or clients are verified. If the verification is completed, then access is granted whereas unauthorized parties are further denied for the data center.

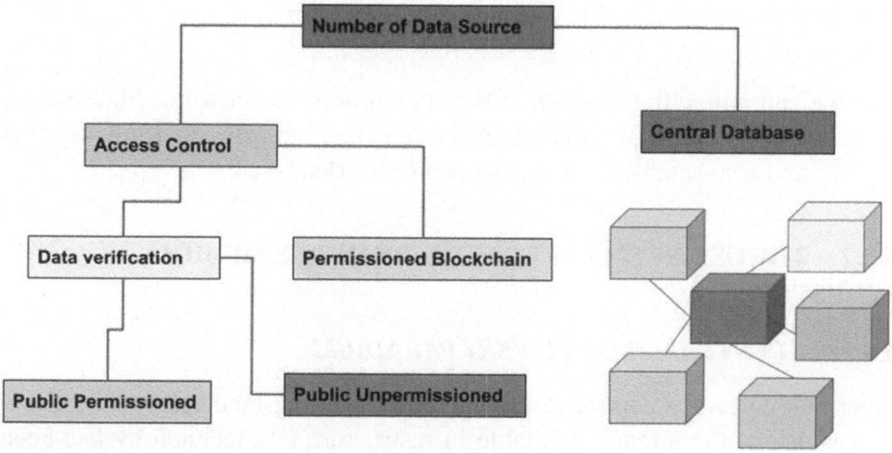

FIGURE 10.2 Blockchain technology selection process.

10.6 ROLE OF SMART CONTRACTS IN THE MEDICAL INDUSTRY

A blockchain is used to maintain the details of a smart contract, which is a contract that is self-enforcing in the form of a code.

Figure 10.3 shows the process of data execution. First, data is encoded within a computer program. It further undergoes automatic execution based on the criteria met by the encoded information. Finally, tamper-proofing is carried out. Some of the benefits that come with using a smart contract are given in Figure 10.4.

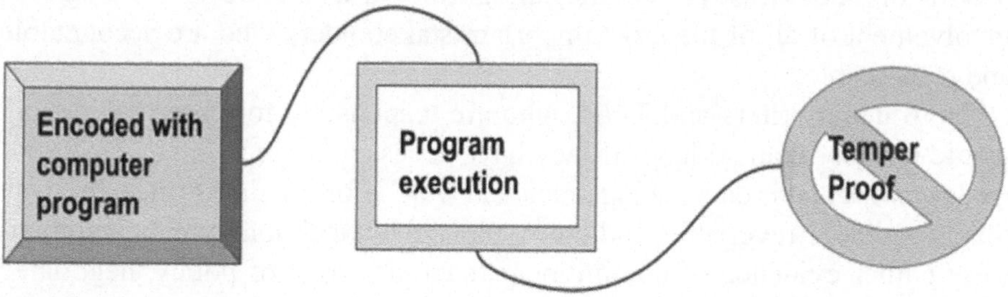

FIGURE 10.3 Data execution process.

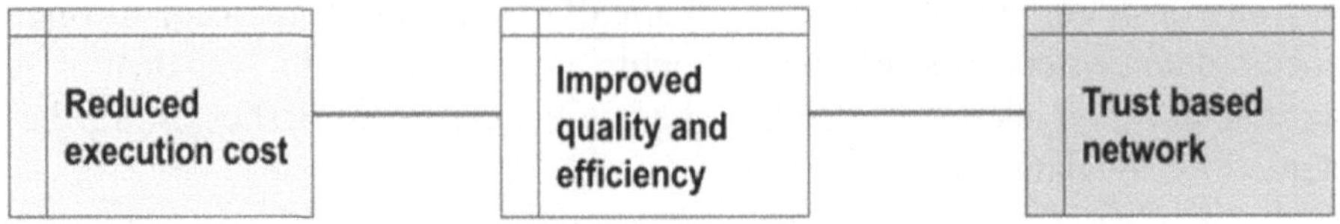

FIGURE 10.4 Smart contract benefits.

One can notice the benefits of smart contracts, as shown in Figure 10.4. Smart contracts help in reducing execution costs, improving efficiency and quality and also establishing trust-based networks.

10.7 THE USE OF SMART CONTRACTS IN THE MEDICAL INDUSTRY

10.7.1 CENTRALIZED DELIVERY PARADIGM

Over many years, a centralized method of providing medical treatment that makes use of the already available infrastructure and technology has been used.

10.7.2 DECENTRALIZED MODEL

Blockchain is now portrayed as one of the most important new technologies due to its distinct business model, which offers a public and reliable method to incorporate management.

10.7.3 BLOCKCHAIN

It has the prospects to revamp some of the most essential processes in the healthcare sector, such as the process of obtaining medical insurance, by making those processes more safe, straightforward, and effective through the involvement of all of the most important stakeholders who are accountable and responsible.

Both underwriters and TPAs, who are responsible for claim validation, would use less manual labor if they have access to an integrated, decentralized network that is data management and well before business rules. In a way that is visible, irreversible, and quasi, blockchain technology may automatically gather evidence of commitments such as terms of policy, negotiated charges, and other pertinent data sets, connect the content and work parallel over smart contracts-based information content. Table 10.1 represent various steps of smart contracts partnership with the industry, while Table 10.2 shows SWOT analysis for the implementation of Blockchain technology.

TABLE 10.1 Smart Contracts Partnership with Industry

Various Steps	Illustration
Identification of the agreements	First, the cooperative opportunities are identified to classify the different outputs with the help of various functions.
Conditional settings	To execute the different contracts, various conditions are executed based on the guiding principles. Smart contracts act as a triggering point to execute the terms and conditions of the contract.
The logic for the business	Blockchain technology has been used to establish business logic.
Encoding and blockchain technology	Blockchain technology plays an important role to execute the encoding.
Effect and operation	The initial contract, verification, and transaction played an important role in blockchain technology.
Networking updation	Once the said contract is executed, then contracts are updated accordingly.

TABLE 10.2 SWOT Analysis for the Implementation of Blockchain Technology

Strength	Weakness	Opportunity	Threats
It is fast and the implementation cost is less.	It is more scalable.	It reduces the complexity.	It is unreliable
Intermediaries are not required for the implementation.	Its performance is very low.	It can address new challenges and opportunities.	Its adoption is very low for new factors.
It is automotive for the new contracts in smart surgeries.	Its energy consumption is very high.	Heterogeneous data is available.	It may be dangerous for the government.
It is accessible globally.	It is autonomous.	It has a competitive advantage.	It's not suitable for all the processes.

10.8 APPLICATION OF BLOCKCHAIN TECHNOLOGY IN THE MEDICAL INDUSTRY

- The use of blockchain technology as an emulsion for the administration of medical data and the interchange of health records has gained wide acceptance worldwide. The implementation of EHRs based on blockchain technology in Estonia is a good example of this.

- The various healthcare systems have electronic medical records (EMRs) solutions that are enabled by blockchain technology in addition to a platform for the interchange of health information. This not only protects the data from external and internal dangers but also makes it possible for organizations in both the public and commercial sectors to communicate and seamlessly share information.
- The electronic health record (EHR) operates much like a centralized, national database. It collects data from several providers, each of whom may be using a unique system, and then provides that data in a standardized manner via the use of an electronic health consumer portal. As the electronic inscription system uses information from the medical care assurance fund, the patient's records on any state medical subsidies to which they are entitled may also be shown.
- Distributed ledger technology (Blockchain) is now being used to guarantee the authenticity of retrieved electronic medical data along with administrative access logs.

10.9 CASE STUDIES

10.9.1 A BIRTH REGISTRATION SYSTEM BASED ON BLOCKCHAIN TECHNOLOGY

Business problem: Every citizen has to have a birth certificate since it contains essential information about their identity. A birth certificate serves as the foundation for various papers that a person may earn throughout his or her lifetime, such as a school diploma, passport, or driver's license, amongst other things. Within the context of a traditional birth registration system, the following issues have been noted as problematic.

1. **Reliability:** If the information on the medical certificate is incorrect, it might have various impacts on the patients.
2. **Authenticity and Certainty:** No system is both unified and resilient that can validate a medical certificate and safeguard information.
3. **Several Sources of Information:** Various collaborators are engaged, and data is provided from a variety of different sources.

4. **Functional Requirement:** The customer expressed interest in developing a birth registration system using blockchain technology but did not want to alter the existing functional flow. In the present setup, two distinct sorts of approvals must be obtained, i.e., approval from the supervisor and administrative officer (AO). Once the AO gives the form final approval, we use application programming interfaces (APIs) that we established to record the information of the birth registration. A transaction hash is returned once the information is stored using blockchain technology and pushed there. This hash will be used in the generation of rapid response (QR) code that will be displayed in the document. Researchers have been working on various mobile-based applications and retrieving information and further used to verify the certificate details.

10.9.6 BUSINESS BENEFITS

The patient would be able to accomplish various information incorporating blockchain technology and other registration technology. Like to on-the-go and safe information storage of digital information; data integrity proof and sanitized source of data; enhancing belief and clarity in the system; efficient protection underlying usage of numerous cryptographic algorithms; mitigation of document validation.

10.9.7 CASUALTY CERTIFICATION BASED ON BLOCKCHAIN TECHNOLOGY

A certificate proving that a death has been registered is important data for every citizen. The issuing of a casualty certification is closely connected to the provision of several benefits by the government for the family of the dead. In a traditional environment for death registration, the following issues have been noted as problematic:

1. **Accuracy:** If the information on the death certificate is not true, it might have significant ramifications for the surviving members of the dead person's family.
2. **Verifiability and Security:** There is no method that is both integrated and reliable for verifying death certificates and keeping death data safe.

3. **Several Sources of Information:** Multiple stakeholders are engaged, and information is provided from a variety of different sources.
4. **Functional Requirement:** The customer expressed interest in developing a blockchain-based system for the recording of deaths without disrupting the existing functional flow. In the present setup, two distinct sorts of approvals must be obtained, i.e., supervisor and AO approval. When the AO gives their approval of the form, we use APIs that we established to get the data of the death registration. A transaction hash is returned once the data is stored in the blockchain and pushed there. The certificate will include a QR code that was generated using this hash after it was printed. We are now working on various smartphone applications which will use scanning code, i.e., QR coding to extract information and be used to validate the same for the casualty certification.
5. **Business Benefits:** The solution provided by blockchain technology adds value by streamlining operations involved with the registration of deaths and all the real-time transactions. It may lead to the emulsion of various benefits, achievements, and goals, verification of the digital documentation, tempered proofing, data resources, accuracy, precision, data integrity and validation of the systems, efficient encryption and decryption underlying use of various cryptographic methods and documents validation.

10.10 A SOLUTION IN PROJECT FINANCE BASED ON BLOCKCHAIN TECHNOLOGY FOR THE ESTABLISHMENT OF A HUMAN CENTER OF EXCELLENCE

10.10.1 BUSINESS PROBLEM

The customer has a strong interest in experimenting with new and safe methods of keeping information on citizens and maintaining their right to personal data privacy. The client's goal for this engagement was to provide a highly regarded social welfare organization with technical help in order to assist the organization in raising money for the establishment of a center of excellence. An application for crowdfunding that is based on blockchain technology has been developed and successfully deployed. This application's goal is to make the contribution process more open and safer. The following specifications were required from the customer:

- The new system needs to be able to facilitate safe financial transactions for project finance and protect the confidentiality of its data.
- Once the transactions have been documented for financing, there should be no room for alterations made by a third party in any way.
- The donors who are helping to facilitate the project should have the ability to examine all of their transactions and should feel safe making payments via the portal that is being used to support such initiatives.
- An ideal system works all the functions independently.

10.10.2 OPERATIONAL NEEDS

In order to achieve clarity, confidence, and stability throughout the process, we needed to develop a contribution management system that was based on blockchain technology and implemented on the Ethereum blockchain platform.

The following is an itemized list of the client's functional requirements:

- The generation of a pseudonym for each contributor, to authenticate the payment made by each contributor following the submission of the registration form in the portal that has been developed.
- After successful payment has been completed using the gateway, every transaction will be recorded on the blockchain. Therefore, this transaction, together with its timestamp, is permanently saved and may be tracked to conduct an audit.
- Providing all entities in the system with a single, unified perspective of the transaction will increase the system's credibility and trustworthiness.
- Providing users with the ability to examine all of their functionalities.

10.10.3 BUSINESS BENEFITS

The following are some of the advantages that have been realized as a result of the created application:

- Enhanced security of transactions as a result of blockchain's immutable ledger.
- Audit trails that are based on cryptographic timestamps rather than traditional ones.
- There is no central authority that can change the data, which increases confidence in the system as a whole.
- There are distributed nodes that have similar information.

10.10.4 MEDICAL ASSURANCE MANAGEMENT USING SMART CONTRACTS

Through the use of a centralized ledger that is distributed over the network, blockchain-based smart contracts will be self-operative and make contract obedience visible across the whole perpetuity. Therefore, it would enable speedier reliable payments by eliminating disputes that normally emerge from ambiguity in the terms and circumstances that are connected to payments in ordinary contracts. Smart contracts will be able to recognize the submission of recurrent false allegations, fake customer credentials, or fake health data, which will result in a reduction in the number of illegal insurance claims. This will be made possible by the accessibility of citizen health information.

Figure 10.5 shows how smart contracts help in maintaining beneficiary records using blockchain technology. It includes transparency, self-execution of smart contracts, records of insurance companies, prevention of ambiguities, contract compliances, EHRs of patients and faster payments, etc.

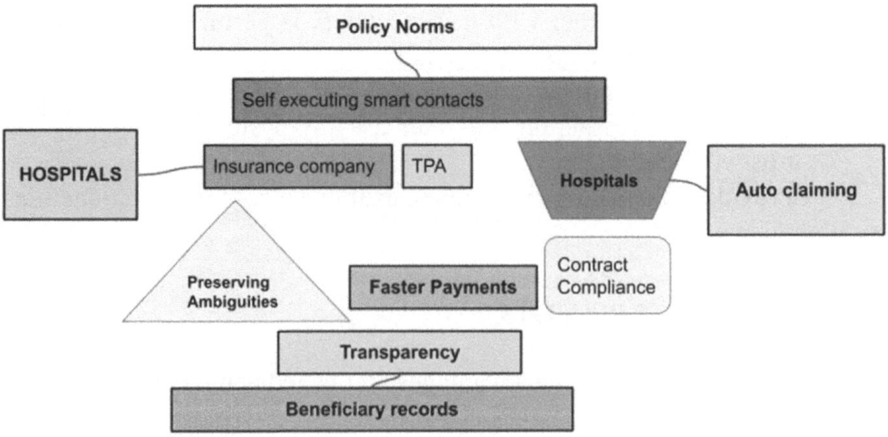

FIGURE 10.5 Beneficiary record.

10.11 THE USE OF ELECTRONIC CONTRACTS IN UNDERWRITING

10.11.1 BENEFICIARY

fills out the proposal form and sends it to the insurance company, together with any necessary documentation on information relating to the patient's medical history.

10.11.2 INSURANCE COMPANY

The proposal is approved by an underwriter or a technological solution. Necessary terms and conditions are prepared.

10.11.3 BENEFICIARY

Makes required deposit. Follow all policy paperwork and associated metadata, along with a list of hospitals participating in the network:

- The use of smart contracts will make it possible to electronically store recommendation forms, medical histories, proclamations, and one-of-a-kind strategy terms of service, such as limits and sub-limits. This applies to every sort of policy, each of which has its distinctive necessity.
- The regulation conditions and the review of participants could be used for the auto-execution of assertions.
- Smart contracts obtain data in an inalienable manner, make it available to key parties, and attempt to prevent any disputes that may arise as a result of the concealment of information or the provision of false information in a manner that is both more accurate and convenient.

10.12 PROCESSING OF INSURANCE CLAIMS VIA ELECTRONIC CONTRACTS

1. **Beneficiary:** After being discharged, the patient begins the process of filing a claim by providing pertinent documents such as the application form, hospital expenses, and tests.
2. **Insurance Company:** A doctor first authorized the claim for further processing, i.e., recommendation and processing. Concerned

authority verified the said claim. Then the transferred amount to the concerned department may raise questions.

3. **Beneficiary:** Then the beneficiary can take the receipt of the claim amount, information, and request for reconsideration and reconciliation as well. Through the seamless implementation of information sharing, smart contracts on blockchain guarantee that all parties have accessibility to a certain set of clinical records. Additionally, each hospital is specific and agreed-upon package costs can be stored in smart contracts, which can be accessed by the necessary parties and automatically carry out predetermined actions.

10.13 REASON FOR SMART CONTRACTS TO BE SUCCESSFUL

Data should be stored in the first place because data kept on a blockchain is not always reliable. In BCT, information is recorded in a centralized database, and the adage "garbage in, garbage out" applies. When data is first being kept in a blockchain system, quality of data, standard protocols, procedures, and stability are essential and must be continuously enhanced. If not, the blockchain can become ineffective and finally disappear. Because the amount of claiming transactions would be vast and enormous, the criteria to build and maintain the blockchain and its infrastructure. As the volume of data increases, the impact on data processing speed will be increased and it is subjected to the frequency of data access. It is estimated that the speed to process data and transactions should be efficient and have powerful computing.

One can see from Figure 10.6 the flow of data. Data is monitored continuously to check the quality and transaction processing speed is evaluated. All the medical results should be processed and kept in electronic form so that any medical center can access them whenever required to examine the patient history. It maintains digital records for a number of healthcare institutions. Corporation data systems, as well as many other communications technology and services, are used to share records. Patients increasingly anticipate fast access to medical records. Moreover, the medical sector needs frequent and faster data access, and it may lead to the various security and privacy loopholes that need to be tackled. Consequently, blockchain technology can help to solve various problems. Blockchain technology has potential and performs better than other traditional centralized database systems, which have serious lags in transparency. This is a distributed technique which was recently introduced to give a different perspective on information network and management performance. This study describes a blockchain technology framework for managing and securing medical information into a data record maintained by the service providers. This framework and technique were created with Ganache and the Ethereum network, as also scripting languages, techniques, and methods like Solidity and web3.js. This platform is used in the ongoing measurement framework technology in this chapter to store patient information and perform various operations in a distributed system based on the blockchain technology smart contracts framework. Once deployed, operations are conducted via the smart contract, which provides data protection characteristics. Moreover, the desired changes to the transaction can be confirmed and communicated to the complete distributed system. There is various blockchain technology framework wallets that contain a centralized, highly confidential system where records may be instantly retrieved and protected by service authorities. Health service providers and users can use the wallet to gain access to the system. Furthermore, all of the doctor and patient data will be secured and handled by this system. This proposed system is intended to accomplish the following tasks: Users may receive the same information at the same time thanks to DLT, which increases efficiency, builds confidence, and lowers obstacles. It allows for secured data storage by restricting access permissions. Furthermore, the proposed method allows for the secure transfer of patient health records. Lastly, this study describes a rapid and secure healthcare system and a new protocol. It improves the medical sector by allowing more transparency and management of critical data to be collected and protected.

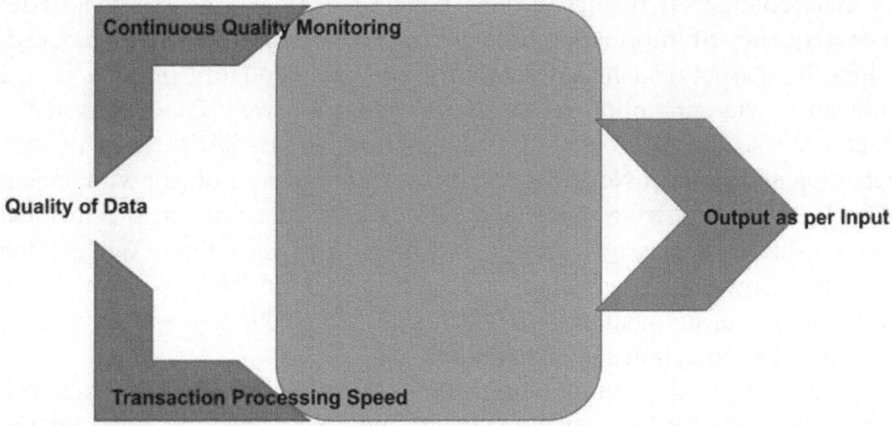

FIGURE 10.6 Data processing.

A blockchain is a distributed network that tracks all operations using peer-to-peer (P2P) technology. It is distributed and lacks a point of contact. Instead, it is a set of nodes that keep things running. Because of the network's components, each operation is incredibly secure. Encryption adds another layer of protection to the interaction. Every component in the network duplicates the digital trail. Before adding a transaction back, each node must verify its legitimacy. A digital ledger is made up of several blocks. Each block contains a thorough record of every transaction. Blockchain has sparked interest in a variety of industries, including academia, industry, and medical. As it is a distributed technology, it benefits the medical sector in a number of ways. ETH, Ethereum's native coin, powers the Ethereum blockchain. Ethereum is a distributed blockchain framework that establishes systems for the secure execution and verification of smart contract coding. It enables distributors and software developers to create new types of ETH blockchain-based tokens that may be utilized to power distribution applications based on smart contracts. Users can do business without depending on trustworthy central authority. A smart contract, as opposed to blockchain technology, is a computer device that acts immediately when certain conditions are satisfied. It adds reasoning to the blockchain from a technology standpoint. Smart contracts are identity transactions which include the terms and conditions of a P2P relationship. It is a compilation of programs and data identified on the Ethereum blockchain at a specified location. In our proposed solution, smart contracts are utilized to transfer records, provide access to health trained and adequately seeing client records, or block access to medical care staff. There are numerous challenges in the healthcare sector, such as keeping track of the massive amounts of data generated by hospitals. With the introduction of smart contracts in medical groups, patient records will be extremely safe. The frequency of information leakage triggered by hackers will be reduced. Blockchain aspects such as decentralization, confidentiality, protection, and robustness via encryption protocols can address current challenges in the healthcare sector. The electronic health sector is crucial in terms of data retention and storage. Nevertheless, it has a significant problem with patient data leaking. Numerous hospital facilities are vulnerable in the medical system due to data access delays and the risk of data theft. Without the patient's knowledge, medical reports can be preserved. There seems to be no investigation or innovation in the healthcare sector due to many difficulties such as data protection and availability.

The suggested solution prioritizes secured information exchange within the network in today's healthcare industry. If applied correctly, the blockchain-based system produces outstanding results in a variety of ways. It is a quick and easy way to protect reliable data. With the smart contract, the information is kept as a ledger characteristic in blockchain technology, managing the patient's access to health information. It ensures the system's safety, easy accessibility, and other key features of management, including its confidentiality, authenticity, and verification. Shortly, the emphasis will be on developing a helpful resource based on blockchain technology that will safeguard all evidence received by physicians and patients. Nonetheless, multiple research studies on the blockchain system in hospitals have been published [1–4].

Technology has progressed over time; technology has made our lives simpler. It has had an impact on the medical sector, boosting the human average lifespan. There are indeed gaps that need to be filled. The medical system lacks openness, which leads to fundamental trust issues between patients and healthcare professionals. A patient today is not sure if he or she will receive appropriate treatment from the clinic for the surcharge. Any insurance provider can repay a patient for hospital expenses. However, the Insurance Provider cannot currently confirm the legitimacy of these bills or medical records. A patient may offer false information in order to obtain economic rewards from an insurance provider. Once again, trust difficulties exist between the patient (i.e., the insurance claimant) and the insurance company. Blockchain combined with smart contracts is a well-known disruptive technology. Technology fosters trust by making the system transparent. In this work, we suggest a BCT Safe and Intelligent Payment System. System of Health. No one can ensure the integrity of all the parties involved in the process, whether they be patients, hospitals, or insurance companies. Trusting one another, the safety and confidentiality of a patient's medical data are also protected. The dissemination of aggregated data to the scientific community for their own purposes. Data that is shared must not be individually identifiable. The obtained data can be linked to the identification of any client or their health information. Blockchain technology (hereinafter referred to as blockchain) has received increased media attention as the technology underlying Bitcoin, a digital payment network that has revolutionized numerous industries, particularly finance. The buzz surrounding the technology has grown in direct proportion to the number of news articles generated by Bitcoin and its accompanying alt-coin ecosystem. Each news story, from the closing of Silk Route to the resistance of Ethereum from the distributed autonomous firm, raises consciousness of different coins and their impact on the technology underpinning Bitcoin can have on numerous industries. Many blockchain firms and fans have targeted healthcare, yet various possibilities provided to the public appear to be specific solutions to the defined problem [5–9].

Due to technological advancement and explosive development in internet communication, medical insurance smart contracts and EHRs for patients are widely used in the medical field. Medical data, i.e., evidence-based medicine (EBM), can be shared securely. To assist patients with optimum clinic care, EBM reviews the research findings and patient knowledge. A clinical decision support system (CDSS) is an artificial intelligence (AI) medical data system which is used to implement EBM. Once the system acquires enough knowledge about a patient, it can medically diagnose with better accuracy. EHR plays an important role in both fields, i.e., CDSS and EBM. Information exchange over the open communication network is considered insecure if the information is in unencrypted form. Various countries have passed rules to secure medical information. Health examination, medical image and medical records, etc., contained in EHR. HIPAA applies to any medical data linked to automation, including healthcare organizations and clearinghouses. HIPAA's data protection standards, which define how to prevent the unlawful breach and untrusted exposure of EHR, are the two primary themes. First, the law states that a person has a right to regulate and understand how his or her medical information is used. In other terms, without the patient's agreement, no EHR information may be shared publicly. Moreover, privacy legislation establishes the de-identification basis. No one, including a medical researcher, has the potential to deduce the real status of a patient from EHR. Second, the protection act includes three measures: regulatory, legal, and technical protections that are used to ensure the secrecy, authenticity, and accessibility of EHR during the retention, accessibility, and transmission procedures. The use of EHR has undoubtedly brought practical answers for physical patient records, such as protection and sloppy calligraphy. It has also improved the clinical data exchange framework in order to enhance the quality of cross-hospital assessment and the efficacy of related research. Because a patient does not have to evaluate the identical medical examination in the case of cross-hospital evaluation with EHR, he or she can save time and keep an accurate diagnosis. Terms of the doctor, he or she is likely to provide an accurate diagnosis by learning the patient's past treatment. The researcher can use the extensive EHRs to investigate a specific ailment for medical research activity. As a result, the patient can receive quality treatment. Nonetheless, with conventional methods, there is still a conflict between healthcare information accuracy and security of health information [10–15]. Multiple password protection of internet information sharing systems was examined. Arbitrary access management, on the other hand, permits users to enhance their privileges over anyone. This could raise the chances of a hacker planting a Trojan. As a result, safe authentication is difficult to execute. Following that, Liu et al. suggested a multi-owner information sharing game that can handle data as per multiple owner authority [11]. The actual data owners and the individual who can analyze information, the so-called user, are two categories of owners. However, once a malevolent cloud server initiates a conspiracy attempt with a suspended user, the actual data will be exposed. As a result, it is unable to maintain the crucial element of secrecy. Later attempted to use a quadratic regression method to send medical information to users in encrypted form. During the exchanging operation, though, the transferred data may be tampered with [12]. To put it another way, an authorized user cannot disclose the right information to fulfill the integrity verification. Following that, Zhu & Jiang [13] proposed an anti-collusion attempt data exchange technique based on the Dolev-Yao model and an asymmetrical encryption algorithm, in which a denied user is unable to retain any information in order to obtain secrecy. Furthermore, Ganesh et al. discovered that the Zhu and Jiang technique is vulnerable to man-in-the-middle and information modification vulnerabilities because the host does not validate the user's enrollment information. Apart from studies, health information leaking is a concern of Healthcare Technology News. Identity, identification number (SSN), postcode, and registration plate are among the information leaked. It's because Universal Healthcare, a non-profit company, failed to configure the central server correctly. The malicious attacker has access to the data of a legitimate user. The attribute of secrecy, in other words, cannot be proven. Because the individual may experience a large financial and personal loss, the desire to share EHR may be lowered. As a result, maintaining the safety and confidentiality of EHR on an information exchange network is a critical and pressing assignment. To summarize, current EHR data exchange methods have concerns with identity, security, secrecy, reliability, and authenticity. As a result, we will present the concepts of blockchain technology to construct a medical blockchain-based EHRs secure channel. Consumers, clinics, and research centers are among their peers. After a patient uploads his or her de-identified EHR to the healthcare blockchain, the university health institute can view it. The implementation of blockchain can ensure the authenticity of health data [16, 17], whereas smart contract governance can maintain the authenticity of a particular patient [18]. In addition, the recommended medical blockchain is HIPAA-compliant. In healthcare blockchain, the EHR must obtain the client's permission. The secrecy of blockchain, in particular, inherits the patient's confidentiality. As per the simulated data, covering examination of potential attacks and intellectual rights, there is no loss of healthcare information, and the dilemma could be identified and resolved without modifying present healthcare equipment. Following that, we'll go over the basic characteristics of a secure data exchange system, which will be tested in a healthcare situation [19, 20]:

1. **Anonymity:** This attribute enables patients to share health data on the blockchain using a pseudonym.
2. **Confidentiality:** This is needed to ensure that data may only be accessed by authorized users.
3. **Availability:** The availability is used to test the system's functionality.
4. **HIPAA Privacy:** It is for validating HIPAA's privacy regulations.
5. **Immutability:** This issue ensures that the data content cannot be tampered with.
6. **Unforgeability:** This feature ensures that a set of data and verification cannot be faked.
7. **Integrity:** This attribute denotes that the information stored cannot be tampered. Furthermore, the cybercriminal will be unable to alter the actual data sent.

10.14 ACCOUNTABILITY OF HEALTH INSURANCE

HIPAA standards govern the integration of medical information and must be followed by all healthcare centers, information exchange hubs, and employees. In the healthcare blockchain ecosystem, data protection standards have become a source of worry since they are due to the individual healthcare system. In addition, the National Institute of Standards and Technology (NIST) has developed a security architecture for upgrading key services [21, 22], which serves as a universal language for organization communication. The Office for Civil Rights (OCR) then released a crossover report that identifies the linkages between both the information security (IS) program and the Security standards rule. It's worth noting that HIPAA-regulated organizations in the healthcare sector are required to follow the security standards rule [23–25].

10.14.1 PRIVACY RULE

The responsibility of a patient to determine how to reveal and then use health records has been declared by this rule. More specifically, the patient must be able to identify and comprehend how private medical data is used. The confidentiality rule has been broken if an organization has published a patient's information without permission. The norm of de-identification, in this instance, has been included in the regulation. No one will be able to relate this information from the original user, even if a person has agreed to accept appropriate EHRs for specified utilization.

10.14.2 SECURITY RULES

To ensure that EHRs are quite well, the security legislation has specified how to maintain, retrieve, and transmit them. Administrative safeguards, physical safeguards, and technical safeguards are among the three measures used to preserve the confidentiality, authenticity, and accessibility of EHRs. Administrative safeguards: This section comprises the government ideology, deploying method, and medical team course of study. To reduce the danger of human error, all participants must adhere to the established method.

10.14.3 PHYSICAL SAFEGUARDS

This refers to the upkeep of technology and the security of the technology. Physical harm and illegal access to EHR can thus be avoided.

10.14.4 TECHNICAL SAFEGUARDS

This applies to all forms of patient records mechanism architecture. The system must be capable of maintaining EHR privacy, authenticity, and accessibility.

In the modern health industry, which is a decentralized method of information preservation, the blockchain has played a major role in confirming patient confidentiality and the data integrity of EHR. Smart grid, dual bidding, and agricultural distribution network are just a few of the industries where blockchain is being used. A node is a term given to each contributor in a blockchain platform. The hash function of transaction information will be published to the network once a trade between servers has begun. We implemented the collaborative blockchain to the new method, which consists of a client, a hospital, and a clinical research organization, in order to maximize efficiency and IS. A patient uploads his or her EHR to the blockchain, which hospitals and other healthcare institutions can use and must provide the computing power to maintain the chain running. An elliptic curve digital signature mechanism is used to create accounts in the blockchain platform. It includes a pair of public and private keys and is used as network identification in activities. The private key is used by a network to encode the transaction information for verification, while the public key is used by others to validate the transaction.

10.14.5 DECENTRALIZED

The transaction information has been validated and saved in blocks; therefore, it is decentralized. Because all nodes have responsibility for preserving block information, an intermediary or centralized node to handle transactions is superfluous.

10.14.6 IMMUTABILITY

Each block holds the hash code of the information of the preceding block. If an individual is trying to manipulate the information, it must be caught quickly since other networks will acquire the delocalized hash values of the following activities.

10.14.7 UNFORGEABILITY

An adversary can't just make up a couple of messages and an associated signature, even without an authorized encryption key.

10.14.8 ANONYMITY

A secret key pair was used to verify a node so that genuine information could not be traced.

10.14.9 TRANSPARENCY

The blocked information has been shared by all nodes, making the data accessible to associated parties.

10.15 SMART CONTACT

The new approach uses a smart contract to consolidate medical data from a single patient. This will allow researchers to keep an eye on the patient at all times. Szabo suggested the concept for the first time in 1997. Szabo urged users to define transfer content in a programming language, which is then executed by a machine. When a smart contract is combined with blockchain, the code described in the contract cannot be improperly altered in order to ensure transactional integrity. The present smart contract's information is developed in the Solidity programming language. The blockchain is used to store the verified material. An externally owned account (EOA) is used as the network identification by a client. The address and specified regulations, like value and jurisdiction, are used to initiate a contract. Contract implementation can be divided into two categories. The first one is a trigger event, such as a transfer of property or information deposition, and the other is to invoke another contract in order to achieve a certain aim. A smart contract can be used in more sophisticated model circumstances, like patent grants, crowdsourcing, and lottery game, without losing its applicability. For example, in the case of a vending machine, a program has been built to calculate the final commodity [24].

The findings will then be released to the general public. People agreeing on the pricing can deposit money in the machine and hit the button. Whenever the contract's terms are met, the system will immediately produce the appropriate beverage; otherwise, it will refund the user's money. This has demonstrated that a payment may be processed efficiently and effectively using a smart contract. Registration and diagnosis are the two most important phases for smart contract medical insurance in a safe and secure environment. A patient (Alice) must first enroll in a smart card with the Healthcare Authority, which is the Ministry of Health and Welfare's health information management department. The smart card enrollment and dissemination are handled by HCA. Each smart card contains a patient's associated patient data. After that, the medical officer can recognize the patient in a hospital using his or her smart card. There are three stages in the diagnosis phase cons:ultation, follow-up consultation, and emergency. A patient's initial consultation refers to his or her first visit to the hospital. The patient can use her smart card to enter the hospital after a successful registration. Username and password, assessment, permission, and validation are the four processes in the first appointment [3, 7].

10.15.1 FOLLOW-UP CONSULTATION

In this service, a patient needs to visit the hospital again to consult the doctor as per requirements.

10.15.2 AUTHENTICATION STEPS

If a patient wants to share her present appointment with research centers, she must keep EHR in her liability account on the hospital computer. The smart card must be inserted into the gadget, and the key must be entered.

10.15.3 EMERGENCY

When a patient is in an emergency circumstance, such as a vegetative state, he or she requires immediate care without the ability to log on. As a result, the health professional can examine the patient's past EHR. It's worth noting that only the authorized emergency health professional gets access to the information. Use of blockchain technologies to improve healthcare processes. Various strategies have been employed in enhancing the efficiency of systems that affect healthcare in order to build a system that improves healthcare processes to meet the difficulties highlighted. In a nutshell, parallelograms represent performance objectives with a value proposition at their foundation. Lower-level functional objectives improve the other, resulting in a tree. Quality goals, which are equivalent to quasi-requirement specifications, are allocated to the performance objectives. It's worth noting that quality objectives are passed down the refining pyramid of functional objectives. Stick men are either real or artificial software agents with the same performance objectives allocated to them and passed along the refined pyramid of the latter.

The key functional objective and value proposition are used to minimize healthcare costs by improving the efficiency of the scheduling and consulting procedures. We need to limit the frequency of visits to the medical practitioner in enhancing the consultation procedure. This is accomplished by giving patients with health concerns for common health conditions, allowing them to avoid visiting the doctor in such circumstances. We use a WebCrawler agent to discover common health risks. We must also ensure that the treatment information offered to patients comes from a reliable source. To create trust, researchers use BCT smart contracts to ensure that only data from reliable sources are being used for medication. The objective of the booking section is to ensure that all clinical document management systems are compatible. No time is wasted in the booking procedure, and only a few hospitals are overburdened with booking requests. Our suggested system leverages a blockchain platform to record booking details from healthcare professionals in order to accomplish scalability [20].

10.15.4 RECOGNITION OF HEALTHCARE PROBLEMS

The first step in the proposed framework is to enhance the patient diagnosis and consultation process to determine the most pressing health concerns that a blockchain technology-based smart contract framework needs to tackle. The technology analyzes health data gathered by computerized web crawlers to determine top health conditions that cause physician advice. The data is then further filtered to produce a list of the most prevalent health problems, along with medical therapies and data about the body part where the medical issue is a concern. A web crawler is a sophisticated tool that travels over website pages, indexes, stores website content, and modifies the domain's pages. It is the important function of any search query on the Web. The process of designing the automatic crawler via the user interface kicks off the process of identifying the top health problems. The crawler's second objective is to seek internet sites for common health problems that require medical assistance, evaluate the gathered data to identify the top common ailments, removing the top common ailments that do not require standard care in order to focus on the top common health problems that do and to save their geolocation data. The crawlers go through the websites of reputable health-care providers, as well as institutions that offer health analysis and reports. Website content with documents and reports gives trustworthy health statistics as well as data on measurement techniques and difficulties. World Wide Web (WWW) documents containing critically reviewed healthcare articles may include data about the most frequent health problems that necessitate medical attention [19].

10.15.5 CONSULTATION AND BOOKING BASED ON SMART CONTRACTS

In the next stage, we integrate the applications and other frameworks. It also discusses operations to address difficulties like quality and processing speed. In a booking process, modern treatment knowledge made available through smart contracts is leveraged to enhance patient temperaments. The patient's data is first evaluated using known right to information, and then a clinical outcome is taken. If a patient needs to see a doctor, explore available slots for doctors with relevant specialization. He can book an appointment if time frames are appropriate and accessible for the patient [17].

If the client does not want to use smart-contract applications, he could use the process for the bookings. As a result, the patient will be referred to the most appropriate person with the least amount of time to wait. The patient's problems, concerns, and health information are described in the consultation with the integrated app. A smart contract application maps the client's input data to accessible medical expertise, and the patient can be requested for extra information if necessary. If the system determines that the contemporary patient's case is frequent, the mapping findings are examined, and if a clinical decision is accessible, the patient is given advice. If no medical decision is provided and the patient's situation is unusual, the review process with a doctor persists [15].

10.15.6 THE MEDICAL KNOWLEDGE UPDATING PROCESS

The final phase in our method is to update the smart contract with new information as it becomes available. If a novel state of research from an authentic source becomes accessible to this area, the data is connected based on data collection, since we have defined previously the top reasons why people desire to visit the doctor. Even though information uploaded into a blockchain is irreversible, our system follows the best possible practice sessions based on the smart contracts systems for management as well as life-spanning and upgrades the available data from clients through the smart technology contract framework.

10.15.7 BLOCKCHAIN TECHNOLOGY MAPPING AND ITS PERFORMANCE

Researchers link blockchain technologies that provide the specified solutions to various core components identified in the previous steps. For the registration process, we leverage blockchain technology, and clinical records are used in the consultation. Smart contracts are often used to make a registration process more interoperable and to give patients access to time frames from several healthcare professionals on one platform. Moreover, smart contracts aid choice during the registration process, reducing health professionals' workload. Smart-contract technologies enable a user with appropriate medical expertise during the review process whenever a doctor is not present [8].

10.16 BENEFITS OF SMART CONTRACTS

10.16.1 STABILITY AND CERTAINTY

Each client to a smart contract recognizes its responsibilities, the method of execution, and the repercussions of compliance or quasi, and translates this information into a code. Post-performance, the data and smart contract cannot be updated. The execution of contracts is automated by the programming. All the settlements are performed irrevocably. Subsequently, the performance of code execution eliminates any doubt that might develop as a result of confusion or disagreement in the contract's provisions written in standard language. It further gives the minimum opportunity for instinctive choice and concerns arising from full or partial quasi-with contractual duties and adherence [23].

10.16.2 REDUCE DELAY

Smart contracts are used to control, verify, and execute the available contracts. It helps in decreasing the completion time and the requirement of contract responsibility. It eliminates the document verification and presentation required for the organization. Once a project is executed in multiple steps, an electronic record is further used to validate the execution of the product and processes.

10.16.3 SAVINGS

Smart contracts help in minimizing the middle person, and automation results in reducing the cost as the involvement of human beings are minimal.

10.16.4 BACKUP

Blockchain technology uses a digital ledger, which means that all data are cloned in many instances, enabling the recovery of data.

10.16.5 SAFETY

Encryption and cryptography can be used to secure information associated with smart contracts.

10.16.6 ACCURACY

All the operations are streamlined and standardized in smart contracts. Inaccuracies can be minimized if manual labor is reduced.

10.17 RESTRICTIONS AND CHALLENGES IN SMART CONTRACTS

10.17.1 TECHNOLOGICAL CHALLENGES

To handle all blockchain activities, a lot of processing power is required. When adopting smart contracts, an organization may run across system limits when it comes to securing the necessary computational capacity. In order for the system to be extended up to form a domestic or foreign system of medical blockchains, information being held by organizations must be standardized and confined to restricted parameters like statistics, age, and ethnicity of patients. Costs of converting to blockchain technology and running it. To transition to a blockchain-based network, a company must either fully revamp its current system or connect its present framework with DLT. The organization may experience transition phase issues since the systems chosen by the organization may not have been capable of handling all services required by the organization, and the organization's reliance on legacy applications for such activities may remain.

10.17.2 LEGAL CHALLENGES

Validity of contract: An offering, transmission of its approval, determination, and legal object for the engagement all constitute a contract underneath the Indian Contract Act, 1872. The Act does not specify a specific form of arrangement. This is not even required that the agreement be documented in writing. Indian courts have ruled that indeed oral commitments are binding contracts. Offering, reception, and compensation are all included in smart contracts, but they are all done electronically. Digital signatures are legally accepted under Sections 5 and 10 of the Indian Information Technology Act, 2000, which determine a contract to be lawful and binding by electronic methods. Contracts digitally signed are acceptable in court, according to Section 65B of the Indian Evidence Act, 1872. As a result, smart contracts can be deemed to be covered by the Indian Contract Act of 1872.

10.17.3 EVIDENTIARY CHALLENGES AND LEGAL REMEDIES

Although smart contracts could be lawful in India, there is no legal framework in place to govern them, and the participants may not have adequate protection in the event of a breach of warranty. While represented as follows the regulation of smart contracts, providing testimony given the mentioned terms and conditions of the agreement, trying to establish the legal implications and plausibility of the contract, and trying to establish the scope or accusation defect in the achievement of the signed contract, parties may face a unique set of challenges.

10.17.4 REGULATORY REGIME RELATING TO CRYPTO-CURRENCIES

On April 5, 2018, the Reserve Bank of India (RBI) released a "Declaration on Developmental and Regulatory Policies" and a circular on April 6, 2018, banning stakeholders from having dealt with blockchain-based or digital currencies, as well as supplying "assistance for enabling any person or organization in interacting with or trying to settle cryptocurrency transactions." The Supreme Court was asked to review the press releases. The Supreme Court, in a ruling dated March 4, 2018, struck down the circular on the grounds of proportion, but just not the Declaration. Following these advancements, there is a lot of confusion about how to regulate the usage of digital currencies, which are an important aspect of smart contracts.

10.17.5 LOCALIZATION

Smart contracts based on blockchain technology store information across a distributed network that isn't limited to a particular geographic region. As a result, smart contracts may be unable to satisfy the state's globalization criteria, which are enforced via laws, regulations, announcements, bulletins, and agreements.

10.17.6 AMENDMENT OF CONTRACTS

Because smart contracts are programs that operate based on specified circumstances and data integrity is a crucial aspect of these contracts, amending them is impossible, even though the parties involved in the contract believe it is required.

10.17.7 JURISDICTION, GOVERNING LAW AND VENUE

Blockchain technology is used to run smart contracts. The agreement is carried out on a decentralized global network that spans multiple jurisdictions. This could make defining the controlling legislation, the venue for conflict resolution, and the jurisdiction of a court with competence over smart contract problems challenging. According to the Ministry of Electronics and Information Technology's Strategic Framework on Cryptocurrency, a strong policy and institutional framework for developing a National Blockchain network as a Public Resource and providing Blockchain as a Service should be developed. It also emphasizes the importance of concentrating on facilities, research, development of India's technology platform, testing and certification, and training programs in order to promote the usage of Blockchain technology.

Parties wanting to use smart contracts might consider it desirable to engage in an agreement to establish their respective ownership terms, duties, perspectives, and purposes till the policy and institutional framework are reinforced and ideally adapted to cope with smart contracts. The code-enabled smart contract might be considered an additional arrangement or a mode of project implementation. If the smart contract fails to repair a condition, the parties are allowed to claim legal avenues depending on the agreement.

10.18 APPLICATION OF SMART CONTRACTS IN THE HEALTH SECTOR

While smart contracts can assist any industry, they are especially beneficial to the healthcare sector. In healthcare, various blockchain transactions look like this.

When a patient engages with a healthcare organization, a new track of his data is created, including his name, identity, and location. The client would be given a secret key, and the data would be kept on a ledger. A customer would be served by the healthcare organization. The client's public ID would contain information on the procedure, the doctor's note, the drug provided by the pharmacy, and so on. The patient-healthcare-organization transaction has been completed and is uniquely determined. Each operation is encoded and assigned a unique identification on the ledger, which includes the participant's public (quasi) ID. Health organizations and institutes can utilize APIs to obtain the data, and the ciphertext can be examined for clinical research using the person's accessible (non-identifiable) ID on the blockchain. New health organizations can utilize the patient's private key to decode his data if he shares it with others. The patient's identity relates to smart contracts data through the private key, and without it, the data is unidentifiable.

10.18.1 MEDICAL INSURANCE

Smart Contracts can allow a patient to purchase healthcare coverage, with the patient's health data being recorded on the ledger. The data might be easily shared only with institutions in which the patient decides to seek medical treatment, depending on the authorization supplied. In the same way, critical information of patient and doctor's prescription is stored based on blockchain technology and also used to communicate with the assurance provider based on clinical and pharmaceutical Medicare. Hospital care and pharmaceutical reimbursement bills for the assurance provider will further process and reduce all the dependencies [1, 2].

10.18.2 TELEMEDICINE AND TELEHEALTH SOLUTIONS

Based on technological progress, doctors can effectively process medical information and use wearable devices to process healthcare information.

10.18.3 TRANSFER OF PATIENTS

People requiring transition to other healthcare provisions as well as future guidelines would be able to exchange hospitals and health service providers without having to exchange their medical files or use several medical documents papers since information is stored on a decentralized blockchain system in smart contracts [3, 4].

10.18.4 MEDICAL RESEARCH

Hospitals, clinics, and drug manufacturers can quickly exchange patient data, allowing medical research organizations to do various studies and tracking of patient information developments.

It may be extremely valuable to deal with medical problems like epidemics and pandemics, as well as monitor and implement effective immunization programs [5, 6].

10.18.5 CONTROL COUNTERFEIT DRUG

Because smart contract exchanges are unchanging and irrevocable, the pharmaceutical industry and drug regulatory agencies can use the techniques to find each drug, verify its truthfulness, and track its path from producer to customer, continuously monitoring and inhibiting its use of falsified medicines.

10.18.6 EFFECTIVE SUPPLY CHAIN MANAGEMENT (SCM)

Among all the medicines, there were 28% legal drugs. Variations in temperature and fault transport account for huge amounts per year. Blockchain technologies help in tamper detection and information about cold chain sensors in multiple steps. Liabilities and financial obligations are responsible to execute the financial obligations and temperature of the device [7, 8].

10.18.7 ROLE OF PATIENT DATA INTEGRITY TO MAINTAIN SMART CONTACTS

The majority of healthcare institutions now employ database management systems to hold patient medical records. Companies also devote a significant amount of effort to establishing surveillance systems that protect information from hostile attacks. Patients, on the other hand, do not always seek medical help from the same institution, and a patient's medical information is dispersed throughout numerous healthcare repositories. Usually, a patient needing treatment from some other medical facility acquires all of his or her documents from multiple agencies and makes them accessible to the new facility. The collection and transmission of data in this manner may result in data loss or inconsistencies. The information in smart contracts is maintained on a blockchain, which is a blockchain platform. The information can be directly shared with some other healthcare organizations. Because each member of the network has a replica of each individual's whole health record, destructive assaults or data breaches on one device or area do not lead to information loss, and information can be recovered and reconstructed from some other node on the blockchain. In addition, any changes to the records are disseminated throughout the network. As a result, smart contracts can better safeguard the integrity of data of health information [9, 10].

10.19 CONCLUSION

Smart contact is an automated process that follows protocols set by authorities. Parties use terms and conditions to make decisions based on a set of conditions, creating a rulebook for implementation. The rulebook contains code stored and processed using blockchain technology on a distributed ledger. Any changes are recorded on the ledger. Medical insurance contracts are also part of smart contracts, where patients claim reimbursement. Smart contracts for medical insurance are crucial in modern insurance technology. Blockchain-based tools have been used by authorities to formalize relationships and achieve objectives. However, challenges may arise during implementation, such as parties not wanting to pursue the smart contract, disagreements on the rulebook, or delays in performance obligations. Despite these challenges, smart contracts have shown promising outcomes. Smart contracts and blockchains are rapidly growing as intelligent systems for various applications that require information exchange across networks. This chapter discusses blockchain-based technology for customers and healthcare companies to execute medical insurance smart contracts. Health standards and semantic webs are used to express smart contracts and individual clients' data. A smart data access policy evaluates smart contracts, while machine learning, AI, and blockchain technology enhance security and prevent attacks on medical insurance smart contracts.

KEYWORDS

- **artificial intelligence**
- **blockchain technology**
- **healthcare problems**
- **jurisdiction**
- **medical insurance**
- **smart contract**
- **supply chain management**

REFERENCES

1. Majumdar, A., Chatterjee, S., Gupta, R., & Rawat, C. S., (2019). *Competing in a New Age of Insurance: How India is Adopting Emerging Technologies*. PwC.
2. Nguyen, D. C., Pathirana, P. N., Ding, M., & Seneviratne, A., (2019). Blockchain for secure EHRs sharing of mobile cloud-based e-health systems. *IEEE Access, 7*, 66792–66806.
3. Androulaki, E., Barger, A., Bortnikov, V., et al., (2018). Hyperledger fabric: A distributed operating system for permissioned blockchains. In: *EuroSys '18: Proceedings of the Thirteenth EuroSys Conference* (pp. 1–15). Porto, Portugal, ACM, New York, NY, USA. https://doi.org/10.1145/3190508.3190538.
4. Skotnica, M., & Pergl, R., (2019). Das contract-a visual domain specific language for modelling blockchain smart contracts. In: *Enterprise Engineering Working Conference* (pp. 149–166). Springer.
5. Hamdaqa, M., Metz, L. A. P., & Qasse, I., (2020). iContractML: A domain-specific language for modeling and deploying smart contracts onto multiple blockchain platforms. In: *Proceedings of the 12th System Analysis and Modelling Conference* (pp. 34–43).
6. Lahiri, S. K., Chen, S., Wang, Y., & Dillig, I., (2018). *Formal Specification and Verification of Smart Contracts for Azure Blockchain*. arXiv:1812.08829.
7. Tan, S., Bhowmick, S. S., Chua, H. E., & Xiao, X., (2020). LATTE: Visual construction of smart contracts. In: *Proceedings of the 2020 ACM SIGMOD International Conference on Management of Data* (pp. 2713–2716).
8. Popovski, P., & Simeone, O., (2019). *Start Making Sense: Semantic Plane Filtering and Control for Post-5G Connectivity*. arXiv:1901.06337.
9. Chen, W., Zheng, Z., Cui, J., Ngai, E., Zheng, P., & Zhou, Y., (2018a). Detecting Ponzi schemes on Ethereum: Towards healthier blockchain technology. In: *Proceedings of the 2018 World Wide Web Conference* (pp. 1409–1418).
10. Zhang, X., & Poslad, S., (2018). Blockchain support for flexible queries with granular access control to electronic medical records (EMR). In: *IEEE International Conference*

on Communications (Vol. 2018, pp. 1–6). Institute of Electrical and Electronics Engineers Inc. http://dx.doi.org/10.1109/ICC.2018.8422883.

11. Omar, I. A., Jayaraman, R., Salah, K., Simsekler, M. C. E., Yaqoob, I., & Ellahham, S., (2020). Ensuring protocol compliance and data transparency in clinical trials using blockchain smart contracts. *BMC Med. Res. Methodol., 20*(1), 1–17.
12. Hirtan, L., Krawiec, P., Dobre, C., & Batalla, J. M., (2019). Blockchain-based approach for e-health data access management with privacy protection. In: *IEEE International Workshop on Computer Aided Modelling and Design of Communication Links and Networks, CAMAD*, (Vol. 2019). Institute of Electrical and Electronics Engineers Inc., http://dx.doi.org/10.1109/CAMAD.2019.8858469.
13. Cui, Y., Che, W., Liu, T., Qin, B., Yang, Z., Wang, S., & Hu, G., (2019). *Pre-training with Whole Word Masking for Chinese BERT*. arXiv preprint arXiv:1906.08101.
14. Esteva, A., Robicquet, A., Ramsundar, B., Kuleshov, V., DePristo, M., Chou, K., Cui, C., et al., (2019). A guide to deep learning in healthcare. *Nature Med., 25*(1), 24.
15. Croce, D., Castellucci, G., & Basili, R., (2020). GAN-BERT: Generative adversarial learning for robust text classification with a bunch of labelled examples. In: *Proceedings of the 58th Annual Meeting of the Association for Computational Linguistics* (pp. 2114–2119).
16. Du, M., Chen, Q., Chen, J., & Ma, X., (2020). An optimized consortium blockchain for medical information sharing. *IEEE Trans. Eng. Manage*, 1–13, http://dx.doi.org/10.1109/TEM.2020.2966832.
17. Zhang, P., Schmidt, D. C., White, J., & Lenz, G., (2018). Blockchain technology use cases in healthcare. *Advances in Computers* (Vol. 111, pp. 1–41). Elsevier.
18. Gerup, J., Soerensen, C. B., & Dieckmann, P., (2020). Augmented reality and mixed reality for healthcare education beyond surgery: An integrative review. *Int. J. Med. Educ., 11*, 1–18. https://doi.org/10.5116/ijme.5e01.eb1a. https://www.ijme.net/pmid/31955150 (accessed on 4 December 2023).
19. O'Reilly, K. *Philips Launches Next Generation Wearable Biosensors for Early Patient Deterioration Detection, Including Clinical Surveillance for COVID-19*. Available online: https://www.globenewswire.com/news-release/2020/05/26/2038736/0/en/Philips-launches-next-generation-wearable-biosensor-for-early-patient-deterioration-detection-including-clinical-surveillance-for-COVID-19.html (accessed on 4 December 2023).
20. Chaudhari, D. A., & Umamaheswari, E., (2020). A new adaptive XOR, hashing and encryption based authentication protocol for secure transmission of the medical data in internet of things (IoMT) Biomed Tech (Berl). 2020 Aug 24:/j/bmte.ahead-of-print/bmt-2019-0123/bmt-2019-0123.xml. doi: 10.1515/bmt-2019-0123.
21. Waltl, B., Sillaber, C., Gallersdorfer, U., & Matthes, F., (2019). Blockchains and smart contracts: a threat for the legal industry? *Business Transformation Through Blockchain* (pp. 287–315). Cham: Springer International Publishing.
22. Gao, F., Zhu, L., Shen, M., Sharif, K., Wan, Z., & Ren, K., (2018). A blockchain-based privacy-preserving payment mechanism for vehicle-to-grid networks. *IEEE Network, 32*(6), 184–192. https://doi.org/10.1109/mnet.2018.1700269.
23. Azim, A., Islam, M. N., & Spranger, P. E., (2020). Blockchain and novel coronavirus: Towards preventing LTDC: COVID-19: RTDC and future pandemics. *Iberoamerican J. Med*. (Epub ahead of print).

24. Hussien, H. M., Yasin, S. M., Udzir, S., Zaidan, A. A., & Zaidan, B. B., (2019). A systematic review for enabling the development of blockchain technology in healthcare application: taxonomy, substantially analysis, motivations, challenges, recommendations, and future direction. *J. Med. Syst., 43*(10), 320.
25. Derhab, A., Guerroumi, M., Belaoued, M., & Cheikhrouhou, O., (2021). Bmc-SDN: Blockchain-based multi-controller architecture for secure software-defined networks. *Wirel. Commun. Mob. Comput., 2021*. http://dx.doi.org/10.1155/2021/9984666.

CHAPTER 11

Remote Patient Monitoring with Blockchain: Powerful and Flexible Patient Observation System

SHWETA KUMARI,[1] VIKASH KUMAR,[2] JYOTIRMAYA SAHOO,[3] MANJEET KUMAR,[4] KAMAL DUA,[5] and SUDHANSHU MISHRA[6]

[1]*T. John College of Pharmacy, Basavanapura, Bengaluru, Karnataka, India*

[2]*Narayan Institute of Pharmacy, Gopal Narayan Singh University, Jamuhar, Sasaram, Bihar, India*

[3]*Sachchidanand Sinha College, Aurangabad Bihar, Under Magadh University, Bodh Gaya, Bihar, India*

[4]*School of Pharmacy, Arka Jain University, Jharkhand, India*

[5]*Faculty of Health, Australian Research Center in Complementary and Integrative Medicine, University of Technology, Sydney, Ultimo, NSW, Australia*

[6]*Department of Pharmaceutical Science and Technology, Madan Mohan Malaviya University of Technology, Gorakhpur, Uttar Pradesh, India*

ABSTRACT

Blockchain is a technique that has the potential to revolutionize healthcare monitoring by stabilizing the shielded way for medical organizations and securing it through a decentralized P2P network. In an attempt to preserve and clarify the interpretation of this cutting-edge patient monitoring (PM) technology. During the COVID-19 pandemic, the illness reaches its highest

Creating Smart Healthcare with Blockchain and Advanced Digital Technology.
Rishabha Malviya and Sonali Sundram (Eds.)

prevalence. As the internet of things (IoT) continues to expand, individuals adopted medical sensors for health monitoring. The immense amount of medical information created by these sensors must be gathered and sent securely to take the necessary measures for patients in critical situations. In addition, the particular details of users must be kept confidential, and fitness data must be managed securely. For the removal of counterfeited activities, the possession data of internet-connected devices must be preserved electronically. The emerging blockchain technology is decentralized with a clarity system that provides a secure, immutable transaction record. Diverse researchers have created a healthcare system using smart contracts on the blockchain that facilitates the enrollment of patients and doctors in a health center; hence, enhancing user participation in PM. This device watches distant patients and generates alerts in case of an emergency. This technology also consists of a legal and safe method of using medical sensors by utilizing smart contracts for device authorization. The patient's fitness details are examined, and timely notifications are sent to patients, health practitioners, and health centers. Blood pressure, temperature, blood oxygen, and brain inflammation monitoring are being used for patients' health monitoring. In addition, for PM, the health contract caller handles information received from the smart device. The primary PM or health contract caller generates a separate contract for each device from which it receives data. The primary contract functions as a container that organizes and establishes connections between all PM devices and subcontracts. Authorized physicians will have access to patient information and will be able to modify monitoring criteria. For instance, if a smart device gets blood pressure data from a patient's body sensor, the data will be delivered to the health contract caller, and then the blood pressure monitor function will be invoked for PM. The device will provide minimum and maximum blood pressure data to this method, which will then generate an object. The blood pressure monitor will next transmit these numbers to its analysis function to examine the obtained data. Subcontracts produce responses to incoming data rather than controlling it under the primary contract. If the analyze function returns a result other than zero (0) or "OK," an alarm (such as high/low blood pressure) is sent to the patient, physician, and health center for treatment. By using blockchain technology in healthcare settings, forgeries and privacy breaches are decreased, consequently boosting public confidence in the blockchain. This technique will also assist the hospitals in better understanding the reputations held by the individual physicians. It is planned to create a prescription review system shortly so that people will be able to provide feedback on their doctors' prescriptions. This chapter intends to incorporate the benefits of blockchain technology into the PM system by developing a secure blockchain-based system.

11.1 INTRODUCTION

A blockchain is a distributed and public digital ledger that prevents any record of a transaction from being altered retroactively without simultaneously changing the following blocks. A lengthy chain is formed by linking each block of the blockchain to the one before it. Blockchain, after all, is the record's name. Every transaction is documented and available for public inspection; transparency is highly ensured by blockchain. Information placed into the blockchain cannot be changed once it has been saved. In the blockchain, data is stored on networks rather than a central database, which enhances stability and reveals its hacker vulnerability if the data is true and constant [1]. The blockchain provides a terrific platform for developing and competing innovative and creative business models with established enterprises. Marketers may utilize the blockchain to keep track of the medical items they're selling. Using blockchain technology, healthcare and pharmaceuticals will eliminate counterfeit drugs, allowing tracking of all medicines. It aids in the investigation of falsifications. Patients' medical histories may be securely stored on the blockchain, where they will be protected from unauthorized access. All of the hospital's standard hardware is connected to this distributed network [2]. Calculating estimates for treatments, medications, and therapies for a wide range of disorders and issues is possible with the use of devices that conserve resources. There can never be any deletions or modifications to the data on a blockchain since it is a distributed ledger network. A blockchain's hash value is calculated by linking newly added data block records with each data block using cryptography [3]. Blockchain's distributed ledger design guarantees that all network users have access to and are responsible for data that is not handled in any single location. A single assault on this decentralized system is thwarted, making the system more secure and robust. Reducing the amount of medical practice and monitoring also helps healthcare providers and patients save time and money while improving health records and patient care. If the patient stores their data on a blockchain, they will be able to keep track of where it is at all times [4]. Using this technique, academics may examine a vast amount of previously undiscovered information on a certain set of people. Longitudinal research is critical to the evolution of precision medicine.

Patients' vital signs, like blood pressure and glucose levels, are stored and updated in real-time using blockchain technology, thanks to the IoT. It can be used by doctors to maintain track of high-risk patients and, in an emergency, advise and notify those patients' relatives and employers. The decentralized nature of the blockchain makes it impossible to compromise a single copy of the information while yet allowing for hacking. The information is kept on the blockchain, called a decentralized network of nodes [5]. Using this technique, you may be certain that your system's sensitive data is well protected as this technology protects data and keeps it safe and secure. All the relevant papers may be stored and securely accessed in one place with this tool. The use of a single patient database and the blockchain accelerates the search for candidates who meet specified trial requirements. Blockchain is a P2P network of computers known as nodes that store and record transaction or history data. It is possible to collaborate with confidence and always be aware of the past and present because all network participants have access to and share information.

Disparate networks may be linked together with this technology, revealing the significance of personalized therapy. As a result, the immutability and security of Blockchain are well-known. The three fundamental concepts of Blockchain are blocks, nodes, and miners [6]. Unlike traditional databases, blockchain does not store any of its data in one central area. Instead, a network of computers replicates and spreads the Blockchain. A new block in the blockchain is reflected on any computer connected to the internet. Cryptocurrencies such as Bitcoin and Ethereum have distributed ledgers that may be used in a variety of ways (Figure 11.1). Each blockchain network has its own set of benefits and weaknesses, which ultimately affects its best use [7].

11.2 BASICS OF BLOCKCHAIN

Before we get into how blockchain technology works, it's important to understand the problems that blockchain technology was created to solve. We consult with the relevant authority to determine whether a document is authentic (such as a dollar bill, a driver's license, or an election ballot). For instance, the bank keeps track of the serial number on each dollar bill, the motor vehicle administration keeps track of each license holder's number, and the election commission maintains a voter registration list. All of these mechanisms - banks, state agencies, or individuals with the power to issue

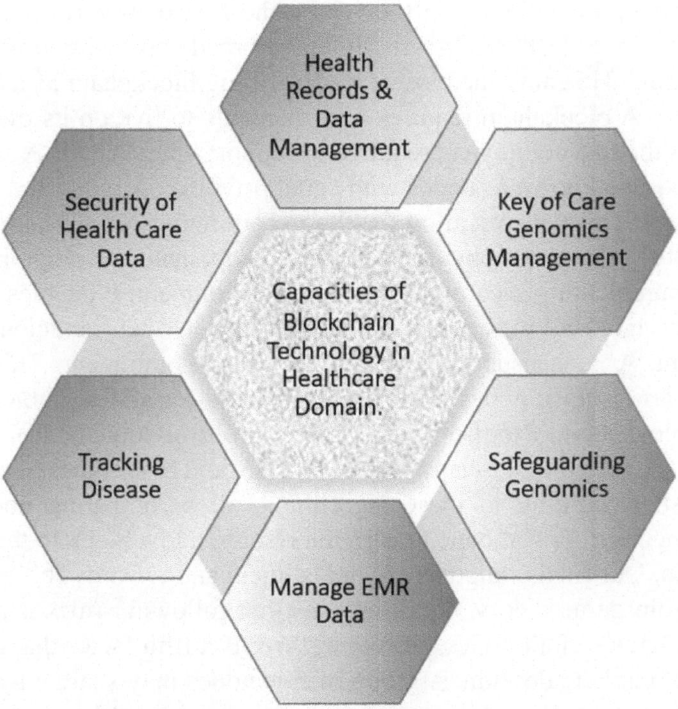

FIGURE 11.1 Capacities of blockchain technology for the healthcare domain.

and validate information have one thing in common: they are all centralized. These central authorities have considerable power and may become corrupt either intentionally or unintentionally. Decentralization lowers the likelihood of corruption, fraud, and manipulation. Blockchain technology is a novel and creative approach to implementing decentralization. In a nutshell, blockchain technology addresses the issue of centralization. It is a system for everyone to keep records without the need for a central authority, a decentralized method of maintaining a ledger that is nearly impossible to falsify [8]. A blockchain is so named because it is simply a chain of blocks. Consider keeping a shared ledger with many pages of records. Each page begins with a summary of the previous page. If the contents of a page are changed, the summary on the following page should also be changed. The pages are thus linked or chained together. Pages are referred to as blocks in technology. And because each block is linked to the data in the previous block, we have a chain of blocks, also known as a blockchain. Many people believe that Satoshi Nakamoto, the enigmatic Bitcoin creator, invented blockchain technology. Technically, he only invented the first real-world implementation, a Bitcoin. Satoshi's original whitepaper made no mention of the term "Blockchain." He came the closest to describing blockchain as a "chain of blocks" [9]. A blockchain requires four elements to live on its own. A P2P network is the first component required to support a blockchain. A network of computers, also known as nodes with equal privilege. Anyone and everyone are welcome. This network allows nodes to communicate and share information remotely. Cryptography is the second component. Cryptography is the art of communicating securely in a hostile environment. It enables a node to verify messages and prove their authenticity even when malicious players are present. A consensus algorithm is the third component. This implies that the participating nodes must agree on rules for adding a block to the existing blockchain. Proof-of-work (PoW), proof-of-stake (PoS), proof-of-authority (PoA), proof-of-elapsed time (PoET), and other types of consensus rules exist. According to these algorithms, all participating nodes must prove something for someone to earn the right to add a block to the existing blockchain. Our final component is punishment and reward. This element is derived from game theory, and it ensures that following rules is always in the best interests of all nodes. However, there is a fifth factor that cannot be combined: market adoption. A group of five nodes may share a ledger with a consensus algorithm. However, it is not decentralized because there are not enough participating nodes in the system. Furthermore, if blockchain technology is not adopted, it has no value, and the fourth element of punishment and reward is ineffective. When a blockchain reaches a critical mass of users, it becomes truly decentralized and, as a result, immutable [10].

11.3 TYPES OF BLOCKCHAIN

The public blockchain is the initial version of blockchain technology, and it is where cyber cash and other virtual currency were created and where distributed ledger technology (DLT) was promoted.

It overcomes the disadvantages of centralization, such as insufficient security and opaqueness. DLT is used to distribute data across a P2P network, as opposed to keeping it centrally. Due to its broadcast nature, the testament is required.

A private blockchain is a blockchain network that runs in a constrained environment, an impenetrable web, or is under the control of a single business. It performs equivalent to a public blockchain network and broadcast, despite its multicasting connectivity performance; however, it is far smaller. The creator of a private blockchain is aware of the network's members from the outset. On the public web, it is impossible to establish permission-based solutions since users are completely anonymous [11].

Sometimes, management who wants in every respect may adopt a hybrid blockchain, a form of blockchain that combines private and public blockchain properties. It authorizes a line of work to construct a non-public authorized-based system in addition to a social and prohibited system, enabling them to enter in certain data that is kept on the blockchain and what information is made public [12].

11.4 BLOCKCHAIN IN THE MEDICAL FIELD

When it comes to the medical management industry, Ethereum is essential. The urgency of progress in medical management is at an all-time high. Superior medical management resources supported by progressive technology are needed nowadays. When it comes to the healthcare industry, blockchain might play a major role. A further patient-oriented approach to the healthcare system is also taking shape, emphasizing the need for readily available resources and enough medical management facilities at all times [13]. Blockchain helps healthcare sectors to deliver enough patient care and excellent healthcare accessories. Another time-consuming and monotonous strategy that raises healthcare costs could be resolved quickly with the help of this advanced technology. With the change of medical knowledge, residents can take part in a medical investigation by using blockchain technology. Better research and exchange of information on public health will also help to boost therapy for various populations. The intact healthcare system and organizations are supervised via the usage of centralized information. Till today, the paramount issues in population health maintenance have been safeguarded to all facts, sharing, and interactivity. Using blockchain to solve this specific issue is a safe bet [14]. A well-executed implementation of this technology improves security and data sharing, as well as interoperability and integrity. Some specialists are concerned about the safekeeping of data in the fields of personalized medicine and wearable technology. Patients and white-collar workers must be able to seize information, pass on, and examine data through networks without the worry of security breaches. This is where blockchain technology comes into play. Blockchain technology has numerous utilizations in healthcare that benefit from its many capabilities [15]. Worldwide, blockchain has a broad variety of uses and capabilities. Patient's medical data may be securely transferred using the ledger technology, which manages the supply chain for pharmaceuticals and facilitates the secure transmission of patient medical details. Figure 11.2 depicts the wide range of blockchain philosophy aspects and important enablers in several healthcare fields and related sectors. Several of the high-tech knowledge-derived and amazing outlooks used to construct and practice blockchain technology include healthcare data protection, management of various genomes, software packages, medical case history, interoperation, capture digitizing and concern outbreak, and so on [16]. Aside from the fact that blockchain technology is completely digital, its usage in healthcare-related applications is a major factor in its acceptance. The blockchain provides the whole transparency to the prescription operation, from manufacturing to the pharmacy counters. IoT and blockchain technology can be used to track choked, freight direction, and speed. To avert interference and scarcity in medical institutions, it produces a chance to organize and buy in a way that minimizes the impact of a particular drug. The application of a blockchain-based automated scheme would aid in guaranteeing that logistical data is not subject to unauthorized changes. As an outcome, additional individuals who want to procure medical-related industry can do so with faith, as the documentation, capital, and medicine themselves are kept guarded. At a reasonable price, the technology may enhance the health of patients while preserving the budget [17]. When it comes to multi-level authentication, it removes all impediments and barriers. Security applications are suitable for blockchain because they can keep an unalterable, distributed, and transparent record of all health data.

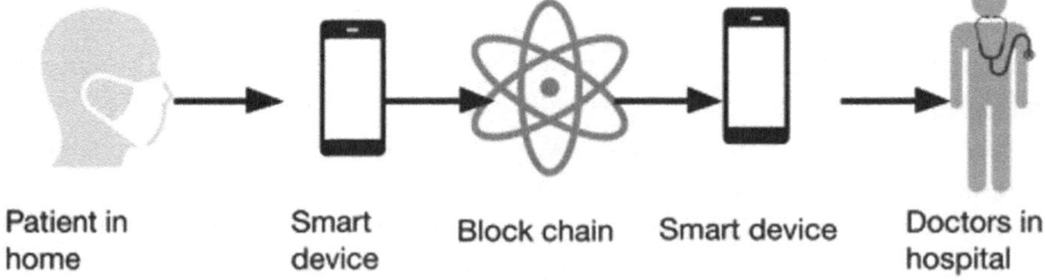

FIGURE 11.2 Health monitoring by blockchain.

Medical data can be kept confidential while still being viewable on the blockchain, thanks to the complex and secure methods used. Modern technology has made it possible for sick people, medical practitioners, and other healthcare workers to access identical details in a decentralized manner. Blockchain technology may help open the door for interoperability by making it easier for patients to exchange their medical records and access legislation. By giving them more control over their personal information, patients' privacy and confidentiality are improved [18]. Quality management and enforcement are difficult to monitor and execute. Blockchain applications have the potential to solve all of these technological challenges in every business. Legal medications may be tracked down using blockchain headlines, which will help regulators. This ensures that all parties who have been permitted to receive it receive the sick-person particulars, digitally. Patients only need to sign a new consent form authorizing the sharing of all their medical information when they switch doctors [19]. The use of blockchain technology in healthcare is on the rise. Preliminary implementers of new health advancements are frequently optimistic. A comprehensive view of blockchain's influence on the pharmaceutical industry in the coming years will concentrate on resolving current structural issues. At any one time, all the relevant information may be accessed by doctors, patients, and pharmacists. Blockchain technology is being researched, experimented with, and discovered in the medical industry 24/7. After medicine, adding up payment alternatives, and decentralizing patient health history data, has shown themselves to be indispensable tool in the field of healthcare [20]. Machine learning (ML) and artificial intelligence (AI), as well as the use of blockchain, are critical to the medical industry. There are several legitimate applications of blockchain in the healthcare sector. The initiative employs blockchain technology to track the medical supply chain and improve efficiency. It is possible to store a person's whole medical history on the blockchain, including all of their diagnoses and results from previous tests and treatments, as well as data from smart sensors. This strategy makes it easy for a doctor to get all the information necessary to make an accurate diagnosis and suggestion. In a single blockchain system, all of the data can't be lost or shifted [21]. Blockchain technology can be used to bypass an organization's internal networks. A large organization made up of many different participants with varying degrees of power over an encrypted blockchain database may shield the firm from external threats and bombard it. Using a blockchain network in healthcare can help to prevent such assaults and other issues, such as computer corruption or hardware failure [22].

Using blockchain technology to handle electronic medical data allows patients to have authority over their information. When the patient (keyholder) dies, such research used various tactics, such as the usage of shared keys, e-medical data maintenance, serialized perspective, secure e-medical records, increased interoperability, proper access, and privacy policy protection measures. Alliance-based referral medical systems used for medical records from Taiwan's national medical record system and clinic e-medical data is one of the few clinically tried blockchain systems which were discovered. To show a functional de-centralized referral system and substantial patient interest in examining their medical data, they took a patient-centric processing approach by constructing an extra blockchain-based de-centralized application [23]. The blockchain required in clinical trial administration has been investigated as a way to enhance accountability and transparency. Clinical trial activities, including voluntary permission, were tracked in a predetermined chronological sequence. The scientist was concerned about medicolegal fraud because the automatic execution might be extended to include clinical permission for operations or treatment. By boosting security and reducing the time it takes to settle claims, a distributed ledger might enhance the claims process in healthcare insurance. Immutable on-chain records of insurance claims may provide the level of openness needed to thwart fraud. This system's viability will be determined by its capacity to communicate with off-chain databases [24].

Blockchain technology has the potential to enhance medical research cooperation, an extreme area of AI development with privacy-securing technologies. AI development and generalization may be improved with the use of federated learning and blockchain technology [25].

Presumed omics technologies (e.g., genomics, proteomics, and metabolomics) and genetics are other areas of blockchain study interest. These issues have sparked an interest in blockchain technology. It analyzes whether or not central databases are capable of handling such sensitive information. To make genetic data more accessible, the platform created a secure trade mechanism using tokens [26].

Pharmaceutical medications have a particularly complicated supply chain because of their vast geographic distribution. Traditional technology, such as universal product code and RF (extremely high frequency) naming have so far given out to stopped faked medication disasters, especially in cost-making areas like Taiwan. Some scientists demonstrated the feasibility of evidence of work consensus using a commercial blockchain platform (GCoin) and proposed the creation of an open-governance surveillance net based on smart contracts. Drug safety is particularly an issue for nations with lower wealth, such as the Philippines. By developing a pharmacovigilance blockchain system, some researchers were able to solve the problem of scalability and flexibility in the standard medicine delivery network by employing either consign evidence of stake or practical Byzantine fault tolerance (PBFT). To keep the pharmaceutical supply chain safe from harmful assaults, blockchain technology is used in these scenarios to provide a trust mechanism for tracking and authenticating medications [27].

COVID-19 is a recent example of a blockchain-based application. In Wuhan, China, a coronavirus-caused pneumonia outbreak (COVID-19) started in December and quickly spread across the city and beyond. The healthcare system throughout the world is today under more strain than ever before. COVID-19 is a pandemic with a devastating impact on the economy and society of the globe. Governments and non-governmental groups throughout the world are working tirelessly to contain the virus and create a vaccine. Finding primary physicians or caregivers is very difficult due to the significant increase in medical patients that most countries are experiencing [28]. Using IoT and wearable devices, remote health monitoring (RHM) has improved the condition of patient care during COVID-19 (RHM). RHM is recommended to give quite long-range treatment outside of hospitals in this pandemic condition. The ability to treat a greater number of people is another benefit. A patient's healthcare provider may be easily accessed via this service. Medical expenditures are reduced, and the quality of service provided is improved as a result [29]. A smartphone with internet access, a health data collection device, and an application are all essential parts of RHM. Due to the use of emerging technologies like blockchain in areas where COVID-19 spreads and information can be continuously monitored, many infected people have been identified. Wearable technology and the IoT play an important role in the development of secure medical records in smart cities [30]. Health monitoring, illness diagnosis, and medicine may all be made easier with the use of wearable gadgets. Microcontroller-equipped smart electronic devices that may be implanted in clothes or worn by people are known as "wearable devices" in the healthcare industry. Their integration with modern features such as wireless data transmission, real-time input, and warning systems makes them easy to operate. Blood pressure, blood glucose levels, and breathing patterns may all be monitored using these devices. Fever, cough, and respiratory activity may be monitored using a new wireless sensor-wearing device that rests comfortably on the throat. The little, flexible, waterproof device, about the size of a postage stamp, is positioned just below the suprasternal notch, the visible dip at the base of the neck. From this vantage position, the device keeps track of respiratory noises, pulse rate, body temperature, and coughing. The first wearable gadget that monitors COVID-19 symptoms has been developed [31]. Medical devices that are fastened to a specific spot are known as fixed devices. Implanted medical devices may be placed within the human body. Physicians (healthcare professionals) may prescribe wearable medical gadgets for patients. Wearable health monitoring gadgets, such as Fitbit and Fuelband, are also popular among consumers. Wearable users may connect and exchange data with IoT devices, which are integrated with software, electronics, sensors, actuators, and networking.

IoT devices combine smart devices and sensors with limited storage and computing capabilities. The city's smartest residents rely on sensors to observe parameters such as temperature, humidity, allergens, noise, traffic conditions, and power grid status. At any given moment, the values of these parameters may be used to offer context for a citizen's current condition. In addition, the strategic use of sensed data is helping to improve healthcare services [32]. The public services can respond more rapidly to medical emergencies and make fast judgments when they have access to real-time COVID-19 data. A pandemic outbreak of COVID-19 is posing several challenges for nations throughout the world, including India, which is scrambling for practical and cost-effective remedies. Currently, practically all problems arise as a result of patients' inability to get vaccines, which is the second most pressing concern after the issue of vaccine manufacturing. When patients can obtain their treatment via the IoT, it helps them recover from their sickness. In addition to collecting data through sensors and smart devices, the IoT may also be used to analyze and process that data in cloud settings. Amid the COVID-19 epidemic, the recommended method for gathering and evaluating patient data is helping to enhance civilizational health. Wearable medical gadgets are essential for monitoring the health of patients at home. Protected and secure transmission of healthcare device data is ensured [33].

Cryptographic primitives will be used to do this. Data is encrypted before being sent to the cloud by IoT devices. The original data's metadata is preserved on the blockchain. A step has been taken toward outsourcing data gathering, processing, and sharing capabilities by merging IoT with the cloud. Trackable, exchange of data, experiment on living, and drug monitoring approaches were all discussed. Blockchain technology might have a positive impact on a wide range of health and wellness industries. Prescription monitoring and insurance coverage also fall under the umbrella of these programs. Throughout the full lifecycle of a system, hospitals may use a blockchain to track their property, network, and patient monitoring (PM). In addition to using post-market analyses to increase productivity savings, the data collected will be used to enhance sick-person welfare [34].

11.5 BLOCKCHAIN APPLICATIONS RELATED TO COVID-19

COVID-19 has spurred extensive data coordination and management efforts. First and foremost, sensitive data must be verified and publicly maintained. If these data management systems gave central authorities full access to data, privacy concerns may be raised, which in turn could be counterproductive. Some scientists created a blockchain-based mobility card that uses smart contracts and tokens (token-based movement cards) that do not need personal information for authentication [31]. Another group of researchers has demonstrated an effective blockchain platform that can desensitize user identity and location information through its hash function, thus protecting the identity of COVID-19 patients as well as the public's private information in a decentralized environment. It is possible to collect sustainability but keep an eye on data using blockchain technology [35].

Second, the development of health, as well as immunity certificates, may be necessary to conduct quick, broad testing and other methods called vaccination. In order to verify whether an individual is COVID-negative or not, blockchain technology can be used [33]. Since critical keys and data shouldn't be tied to any one individual; therefore, another researcher developed an Ethereum-based consortium blockchain architecture and mobile app to instantly verify tamper-proof tests [36].

Third, supply chains for critical products including personal protective equipment, life-saving pharmaceuticals, and COVID-19 vaccinations are under more scrutiny than ever before. Respective vials and packages are monitored using oracles, IoT, and other application programming interfaces (APIs). End-to-end monitoring of COVID-19 vaccination distribution data was ensured by combining IoT self-enforcing sensor devices with smart contracts on the Ethereum blockchain platform by a scientist. To further address a critical issue, the suggested vaccination tracking system also included on-chain reporting of adverse events and the use of blockchain to handle a supply chain and manage waste for COVID-19-related medical goods and some other equipment [37].

Fourth, to develop a blockchain-based consortium network for the distribution of COVID-19-related information (e.g., CT scans of the chest), filtered reports that are not related to COVID-19 and the blockchain compares each report's noncognitive hash to those recorded on-chain, which can identify and validate them before they're stored [38].

Fifth, the "proof-of-authority" consensus was used by some researchers to develop a worldwide global patient details electronic medical data system.

API, as well as fast healthcare interoperability resources (FHIR), were used to enable real-time uploads from clinic EMR systems. Thus, they may give rapid public updates, aid the government in dynamically adjusting healthcare policy, and promote pandemic research via this method [39].

11.6 BLOCKCHAIN FAVORS REMOTE MONITORING

IoT system was built to capture the patient's ECG signals, which were recorded at home, and communicate the data to the medical facility to reduce the patient's need to visit a medical facility for a health checkup. A Bluetooth component was included in the ECG. Because of this, data could be sent to a facility for processing using a laptop or smartphone with internet connectivity. Since the method designed is cost-effective, the accuracy of the ECG signals was a restriction of the data, according to the author. It was also claimed that a GSM mobile signal would require additional components, such as more powerful computers, raising the cost and limiting the devices' capacity to connect through Bluetooth to their service provider [40].

Similarly, another technique looked into how a modular monitoring system for ECG, SpO_2, temperature, and movement data could "enable" quicker and better medical actions in emergency scenarios. The study's primary goal, according to the chapter, is to cover the time between monitoring a patient's vital signs in the intensive care unit (ICU) and discharge from the hospital. In contrast to the earlier research, the monitoring system for this utilizes a gateway based on a Raspberry Pi B+ system as the primary component. Android-based medical personnel may access the patient's ECG or SpO_2 through a RESTful-based web interface given by a sensor node (a mobile device equipped with IEEE, rather than Bluetooth). Despite the system's performance, it is now only accessible to Android smartphones. There was some discussion on the need of strengthening data security, but no more investigation was done. Additionally, none of these articles mentions the importance of correctly using these devices, such as ensuring a reliable ECG signal [41].

Experiments were performed to examine how environmental factors such as proper gadget functioning and proper use affect the device's overall performance. Patients' environments and their ability to operate tests have an impact on the test outcomes, according to the research (compared to a qualified operator). According to the article's author, hospital environments are standardized, strictly regulated, and easily accessible settings operating under strict professional supervision. There is no one-size-fits-all treatment plan for patients in their own homes. Because of the lack of control, it's possible that accurate and precise testing may be hampered. Because of this, Bitterman feels that a well-defined home environment is essential for avoiding mistakes and achieving exact outcomes. Increasing the number of people who use remote services will result from this. Medical professionals must educate and teach patients in a non-threatening manner and build an automated system that will alert them when they are using the medication in an unsuitable way. This might be a warning if a patient's desire to use the device has waned, or if an inaccessible data set is observed [42].

Reflex syncope is the most prevalent reason for syncope, on distant control of patients with this condition. There are issues with employing Holter systems for remote monitoring of such situations, as well as issues with an implanted monitor that he explains in this chapter. However, both types of monitoring devices present challenges for implanting because of the prolonged use or invasive procedures needed. A wireless, congenital remote monitoring system was put to the test in this investigation. Implanting the wearable inside the clothing allowed for the patient to be monitored. The average age of the people who took part in the study was 46 years old. The data from the wearable were compared to those from a traditional monitoring system in the research. For patients with reflex syncope, the Holter system had a great agreement with traditional EKG (ECG) monitoring methods, according to the findings. According to the research, this wearable has a 3-axis accelerometer, which allows for real-time tracking of the patient's posture, which will aid in assessing how effective it is for patients. There are no known limitations to this research; nevertheless, the author did not specify that certain positions (wrong size, not wearing correctly) might indicate an inaccurate usage of the wearable (accelerometer) and warn the physician of possibly unreliable data, as detected by the accelerometer [43].

In order to correctly monitor a patient's health, the patient must be motivated to do tests as instructed by their doctor or other healthcare practitioners. Financial incentives may be used to encourage people to stick to their medication regimens at home. In a three-month test period, three home-monitoring devices were used every day with a three-month follow-up period. When conducting this research, researchers employed gadgets that enabled patients with uncontrolled diabetes to self-monitor blood glucose, blood pressure, and weight. After each usage, the subjects were given a gadget that automatically sent their findings to a website (once daily). In addition, the patient was asked to verify that the data had been sent successfully.

Study evaluations indicated that the variable number of people involved with an economic impulse was greater than the control group, and that group's compliance with the encouragement was higher than the control group after three months [44]. According to the research, all candidates came from one primary medical center, which restricted this study to a certain geographic area. It's also possible that the three-month incentive payment period wasn't long enough for research participants to form a new habit. Incorporating financial incentives, like cash prizes, may seem like it would be a good idea in a study environment, but it is challenging in the real world when a sick person must travel great distances to get the promised reward or when the institution must deliver checks regularly [45].

Wearable sensors for remote monitoring have a number of drawbacks, including the need to manage enormous amounts of data collected by sensors, battery life for prolonged use, low signal-to-noise ratio (SNR), and the need for a secure connection channel to protect sensitive individual health information when transferred online. Additionally, these devices must be easy to use, affordable, and unobtrusive, all of which pose issues, as does their compatibility across various sensors and applications. The limits of camera-based home monitoring systems are explored in various articles. These systems are expensive and complicated and limit the user's mobility to a specific area. It also goes into detail on how accelerometers, gyroscopes, and magnetometers have grown in popularity because of their low cost and wide range of applications. When used in conjunction with position tracking motion sensors, wearables, and home medical equipment may be able to be evaluated and identified for good use even when the user only had little training. If the patient's location isn't precisely detected by an accelerometer, gyroscope, or magnetometer, it's because the little devices aren't as exact and precise as they should be [46].

The use of blockchain-based smart contracts, which execute orders following the judgment of the originator, is one possibility for establishing the correct usage of these gadgets. A patient's weight, for example, may be tracked in a smart contract technique. Once the data has been received and validated, such as the weight, the software sends the data out on its own [47].

To provide remote PM services including, heart, observe sleep apnoea testing, and electroencephalogram (EEG) monitoring, blockchain technology with medical IoT, On-chain (public blockchain for confirmation and evidence charge), and off-chain solutions were used in the research to solve the inherent blockchain and IoT challenges, such as confidentiality and expandability. The IOTA protocol is an affordable dais particularly developed for computationally lightweight IoT, instead of Ethereum or Hyperledger. They were able to send, get validated, and encode activity data from a wearable gadget using this blockchain technology. In the future, distant control and mobile health might be used for clinical or research reasons if this feature is implemented [48].

11.6.1 THE ESSENTIAL PART OF DATA USABILITY IN WEARABLES, HEALTH RECORDS, AND HOME PHARMACEUTICAL EQUIPMENT

Providers must depend on the patient's desire to use and wear the device following the manufacturer's instructions when patients are being treated at home. The user may find it difficult to establish a new habit. It's possible to misinterpret data if a single data connection is absent. To encourage patients to stick with their new habits, a system that rewards them for their continuing engagement would be ideal [49].

Telehealth (the use of virtual services to improve the health of patients) or other methods of remote monitoring are required. In order to depend only on the patient's ability to utilize the device following the provider's instructions, this is essential.

Patients will be using these gadgets on their own, thus, a human-centered design approach must be taken into consideration while designing them. As a result, the user will no longer be reliant on the manual, customer service, or healthcare professionals to complete the task. Not only would this fail to meet its stated goal of providing home-based patient care, but it will also pose significant difficulties in the implementation of value-based care [50].

Health Level 7 (HL7's) FHIR standard, for example, may be used to copy generated data into the appropriate data fields in the provider's electronic health record (EHR), commonly referred to as electronic medical record (EMR) FHIR. Data security and privacy, as well as legal responsibility: The Health Information Trust Alliance (HITRUST) and Health Insurance Portability and Accountability Act (HIPAA) 1996 compliance with encrypted data is the basic necessity of the Resources Information Security (IS) Department [51].

A secure log-in is required by most devices and wired dashboards (which keep the patient's produced data) in order to verify the user's identity. This is a laborious and time-consuming procedure that necessitates the creation of several strong passwords, each of which must meet certain criteria, such as the inclusion or exclusion of specific letters and symbols [52].

Patient approval: The procedure of exchanging medical information with a new physician, pharmacy, or payer is still quite time-consuming as every time a patient has to grant their consent. As a patient, you should have an option to access a database, provide your permission to share certain information with a specific contact (such as your insurance company, a doctor, or a pharmacy), and do so securely and encrypted [53].

In order to minimize data fatigue in patients and employees, all patient-produced information must be structured and excavated appropriately, giving valuable data without overload. The produced data should be filtered so that only related data is delivered to the EHR since this information will later be needed to fill the patient's EHR. Exchange of data, interoperability: if a sick person uses a Japanese smart scale to track their improvement in a weight-loss program, a German smart blood pressure cuff, or a United States vendor's smart glucose meter, a common protocol is needed to equalize results and data attainability after removing exclusive and achieved data structures. All three devices need to be able to parse each other's findings in order for patient-generated data to make sense. This must be done before the data is sent to the EHR of the provider. Progress in therapy may only be confirmed if no more physical labor is required [54].

Big data and social media have made it possible for patients to securely and reliably access their particular medical assessment at any time. The inmate should also be able to provide access to his or her followers. The purpose of this research is to find out whether blockchain technology can help solve these usability issues [55].

As mentioned in the chapter, sensors on wearables connect with service providers via blockchain smart contracts to record events in an immutable transaction log. This setup also enables the transfer of data to any EMR database of one's choosing and the pre-setting of anticipated values for a patient's use of a device. If the system detects abnormal data or "unusual behavior," it will alert the user or their healthcare professionals. If you are using a wearable device, the data is delivered to your phone or tablet, which is then used to gather and prepare the raw data.

In order to match and format data from various manufacturers, interfacing communication methods, which may be seen as a restriction, may be necessary. As far as we know, this is not referenced elsewhere in the study. When data is sent through an open channel (such as a patient's Wi-Fi), ensuring security at every node is the largest difficulty. A final problem is that it takes longer than real-time data transmission to validate each new block before it can be sent across the network [56].

Geospatially enabled blockchain systems to have the ability to "not only provide the entire information about an entry's particular time but also need and validate its related evidence of place, thereby permitting the exact configurational mapping of real-world occurrences." It is now possible to remotely monitor and analyze the impact of certain locations (such as a workplace, a family activity, or even a doctor's office waiting room) on the heart rate recorded by a wearable device using geospatially enabled blockchain [57]. Blockchain's interoperability and security are also listed as challenges by the researcher, who is concerned about the adoption of blockchain in light of GDPR's severe privacy requirements in the European Union (EU). This information will be overlooked since the research will only be conducted in the United States [58]. Women undergoing breast cancer therapy may benefit from the use of telemedicine and remote PM. An ultrasound scan captured at a distant place and delivered to a physician through blockchain is discussed by the author, who recommends a paradigm for telemedicine that uses this technology. Since photos of the patient can be checked for fidelity through remote monitoring and blockchain integration, the author claims that this method provides "a fully accurate portrayal of the condition." Also on the table is the topic of EHRs and the issue of pictures being dispersed throughout various health networks [59]. "Interoperability solutions that would correlate facts management and exchange," he adds when the necessity arises for sharing data and managing authentication. Image file interoperability and integrity are two problems that blockchain aims to solve. Patients will have access to their medical records under certain conditions, and providers may interact with and share data through smart contracts [60].

Although ultrasound imaging generates fewer data sets than MRI or CT imaging, ultrasound picture files are large and are controlled by a blockchain based on the number of images received. This is one of blockchain's limitations. An ultrasound breast image exchange may give an accurate portrayal of the issue by giving an integrity check on patient images. However, it is considered that the issue lies more in the interchange of images than anything else. A non-proprietary picture archiving communication system (PACS) may only be used to store and exchange images if many providers utilize the same PACS vendor, which is frequently the case.

These silos may be broken down with the use of vendor-neutral archives (VNA). However, since this technology is still in its infancy, it is being embraced at a glacial pace [61].

11.7 VARIOUS APPLICATIONS OF BLOCKCHAIN IN THE MEDICAL FIELD

11.7.1 RESERVE DETAILS OF A PARTICULAR CASE

A considerable number of patient data and information is created both preliminary and during the various stages of a clinical investigation. Numerous people's blood tests, quality evaluations, and estimations, as well as wellness surveys, are available for comparison. A document or record's existence may be shown using the search results. Healthcare practitioners will be able to verify the veracity of recorded data by comparing it to the original records kept on the blockchain system, and this will be done smoothly. Existing cryptographic methods are used to build the blockchain, including a framework for data exchange encryption. Healthcare providers record the patient's name, date of birth, diagnoses, and treatments in EHR format during patient details. Cloud computing or contemporary databases are used to store this data [62].

11.7.2 EXAMINE THE OUTCOMES OF A SPECIFIC PROCEDURE

Researchers have confirmed access to patient data, which allows them to efficiently analyze any operation on a substantial portion of the patient population. As a consequence of these findings, patient care for these populations will be improved. It is now feasible to acquire real-time data from the blockchain infrastructure to supply a broad choice of precisely customized pharmaceuticals for patients. Pharmacies' work is made easier by blockchain, which has all of the relevant data stored on top of it. They will be able to effectively communicate with patients based on these findings. Real-time updates on the patient's condition and any emergencies will be given to doctors through the wearable data they collect [63].

11.7.3 VALIDATION

Until they are joined to the chain, all transactions in a blockchain are confirmed using algorithms. Once the content is encrypted, digitally signed, and preserved, it cannot be authenticated. Technology and healthcare firms are always looking for new ways to make healthcare safer and more affordable, both today and shortly. When healthcare organizations can effectively authenticate their outcomes, blockchain might be a revolutionary in the health ecosystem.

11.7.4 ACCURACY AND SECURITY

It enables doctors to spend more time treating patients while maintaining high levels of safety and transparency. Providing funding for clinical studies and therapies for any uncommon condition would be possible as well. Data interchange across medical solution providers may improve diagnosis accuracy, treatment efficiency, and cost-effective healthcare ecosystems. The blockchain enables communication and information sharing between various health ecosystem organizations for increased protection and clarity. When employing such a system, users don't have to worry about compromising their data's integrity or secrecy by looking for other methods of communication [64].

11.7.5 HEALTH RECORD KEEPING

A blockchain is an ideal tool for medical record-keeping. A few of the things it may be used include data exchange, electronic recordkeeping, insurance management, and other administrative errands. Using an app, patients may upload their medical records to a blockchain network. Digital blockchain contracts make it possible for sensors and intelligent devices to work together. The majority of the time, EHRs are shared throughout several different healthcare facilities. In the future, patients will be able to view their medical records thanks to blockchain technology. If all the information is gathered in one location, we will learn new things about the health of the patient. The blockchain paradigm would therefore ensure information's legitimacy and authenticity while also preserving customers' privacy [65].

11.7.6 CLINICAL TRIAL

Wrong results and data disintegration in clinical studies may be addressed with blockchain technology, which is a distributed ledger system. Clinical trials will benefit from the increased transparency and accountability afforded by the blockchain. The medical management production can better comprehend the possibilities by using the business analysis platform's examination of swap retail kinetics. The use of the blockchain to handle pharmaceuticals is merely a second chance to create and observe the supply chain from the producer to the end user [66].

11.7.7 DISPLAY INFORMATION

To assure the quality and supply of the drug, the blockchain system will reveal information about the medication's sources. If implemented properly, blockchain may offer greater protection for delicate data than ever before. Several fabrications, including bank retail, and the confinement sector, have started to use the blockchain app trend to display information and benefit from it in many ways. Complexity and nuance are also regarded to be part of healthcare. This announcement is certain to create a firestorm of controversy. The market has seen major changes in several industries because of its intricacy and complexity, such as pharmaceuticals, treatments, vaccinations, clinical trials, and the use of cloud computing [67].

11.7.8 DETECTION OF FAKE CONTENT

Blockchain will increase transparency and erroneous spotting;-experiments for subjects and patients should continue to be straightforward to confirm. A brilliant accord is ideal for getting approval and maintaining the transparency of the protocol and findings. First, the public was able to closely follow a clinical trial thanks to technology. This technology's user-friendliness and tight real-time access to patient's medical and insurance records are its main objectives [68].

11.7.9 DECREASE NEEDLESS OVERHEAD COSTS

Blockchain facilitates the right use of health data by reducing administrative costs that would otherwise be incurred. Additionally, the need for several middlemen to keep track of vital health information will be reduced by this technology. Providing timely, effective, and appropriate healthcare services to patients may thus be simplified.

Patient's medical records will be available to service providers at all times using blockchain-based healthcare technology. Interworking, statement finalization, stealing, and even catastrophic facts defeat are just a few of the many issues plaguing the healthcare system that may be addressed [69].

11.7.10 PATIENT MONITORING (PM)

Medical professionals may rely on the blockchain's security to ensure that, if needed, they will have access to pharmaceutical equipment. The medical practitioner may also find it more time-consuming to monitor patients and respond to fitness-related problems from afar. Using blockchain and healthcare, it is possible to monitor patient room temperatures, bed occupancy, and supply availability. Healthcare organizations and providers may establish and maintain a digital identity on the blockchain. As a result, healthcare logistics will become clearer for the correct monitoring of the patient [70].

11.7.11 CREATE RESEARCH INITIATIVES

A trustworthy source of information may be provided through the blockchain. For membership claims and disputes, blockchain technology has the potential to replace the current manual procedure. Using blockchains to facilitate the exchange of patient data might lead to new and innovative research projects. An unprecedented collaboration between participants and researchers may be sparked by a more thorough sharing of patient results. The management of patient referrals may also benefit from the use of this technology. It will be applied to the patient's treatment record on the blockchain as soon as the patient interacts with the doctor and prepares a therapeutic plan [71].

11.7.12 MAINTAIN FINANCIAL STATEMENTS IN THE HOSPITAL

An accurate accounting record is essential for a successful bookkeeping procedure. The test on animal practice is applicable for efficient surgical procedures and accurate evaluations. The accounting and reporting procedure has been simplified thanks to the work of blockchain enterprises. Anyone may prepare for a medical appointment by filling out the necessary papers in advance using this app. Because they won't have to wait in line, it will save time. However, the real-world applications of blockchain and the kind of issues it resolves in the healthcare system may teach us about the dangers and advantages of this technology [72].

11.7.13 IMPROVES SAFETY

Increases patient protection by direct pharmaceutical validity and traceability issues as well as providing safe interworking in the healthcare industry. No other method of supply chain management (SCM) can replace the current one and prevent counterfeit pharma producers from bringing inferior products to market. No matter how many hospitals and organizations there are, it would be possible to keep all data in a single place using blockchain technology. For physicians, the interoperability of blockchain technology will make it easier to access thorough medical information so that they may better understand their diagnosis and plan a more exact procedure.

11.7.14 MINIMIZE THE HOUR AND CASH ON DATA TRANSFER

Blockchain networks reduce the amount of time and money needed to change data. Using blockchain technology, medical qualifications may be verified quickly and effectively. The anonymity and safety of patients are guaranteed by blockchain networks. This might lead to a substantial shift in the way healthcare is delivered throughout the globe. The use of blockchain will lead to monetized data sharing networks that are lucrative and respect privacy. Transaction history and documentation may be stored with time stamps on the blockchain, which is a distributed network computing platform. Data is verified and recorded by each node in this network as it enters and exits it [73].

11.8 CHALLENGES

There are various challenges faced during the application of blockchain technology in healthcare systems:

1. **Authority:** The proposed blockchain-based healthcare system needs public and private blockchains to communicate with one another. This demonstrates the value of globally coordinated standards and agreements that cut across national boundaries and legal systems [74].
2. **Absence of Law:** The proposed blockchain-based healthcare system faces difficulties in creating appropriate regulations to control ownership rights in medical transactions globally. Data ownership

and the current medical law of the traditional healthcare system are crucial issues that must be appropriately addressed due to the presence of numerous stakeholders. Concerning the new administration's policy goals governing the digitally described automated, and global nature of blockchain, it will be challenging to change the existing regulatory framework. It is important to fully understand the distributed storage structure, granted access rights, and record ownership in blockchain [75].

3. **Clarity and Confidentiality:** Transparency is emphasized by blockchain technology, which isn't always a good thing in the healthcare industry. Healthcare stakeholders view the accessibility of a database, even in encrypted form, as a critical issue, even though it offers security through encryption. Access control in the context of blockchain, therefore, needs to be properly addressed.
4. **Sustainability:** In the blockchain, the encryption key is essential. It is impossible to retrieve the private encrypted key. This makes healthcare data more complex due to its longevity. The reliability and worth of a patient's health record are significantly diminished when pieces are missing. Furthermore, access to a user's private encryption key can be gained by hacking or stealing the user [76].
5. **Expandability:** As users add data, the blockchain grows by storing all of the hashes related to the newly added data. This increases the need for storage and computing power, which could result in fewer nodes on the network having enough processing power to process and validate blockchain data. The probability of increased centralization and slower data validation and confirmation increases if health professionals are unable to meet storage and computational power demands [77].
6. **Adoption for Participation:** A network of interconnected computers is required for blockchain technology to provide the necessary computing power for both the creation of transaction blocks and cryptocurrencies. Utilizing incentive mechanisms, participants should be urged to contribute computing power. Additionally, it might be necessary to motivate health organizations to use blockchain technology and sign up for the shared network. The more parties involved, the greater the impact of the blockchain will be [78].

11.9 FUTURE BLOCKCHAIN RESEARCH DIRECTIONS

New features have been added as the blockchain has developed in order to increase certainty and expandability. The multi-channel blockchain network, which enables users to access data and communicate privately, is a key component. Each channel in this network corresponds to a separate chain of transactions. A concept like this enables hospitals and groups of patients to share information while confirming sealed data access and system expandability. Data privacy worries are not completely dispelled by blockchain technology. Threatening actors stealing private keys could still jeopardize data security and patient privacy. Governance issues are also brought up by the small number of links in a federation or trade healthcare blockchain. The risks posed by these vulnerabilities will necessitate the use of complete internet safety analysis, namely probing testing. Finally, storing massive amounts of health information on a blockchain is simply not a viable option. To keep this data on the blockchain, every node would have to access it, severely limiting the use of healthcare apps on a decentralized network. Unresolved cache options, such as a central fact or decentralized entrepot, such as the cloud must be investigated.

11.10 CONCLUSION

Blockchain has the potential to completely transform the healthcare ecosystem through secure data sharing. We conclude that a new electronic health system generates efficient, expansive, and cooperative systems capable of delivering top-notch patient care and making important strides in the treatment of diseases. The proposed system combines blockchain and edge computing to allow for the exchange of massive amounts of medical data produced by various healthcare organizations while preserving patient privacy. In this study, we also discussed the application of blockchain technology in the fight against the COVID-19 pandemic. By offering better solutions, outbreak tracking, user privacy protection, medical supply chain performance, donation tracking, and secure day-to-day operations, this technology can help during this pandemic crisis. Blockchain technology should be applied in a way that decreases network latency and offers a secure environment for transferring and stowing important data. The most effective way to combat deadly pandemics like the coronavirus is by combining blockchain technology with other cutting-edge technologies like AI, big data, and cloud computing. Additionally, in order to guarantee a swift response, scalability, and secure medical data transmission within the blockchain network, we defined a novel mechanism. The performance of the health system as a whole can be markedly improved while satisfying the needs of various applications by mapping the characteristics of the collected data onto an appropriate blockchain configuration.

ACKNOWLEDGMENTS

I would like to thank my co-authors for contributing their time, support, and knowledge to the execution of the work.

CONFLICTS OF INTEREST

The authors declare no conflict of interest.

KEYWORDS

- **blockchain**
- **COVID-19**
- **data transfer**
- **health contract caller**
- **medical sensors**
- **patient monitoring system**
- **validation**

REFERENCES

1. Aujla, G. S., & Jindal, A., (2020). A decoupled blockchain approach for edge-envisioned IoT-based healthcare monitoring. *IEEE Journal on Selected Areas in Communications*, *39*(2), 491–499.
2. Attaran, M., (2022). Blockchain technology in healthcare: Challenges and opportunities. *International Journal of Healthcare Management*, *15*(1), 70–83.
3. Vahdati, M., Gholizadeh, H. K., & Saghiri, A. M., (2021). IoT-Based healthcare monitoring using blockchain. In: *Applications of Blockchain in Healthcare* (pp. 141–170). Springer, Singapore.

4. Barka, E., Dahmane, S., Kerrache, C. A., Khayat, M., & Sallabi, F., (2021). STHM: A secured and trusted healthcare monitoring architecture using SDN and blockchain. *Electronics*, *10*(15), 1787.
5. Jeong, S., Shen, J. H., & Ahn, B., (2021). A study on smart healthcare monitoring using IoT based on blockchain. *Wireless Communications and Mobile Computing, 2021.*
6. Tan, H., Kim, P., & Chung, I., (2020). Practical homomorphic authentication in cloud-assisted vanets with blockchain-based healthcare monitoring for pandemic control. *Electronics*, *9*(10), 1683.
7. Narayana, V. L., Gopi, A. P., & Chaitanya, K., (2019). Avoiding interoperability and delay in healthcare monitoring system using block chain technology. *Rev. D'intelligence Artif.*, *33*(1), 45–48.
8. Sharmila, A. H., & Jaisankar, N., (2021). Edge intelligent agent assisted hybrid hierarchical blockchain for continuous healthcare monitoring & recommendation system in 5G WBAN-IoT. *Computer Networks*, *200*, 108508.
9. Ratta, P., Kaur, A., Sharma, S., Shabaz, M., & Dhiman, G., (2021). Application of blockchain and internet of things in healthcare and medical sector: Applications, challenges, and future perspectives. *Journal of Food Quality*, *2021.*
10. Hathaliya, J., Sharma, P., Tanwar, S., & Gupta, R., (2019). Blockchain-based remote patient monitoring in healthcare 4.0. In: *2019 IEEE 9th International Conference on Advanced Computing (IACC)* (pp. 87–91). IEEE.
11. Awotunde, J. B., Chakraborty, C., & Folorunso, S. O., (2022). A secured smart healthcare monitoring system using blockchain technology. In: *Intelligent Internet of Things for Healthcare and Industry* (pp. 127–143). Springer, Cham.
12. Haleem, A., Javaid, M., Singh, R. P., Suman, R., & Rab, S., (2021). Blockchain technology applications in healthcare: An overview. *International Journal of Intelligent Networks*, *2*, 130–139.
13. Chen, H. S., Jarrell, J. T., Carpenter, K. A., Cohen, D. S., & Huang, X., (2019). Blockchain in healthcare: A patient-centered model. *Biomedical Journal of Scientific & Technical Research*, *20*(3), 15017.
14. Griggs, K. N., Ossipova, O., Kohlios, C. P., Baccarini, A. N., Howson, E. A., & Hayajneh, T., (2018). Healthcare blockchain system using smart contracts for secure automated remote patient monitoring. *Journal of Medical Systems*, *42*(7), 1–7.
15. Bay, J., Kek, J., Tan, A., & Hau, C. S., (2020). BlueTrace: A privacy-preserving protocol for community-driven contact tracing across borders.
16. Idrees, S. M., Nowostawski, M., & Jameel, R., (2021). Blockchain-based digital contact tracing apps for COVID-19 pandemic management: Issues, challenges, solutions, and future directions. *JMIR Med. Inform., 9*, e25245.
17. Garg, C., Bansal, A., & Padappayil, R. P., (2020). COVID-19: Prolonged social distancing implementation strategy using blockchain-based movement passes. *J. Med. Syst., 44*, 165.
18. Xu, H., Zhang, L., Onireti, O., Fang, Y., Buchanan, W. B., & Imran, M. A., (2020). "BeepTrace: Blockchain-Enabled Privacy-Preserving Contact Tracing for COVID-19 Pandemic and Beyond." *IEEE Internet of Things Journal, 8*(5), 3915–3929, 1 March1, 2021, doi: 10.1109/JIOT.2020.3025953.
19. Eisenstadt, M., Ramachandran, M., Chowdhury, N., Third, A., & Domingue, J., (2020). COVID-19 antibody test/vaccination certification: There's an app for that. *IEEE Open J. Eng. Med. Biol., 1*, 148–155.

20. Hasan, H. R., Salah, K., Jayaraman, R., et al., (2020). *Blockchain-Based Solution for COVID-19 Digital Medical Passports and Immunity Certificates*. TechRxiv.
21. Bansal, A., Garg, C., & Padappayil, R. P., (2020). Optimizing the implementation of COVID-19 "immunity certificates" using blockchain. *J. Med. Syst., 44*, 140.
22. De Aguiar, E. J., Faiçal, B. S., Krishnamachari, B., & Ueyama, J., (2020). A survey of blockchain-based strategies for healthcare. *ACM Computing Surveys (CSUR), 53*(2), 1–27.
23. Agbo, C. C., & Mahmoud, Q. H., (2020). Blockchain in healthcare: Opportunities, challenges, and possible solutions. *International Journal of Healthcare Information Systems and Informatics (IJHISI), 15*(3), 82–97.
24. Ben, F. R., & Lahami, M., (2020). Application of blockchain technology in healthcare: A comprehensive study. In: *International Conference on Smart Homes and Health Telematics* (pp. 268–276). Springer, Cham.
25. Siyal, A. A., Junejo, A. Z., Zawish, M., Ahmed, K., Khalil, A., & Soursou, G., (2019). Applications of blockchain technology in medicine and healthcare: Challenges and future perspectives. *Cryptography, 3*(1), 3.
26. Abu-Elezz, I., Hassan, A., Nazeemudeen, A., Househ, M., & Abd-Alrazaq, A., (2020). The benefits and threats of blockchain technology in healthcare: A scoping review. *International Journal of Medical Informatics, 142*, 104246.
27. Kordestani, H., Barkaoui, K., & Zahran, W., (2020). HapiChain: A blockchain-based framework for patient-centric telemedicine. In: *2020 IEEE 8th International Conference on Serious Games and Applications for Health (SeGAH)* (pp. 1–6). IEEE.
28. Kumar, T., Ramani, V., Ahmad, I., Braeken, A., Harjula, E., & Ylianttila, M., (2018). Blockchain utilization in healthcare: Key requirements and challenges. In: *2018 IEEE 20th International Conference on e-Health Networking, Applications and Services (Healthcom)* (pp. 1–7). IEEE.
29. Rakic, D., (2018). Blockchain technology in healthcare. In: *ICT4AWE* (pp. 13–20).
30. Faruk, M. J. H., Shahriar, H., Valero, M., Sneha, S., Ahamed, S. I., & Rahman, M., (2021). Towards blockchain-based secure data management for remote patient monitoring. In: *2021 IEEE International Conference on Digital Health (ICDH)* (pp. 299–308). IEEE.
31. Khezr, S., Moniruzzaman, M., Yassine, A., & Benlamri, R., (2019). Blockchain technology in healthcare: A comprehensive review and directions for future research. *Applied Sciences, 9*(9), 1736.
32. Zhuang, Y., Sheets, L., Shae, Z., Tsai, J. J., & Shyu, C. R., (2018). Applying blockchain technology for health information exchange and persistent monitoring for clinical trials. In: *AMIA Annual Symposium Proceedings* (Vol. 2018, p. 1167). American Medical Informatics Association.
33. Soni, R., & Kumar, G., (2019). A review on blockchain urgency in the internet of things in healthcare. In: *2019 International Conference on Intelligent Sustainable Systems (ICISS)* (pp. 578–583). IEEE.
34. Kumar, R., Kumar, P., Tripathi, R., Gupta, G. P., Islam, A. N., & Shorfuzzaman, M., (2022). Permissioned blockchain and deep-learning for secure and efficient data sharing in industrial healthcare systems. *IEEE Transactions on Industrial Informatics*.
35. Namasudra, S., & Deka, G. C., (2021). *Applications of Blockchain in Healthcare*. Singapore: Springer.

36. Hasselgren, A., Kralevska, K., Gligoroski, D., Pedersen, S. A., & Faxvaag, A., (2020). Blockchain in healthcare and health sciences—A scoping review. *International Journal of Medical Informatics, 134*, 104040.
37. Kazmi, H. S. Z., Nazeer, F., Mubarak, S., Hameed, S., Basharat, A., & Javaid, N., (2019). Trusted remote patient monitoring using blockchain-based smart contracts. In: *International Conference on Broadband and Wireless Computing, Communication and Applications* (pp. 765–776). Springer, Cham.
38. Engelhardt, M. A., (2017). Hitching healthcare to the chain: An introduction to blockchain technology in the healthcare sector. *Technology Innovation Management Review, 7*(10).
39. Yaeger, K., Martini, M., Rasouli, J., & Costa, A., (2019). Emerging blockchain technology solutions for modern healthcare infrastructure. *Journal of Scientific Innovation in Medicine, 2*(1).
40. Pilkington, M., (2017). Can blockchain improve healthcare management? Consumer medical electronics and the IoMT. *Consumer Medical Electronics and the IoMT.*
41. Giordanengo, A., (2019). Possible usages of smart contracts (blockchain) in healthcare and why no one is using them. In: *MEDINFO 2019: Health and Wellbeing e-Networks for All* (pp. 596–600). IOS Press.
42. Hölbl, M., Kompara, M., Kamišalić, A., & Nemec, Z. L., (2018). A systematic review of the use of blockchain in healthcare. *Symmetry, 10*(10), 470.
43. McGhin, T., Choo, K. K. R., Liu, C. Z., & He, D., (2019). Blockchain in healthcare applications: Research challenges and opportunities. *Journal of Network and Computer Applications, 135*, 62–75.
44. Kazmi, H. S. Z., Nazeer, F., Mubarak, S., Hameed, S., Basharat, A., & Javaid, N., (2019). Trusted remote patient monitoring using blockchain-based smart contracts. In: *International Conference on Broadband and Wireless Computing, Communication and Applications* (pp. 765–776). Springer, Cham.
45. Pirtle, C., & Ehrenfeld, J., (2018). Blockchain for healthcare: The next generation of medical records? *Journal of Medical Systems, 42*(9), 1–3.
46. Alam, T., (2020). *Internet of Things and Blockchain-Based Framework for Coronavirus (COVID-19) Disease.* Available at SSRN 3660503.
47. Fernández-Caramés, T. M., Froiz-Míguez, I., Blanco-Novoa, O., & Fraga-Lamas, P., (2019). Enabling the internet of mobile crowdsourcing health things: A mobile fog computing, blockchain and IoT based continuous glucose monitoring system for diabetes mellitus research and care. *Sensors, 19*(15), 3319.
48. Bhalaji, N., Abilashkumar, P. C., & Aboorva, S., (2019). A blockchain-based approach for privacy preservation in healthcare IoT. In: *International Conference on Intelligent Computing and Communication Technologies* (pp. 465–473). Springer, Singapore.
49. Rathore, H., Mohamed, A., & Guizani, M., (2020). Blockchain applications for healthcare. In: *Energy Efficiency of Medical Devices and Healthcare Applications* (pp. 153–166). Academic Press.
50. Fetjah, L., Azbeg, K., Ouchetto, O., & Andaloussi, S. J., (2021). Towards a smart healthcare system: An architecture based on IoT, blockchain, and fog computing. *International Journal of Healthcare Information Systems and Informatics (IJHISI), 16*(4), 1–18.
51. Pandey, S., Vanshika, Anshul, & Dwivedi, R. K. (2023)"A Secure Design of Healthcare System with Blockchain and Internet of Things (IoT)," *2023 International Conference*

on Intelligent Data Communication Technologies and Internet of Things (IDCIoT), Bengaluru, India, 2023, pp. 105–111, doi: 10.1109/IDCIoT56793.2023.10053491.

52. Ratta, P., Kaur, A., Sharma, S., Shabaz, M., & Dhiman, G., (2021). Application of blockchain and internet of things in healthcare and medical sector: Applications, challenges, and future perspectives. *Journal of Food Quality, 2021*.
53. Enescu, F. M., Bizon, N., Cirstea, A., & Stirbu, C., (2018). Blockchain technology applied in health is the study of blockchain application in the health system (I). In: *2018 10th International Conference on Electronics, Computers and Artificial Intelligence (ECAI)* (pp. 1–4). IEEE.
54. Heston, T., (2017). *A Case Study in Blockchain Healthcare Innovation* (November 24, 2017). Authorea Working Paper No AUTHOREA_213011_3643634, Available at SSRN: https://ssrn.com/abstract=3077455.
55. Ben, F. R., & Lahami, M., (2020). Application of blockchain technology in healthcare: A comprehensive study. In: *International Conference on Smart Homes and Health Telematics* (pp. 268–276). Springer, Cham.
56. Bhargava, R., (2019). Blockchain technology and its application: A review. *IUP Journal of Information Technology, 15*(1).
57. Baygin, N., Baygin, M., & Karakose, M., (2019). Blockchain technology: Applications, benefits, and challenges. In: *2019 1st International Informatics and Software Engineering Conference (UBMYK)* (pp. 1–5). IEEE.
58. Kumar, T., Ramani, V., Ahmad, I., Braeken, A., Harjula, E., & Ylianttila, M., (2018). Blockchain utilization in healthcare: Key requirements and challenges. In: *2018 IEEE 20th International Conference on e-Health Networking, Applications, and Services (Healthcom)* (pp. 1–7). IEEE.
59. Maesa, D. D. F., & Mori, P., (2020). Blockchain 3.0 applications survey. *Journal of Parallel and Distributed Computing, 138*, 99–114.
60. Lee, C. K., (2019). Blockchain application with health token in medical & health industrials. In: *2nd International Conference on Social Science, Public Health, and Education (SSPHE 2018)* (pp. 233–236). Atlantis Press.
61. Srivastava, S., Singh, S. V., Singh, R. B., & Shukla, H. K., (2021). Digital transformation of healthcare: A blockchain study. *International Journal of Innovative Science, Engineering & Technology, 8*(5).
62. Sharma, Y., Balamurugan, B., & Khan, F., (2020). Blockchain and big data in the healthcare sector. In: *Blockchain, Big Data and Machine Learning* (pp. 207–231). CRC Press.
63. Rejeb, A., Keogh, J. G., & Treiblmaier, H., (2019). The impact of blockchain on medical tourism. In: *Workshop on E-Business* (pp. 29–40). Springer, Cham.
64. Fatima, N., Agarwal, P., & Sohail, S. S., (2022). Security and privacy issues of blockchain technology in health care—A review. *ICT Analysis and Applications*, 193–201.
65. Laroiya, C., Saxena, D., & Komalavalli, C., (2020). Applications of blockchain technology. In: *Handbook of Research on Blockchain Technology* (pp. 213–243). Academic Press.
66. Reegu, F. A., Mohd, S., Hakami, Z., Reegu, K. K., & Alam, S., (2021). Towards trustworthiness of electronic health record system using blockchain. *Annals of the Romanian Society for Cell Biology, 25*(6), 2425–2434.
67. Yfantis, V., Leligou, H. C., & Ntalianis, K., (2021). New development: Blockchain—A revolutionary tool for the public sector. *Public Money & Management, 41*(5), 408–411.

68. Nwosu, A. U., Goyal, S. B., & Bedi, P., (2020). Blockchain transforming cyber-attacks: Healthcare industry. In: *International Conference on Innovations in Bio-Inspired Computing and Applications* (pp. 258–266). Springer, Cham.
69. Sun, B., Lv, Z., & Li, Q., (2021). Obstetrics nursing and medical health system based on blockchain technology. *Journal of Healthcare Engineering, 2021.*
70. Mackey, T. K., Kuo, T. T., Gummadi, B., Clauson, K. A., Church, G., Grishin, D., & Palombini, M., (2019). 'Fit-for-purpose?'–challenges and opportunities for applications of blockchain technology in the future of healthcare. *BMC Medicine*, *17*(1), 1–17.
71. Pandey, P., & Litoriya, R., (2021). Securing e-health networks from counterfeit medicine penetration using blockchain. *Wireless Personal Communications*, *117*(1), 7–25.
72. Prokofieva, M., & Miah, S. J., (2019). Blockchain in healthcare. *Australasian Journal of Information Systems*, *23*.
73. Gupta, M., Tanwar, S., Badotra, S., & Rana, A., (2022). A systematic review on blockchain in transforming the healthcare sector. *Transformations Through Blockchain Technology*, 181–200.
74. Premkumar, A., & Srimathi, C., (2020). Application of blockchain and IoT towards pharmaceutical industry. In: *2020 6th International Conference on Advanced Computing and Communication Systems (ICACCS)* (pp. 729–733). IEEE.
75. Narikimilli, N. R. S., Kumar, A., Antu, A. D., & Xie, B., (2020). Blockchain applications in healthcare–A review and future perspective. In: *International Conference on Blockchain* (pp. 198–218). Springer, Cham.
76. Ghazal, T. M., Alshurideh, M. T., & Alzoubi, H. M., (2021). Blockchain-enabled internet of things (IoT) platforms for pharmaceutical and biomedical research. In: *The International Conference on Artificial Intelligence and Computer Vision* (pp. 589–600). Springer, Cham.
77. Unnithan, C., Houghton, A., Anema, A., & Lemieux, V., (2019). Blockchain in global health: An appraisal of current and future applications. In: *Essentials of Blockchain Technology* (pp. 189–204). Chapman and Hall/CRC.
78. Quasim, M. T., Algarni, F., Radwan, A. A. E., & Alshmrani, G. M. M., (2020). A blockchain based secured healthcare framework. In: The *2020 International Conference on Computational Performance Evaluation (ComPE).*

CHAPTER 12

Secure Data Transmission Based on Deep Q-Learning Architecture with Internet of Things Module in Healthcare Application

B. SATHIYAPRASAD[1] and B. SATHEESH KUMAR[2]

[1]*Department of Computer Science and Engineering, Sathyabama Institute of Science and Technology, Rajiv Gandhi Salai, Chennai, Tamil Nadu, India*

[2]*Department of Computer Science and Engineering, Galgotia University, Yamuna Expressway, Greater Noida, Uttar Pradesh, India*

ABSTRACT

Intelligent healthcare intends to provide a platform to remotely monitor users' health-related data based on wearable devices as the Internet of Things (IoT) develops. The development of blockchain and AI technologies also supports the advancement of secure, intelligent healthcare. Data is still susceptible to attack and privacy leaks because they are kept on a cloud server. In order to ensure patient safety and privacy when utilizing medical equipment, patient information, such as health status, must be protected. Experts securely exchange information about healthcare in order to analyze healthcare and give patients timely care. Deep Learning (DL) algorithms and other recent cryptographic and biometric systems have been widely employed to authenticate and detect abnormalities in order to ensure protection for healthcare systems. Since the grid's sensors are energy-constrained procedures, a security mechanism based on DL techniques has been

Creating Smart Healthcare with Blockchain and Advanced Digital Technology.
Rishabha Malviya and Sonali Sundram (Eds.)

implemented. Security and efficiency must be balanced. In order to protect data transmission from exterior extortions with minimal encryption and decryption time, a novel framework known as deep Q-learning based neural network with privacy preservation technique (DQ-NNPP) was developed in this work. Comparatively, the suggested model performed better than various conventional methods. Parametric analysis has been carried out in terms of accuracy, sensitivity, specificity, communication overhead, encryption time, and decryption time.

12.1 INTRODUCTION

The internet of things (IoT) utilizes IP-based communication for connecting the internet with sensors and a multitude of procedures. For instance, healthcare sectors with IoT can achieve remote monitoring, early diagnosis, treatment, and prevention [1]. Moreover, objects or people can be furnished with sensors, such as radio-frequency identification (RFID) tags, and actuators, in IoT to monitor the status. RFID tags or personal medical devices of patients are comprehensible, locatable, identifiable, and well-regulated using IoT applications [2]. Several smart applications and services can overcome the challenges faced by individuals and the healthcare industry [3]. Machines, humans, dynamic systems, and smart devices are intellectually connected to ensure the efficiency of the healthcare system [4].

In general, the structure of IoT is comprised of three layers, namely perception, network, and application layers. The perception layer is responsible for collecting healthcare data using several devices [5]. The role of the network layer, which consists of wired, wireless, and middleware systems, is to process and transmit the input from the perception layer. When designed efficiently, transport protocols can improve the efficiency of data transmission, decrease energy consumption, and make sure security and confidentiality [6]. The application layer combines sources of medical data and offers medical services that satisfy the needs of the user based on the current situation and demand. Security and privacy of information related to patients are the most essential concepts in an IoT-based environment [7].

Data security can be achieved by storing and securely transferring data, ensuring integrity, authenticity, and validity. Privacy of data is achieved when data are accessed only by authorized individuals [8]. Based on the demands, purposes, and needs, protection strategies can be reasonably developed.

Although widely used IoT devices can help improve the health of patients, securing and protecting human information must be achieved at the same time. As attacks have increased on the next-generation systems, IoT devices are vulnerable to both known as well as unknown attacks [9]. Data that flow IoT domain to the cloud and visualization domains get altered at several points in the hierarchy of the cloud.

The conventional systems based on signature or machine learning (ML) approaches are not capable of dealing with the current situation due to the frequent occurrence of unknown attacks. Deep neural networks (DNNs) can detect a virtualized communication network failure by recognizing the normal data flow and reconstructing it to produce higher accuracy [10]. However, the major challenge faced with these models is that it takes more time for training complex DNNs in the core clouds compared to existing traditional methods. Hence, it is necessary to develop innovative approaches that reduce the training time without compromising detection accuracy.

The objectives of this work were to:

- Construct a systematic framework using the deep Q-learning method for processing patient data, which further reduces the traffic in a network.
- Adopt the Ciphertext-Policy Attribute-Based Privacy Preservation (Cip-PolAttPrivPre).
- Communicate with diagnosed patients in a securable way with less communication cost and error.

12.2 RELATED WORKS

Ahmad et al. [11] used advanced counterfeit savvy ways to develop a model that preserves information security in the cloud. This model consists of two main stages: sterilization and recovery of information. The process of sterilization depends on the generation technique. A multi-objective capability was determined with the ratio of a boundary to generate the optimal key. Deebak et al. [12] developed a Solid and Unknown Biometric Based-Client Verification Plan, which ensures secure communication in the healthcare industry. Results showed that a fraud cannot act as a genuine client to access or manipulate a handheld smart card. Wang et al. [13] designed a forward security protection method for healthcare systems based on IoT. This scheme includes a hidden gateway stage for exchanging the status counter, making it difficult for the enemy to determine the valid status counter of the record with just the user's public key.

Kwabena et al. [14] developed an intelligent framework called MSCryptoNet that enables a flexible implementation approach to approximate an activation function that is commonly used in Sigmoid and ReLU of CNNs with low-degree polynomials. Keshavarzian et al. [15] designed a Modified Deep Residual Network, in which new smooth pooling layers are defined to enhance the performance of the model. The researchers also proposed a method to recognize human activities in an IoT cloud environment, thus enabling users to create scenarios based on their actions at home. Functionality as a Service architecture was employed to solve the problem of scalability, whereby each functionality was implemented in a distinct container. Zhang et al. [16] developed the Privacy Preserving Disease Prediction method to efficiently encrypt and then store patients' medical data in a cloud server for further processing. Prediction models were trained with the Single-Layer Perceptron learning method.

Although the review of related works reveals that much focus has been directed towards developing secure and privacy models for the healthcare sector, improved security and privacy have yet to be achieved. Conversely, several privacy systems are not suitable for providing effective security measures. To overcome these problems [17].

12.3 SYSTEM MODEL

Private patient data, which is essential for hospital applications, is uploaded to centralized locations. Then, ML techniques utilize this data to extract unique patterns for developing models. When such private data becomes visible to the members of the company or if the company dataset is hacked, insider and outsider threats occur, respectively.

As shown in Figure 12.1, the constructed model applies neural network techniques for maintaining the security and privacy of healthcare information. Here, several intermediate attacks are encountered by the system, and hence, unauthorized access to the cloud storage must be eliminated. Once user data is obtained, for every request made, the features are extracted and stored to analyze the malware activities and issues related to security and privacy. From these features, the quality value of data can be determined with the use of feature states, and their corresponding actions help to determine the data quality.

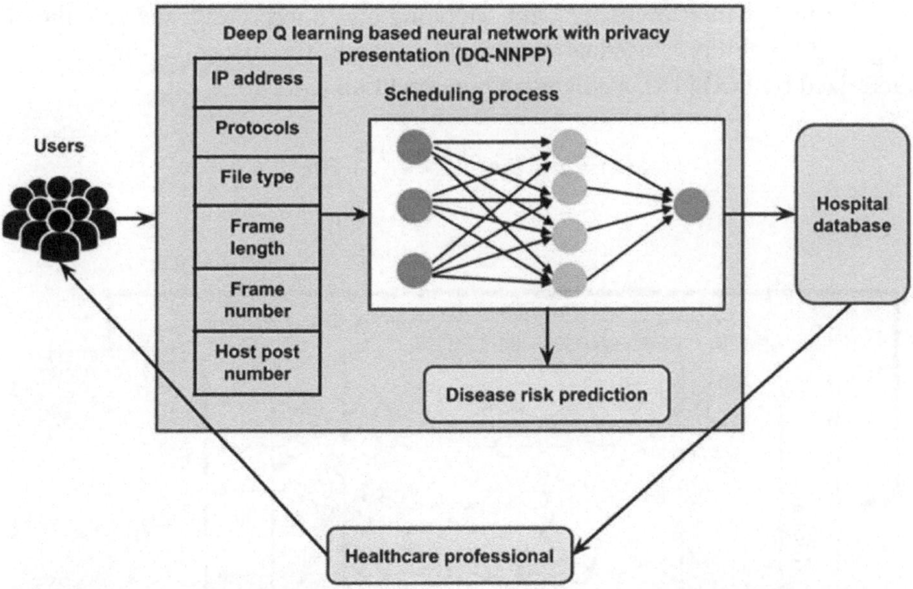

FIGURE 12.1 System architecture of privacy preservation method in IoT healthcare infrastructure.

12.3.1 DEEP Q-LEARNING-BASED SCHEDULING AND DATA TRANSMISSION

Input = [a_1 to f_1, a_2 to f_2, …, a_n to f_n] addresses information of a framework state, and a+b demonstrates number of neurons in layer. The result layer addressing data of the choice activity is represented in Figure 12.2, which contains channel (m) in correspondence mode j and support k with a+b+J neurons. The secret layer is made out of a few layers, and the quantity of neurons is assessed utilizing conditions (1) and (2):

$$N(h) = \sqrt{n(i)} + n(o) + con \tag{1}$$

$$W = \{w_{ij}\} \in (n * m)\} \tag{2}$$

where; n(i), n(o), and N(h) are quantities of information, yield, and secret layers separately; Con demonstrates a steady restricted in Con [1,10], and w_{ij} addresses the load between the ith visible and j^{th} stowed away cells.

For the method involved with encoding and interpreting, the calculated sigmoid capability is used as an exchange capability. Cost capability is characterized by L(x) [18], as displayed in condition (3):

$$L(x) = arg\ min \sum_{i=1}^{n} \frac{xi - fi}{2} + j(m) \tag{3}$$

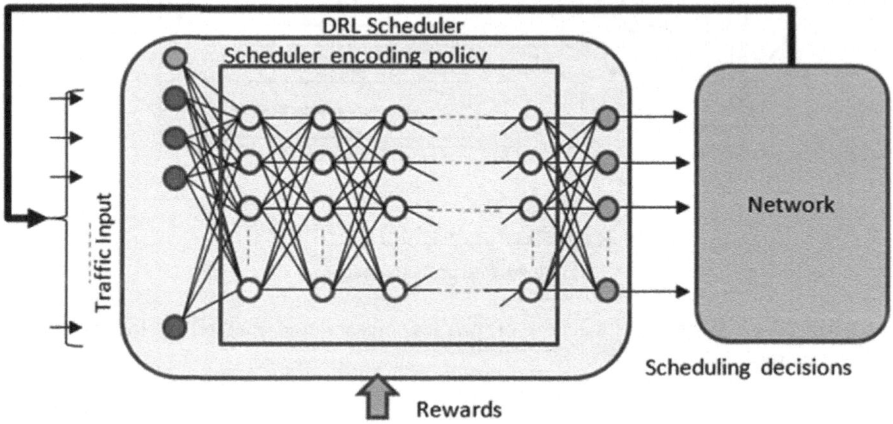

FIGURE 12.2 Data scheduling from patients using deep Q-learning.

where *J*(*m*) is the weight decay that reduces the weight, thereby preventing over-fitting during training. To update the weight and bias vector, the rules in Eqns. (4) and (5) are used:

$$W(k+1) = W(k) - \beta \tag{4}$$

$$b(k+1) = b(k) - \beta \tag{5}$$

where β is the learning rate.

Backpropagation of residual error is δ, which is given in Eqns. (6) and (7):

$$\Delta im = \Delta im + 1 \times W_{ij} \times fm \tag{6}$$

$$A = \{bi \in Rn\} \tag{7}$$

where; bj is the bias threshold of jth visible cell. Consider that the noticeable and secret layers follow Bernoulli circulation, then the request for (v,h) is addressed as displayed in condition (8):

$$E(v,h \mid \theta) = -\sum n_i = 1 a_i v_i - \sum m_j = 1 b_j h_j - \sum n_j = 1 \sum n_j = 1 v_j w_{ij} h_j \quad (8)$$

where; $\theta = \{W_{ij}, a_i, b_j\}$; what's more, the energy capability demonstrates the energy assessed in each hub of the apparent and secret layers.

12.3.2 *SYSTEM MODEL FOR SECURITY*

Here, the security of medical record datasets and preserving the privacy of patients and hospitals are achieved. This model contains a trusted authority (TA), Hospitals with healthcare professionals, patients (USER), and Servers, as shown in Figure 12.3.

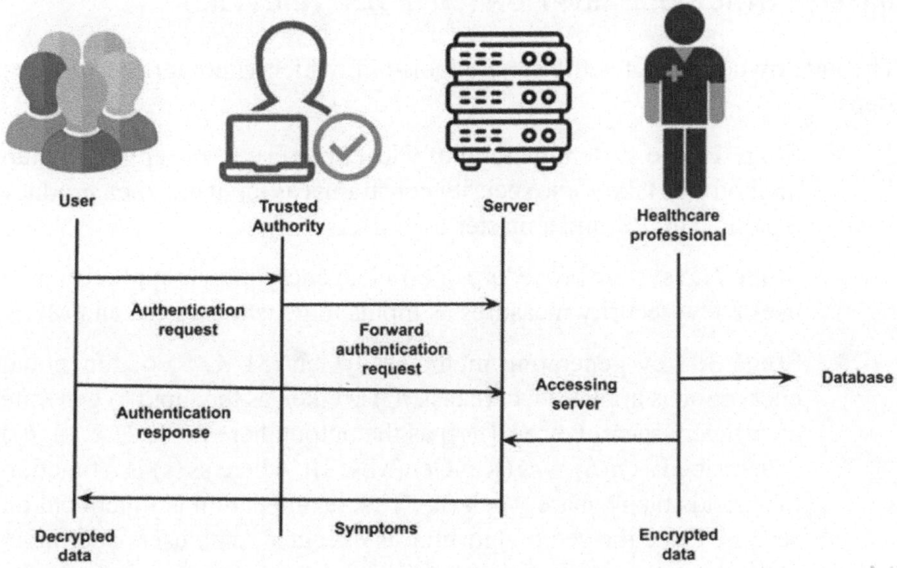

FIGURE 12.3 System model for securable data transmission to the healthcare provider.

The roles of each entity in the system model are described below:

- TA generates the parameters and deals with registration.
- Hospitals supply patients' medical information to the servers.

- The USER queries the doctors about the source and destination stages.
- Interaction between the servers generates a portion of the clinical pathway, which in turn is returned to the USER. Multiple interactions are allowed to occur with other interactions instead of between the hospital and USER, thereby effectively reducing the local communication overhead and computational cost.

In this model, data (k = 1, 2, 3, …, m) of clinical datasets incorporate subtleties of the patients, like name, age, orientation, costs, other files, drug, and season of arrangements. These subtleties are shared and safeguarded by the Ciphertext-Policy Attribute-Based Privacy Preservation approach. In light of these protection approaches, the server makes a coordinated directional associated network.

12.3.3 GENERATION OF KEY ON CIPHERTEXT-POLICY ATTRIBUTE-BASED PRIVACY PRESERVATION (CIP-POLATTPRIVPRE)

The data owner executes the setup algorithm, which is comprised of three steps:

- **Stage 1:** The system method of Cip-PolAttPrivPre is applied, setup method will take some security constraints as input and then produce a public key PK and a master key MK.
- **Stage 2:** A system procedure of efficient encryption is applied, which uses a few security measures as inputs to generate a PKF and MKF.
- **Stage 3:** Key generating method KeyGen (M K, S) of functional encryption is applied, where task $f(i)$ is taken as the input to generate an efficient secret key SK[f(i)] as the output, here i = 1, 2, …, n. $f(i)$ is described as $fi(S) = ss_i(\text{KeyGen(MK,S)})$, where $ss_i(s)$ is a function that yields the ith share when (n, k) secret allocation is functional on secrets. Once the setup algorithm is executed, data users and the ith authority receive PK_F and SK [f_i] sent by the data owner over the secure channel, respectively.

In this process, a large number of subkeys are used, which are pre-computed before the encryption or decryption process. P-array contains 18 to 32-bit subkeys: *P1*, *P2*, …, *P18*.

Algorithm for Generating Subkeys

Input-plain text

Output-sub-keys

Strings(x)=P1, P2, P3, …, Pn

if

A= P1(XOR) P2

(P1 = n; P1 < n+1)

B= P2(XOR) P3

(P2 = n;P2<n+1)

C= P3(XOR) P4

(P1 = n;P1<n+1)

N= Pn(XOR) Pn

(P1 = n;P1<n+1)

End if

*A1 = M*N* (D mode)*

*A2 = S*W*(Q mod X)*

*A3 = Y*X*(C mod G)*

*βA1 = α2 (C*V* (B mod X))*

*βA2 = α2 (Y*H*(K mod L))*

*βK3 = α2 (Q*W*(M mod N))end*

12.3.4 ENCRYPTION PROCESS

Parameter A is assigned a positive numeral value, such that $A \neq k \times 257$, where k ranges from 1 to n. Consider an array T taking values from 0 to 255, thus a total of 256 unique integers. A new array R is obtained based on A and T, which follows linear mapping [20] as given in Eqn. (9):

$$R(i) = mod\left(\left(A \times (T(i)+1)\right)\right).257 \tag{9}$$

where; 'I' range from 1 to 256; $T(i)$ takes values from 0 to 255; the positive integer A satisfies $A \neq k \times 257$; and k takes up an integer greater than 0. ($A/257$) and ($T(i)$+1)/257 yield non-integer values, such that they are not exactly divisible by 257. Thus, mod (($A\times(T(i)+1)$), 257) is non-zero. Consider $R(i) \leftarrow R(i) - 1$, then $R(i)$ ranges from 0 to 255, where is 1 to 256. The 1D array $R = \{R(i)\}$ is then transformed into a 2D matrix R_b, which is the initial S-Box.

The tent – the logistic map is then repeated *L* times for generating a chaotic series with length *L*. The sensitivity of the chaotic series is improved, as the first (*L*-256) elements are discarded from the actual chaotic series, therefore obtaining a new chaotic series with length 256 denoted as *X*. By sorting *X*, a key group $J = \{J(1), J(2), \ldots, J(256)\}$ is obtained. As the chaotic series is non-periodic and ergodic, it certainly gives $J(i) \neq J(j)$ provided that $i \neq j$.

12.3.5 COMMUNICATION WITH DIAGNOSED PATIENTS

A unique ID is generated by each hospital based on the logic and node distance, as shown in Eqn. (12.10):

$$d_i\left(H_i, H_j\right) = \frac{\sum_{p,q \in \{Hi \cup H_j - H_i \cap H_j\}} \left(x_{pq}^{H_i} + x_{pq}^{H_j}\right)}{\sum_{pq \in H_i \cup H_j} \left(x_{pq}^{H_i} + x_{pq}^{H_j}\right)} \tag{10}$$

where; H_i and H_j are nodes with IDs of $H_i(id)$ and $H_i(id)$, respectively; p is the source; and q is the destination.

Data privacy is secured in a decentralized way [20] using a randomized approach for two nodes of hospitals, as shown in Eqn. (12.11):

$$Hr[(R0) \in S] \leq \exp(\in).Hr[R') \in o] \tag{11}$$

where; *R* and R_0 represent adjacent data records; and O indicates the set of data received as output. $R \in S$ achieves data privacy, but for several hospitals, Laplace is applied to the local training model m_i, as shown in Eqn. (12.12):

$$\overrightarrow{m_1} = m_i + Laplace\left(\frac{s}{\in}\right) \tag{12}$$

where; *s* stands for sensitivity; and $\in$ indicates the total cost for transmission.

For the preservation of data privacy in hospitals, encryption is provided on every data by public and private keys (PK_i, PK_i) . MAE (mean absolute error) estimates every transaction and broadcasts H_j via *MAE* (m_i) and *MAE* (H_j). Every record of the approved transaction is maintained in the distributed ledger. MAE is given in Eqn. (12.13):

$$MAE\left(m_i\right) = \frac{1}{n} \sum_{i=l}^{n} | y_i - f\left(x_i\right) | \tag{13}$$

where; 'n' represents the total number of users; and $MAE\ (x_i\ and\ y_i)$ indicate communication and transaction cost, respectively. Sharing personal data is a risk for data providers due to some specific security attacks. This can be defeated by simply transmitting data to the user with valid details to the requester and preserving the data privacy of the holders. Rather than sharing the actual data, learned models alone can be exchanged by the data provided like hospitals with the requester.

12.4 PERFORMANCE ANALYSIS

For analysis, accuracy, sensitivity, specificity, communication overhead, encryption time, and decryption time were selected as the parameters. The proposed DQ-NNPP was compared with three standard methods, namely SAB-UAS (secure and anonymous biometric based-user authentication scheme), MSCryptoNet, and Privacy-PPDP, based on these parameters.

Precision defines the limit of the total assumption made through the proposed architecture. The definition for precision is given in condition (12.14):

$$Accuracy = \frac{TP + TN}{TP + TN + FP + FN} \tag{14}$$

Figure 12.4 illustrates SAB-UAS, MSCryptoNet, PPDP (privacy-preserving disease prediction) methods and the proposed DQ-NNPP technique. While related, existing SAB-UAS, MSCryptoNet and PPDP technique achieved an accuracy of 92.02%, 94.3%, and 93.04%. The proposed DQ-NNPP method achieved 93.74% accuracy, which is 1.76% better than SAB-UAS, 0.7% better than PPDP method but only slightly worse (1.24%) than MSCryptoNet.

1. **Sensitivity:** It states the effectiveness of the scheduling technique. It is measured as the possibility of the optimistic calculation of recognized features and defined by true positive rate (TPR), as given in Eqn. (12.15):

$$Sensitivity = \frac{TP}{TP + FP} \tag{15}$$

Figure 12.5 illustrates comparison of sensitivity between existing SAB-UAS, MSCryptoNet, and PPDP techniques and proposed DQ-NNPP strategy. X-pivot presents number of ages utilized for examination, and

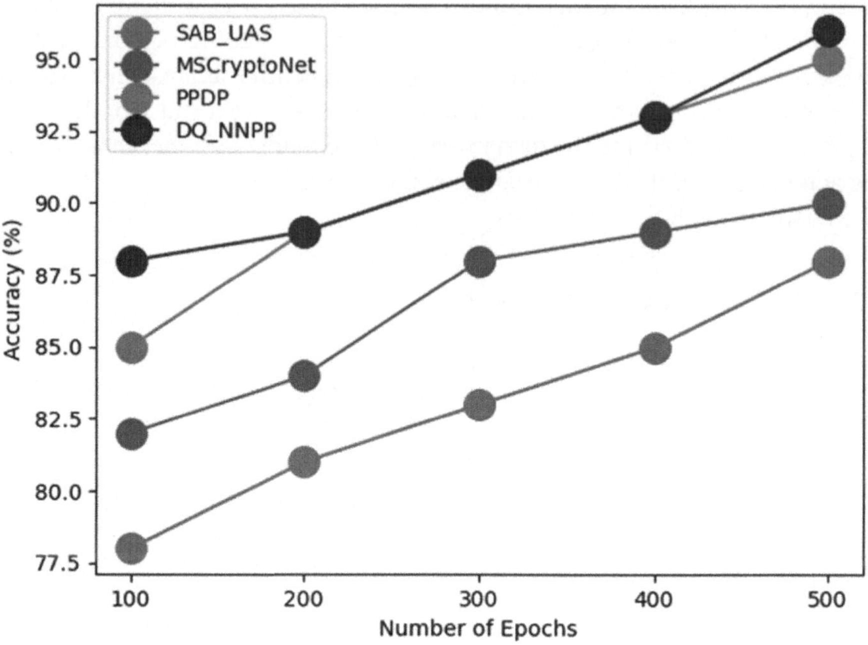

FIGURE 12.4 Comparison of accuracy.

Y-hub shows responsiveness values acquired in rate. The current SAB-UAS, MSCryptoNet, and PPDP techniques achieved a sensitivity of 79.4%, 84.72%, and 86.42%. Comparatively, the proposed DQ-NNPP method achieved 92% sensitivity, which is 13.4%, 8.72%, and 6.42% better than SAB-UAS, MSCryptoNet, and PPDP methods, respectively.

Explicitness is the likelihood of genuine negatives that are suitably recognized and is additionally named True Negative Rate (TNR). The recipe for explicitness is given in condition (12.16):

$$specificity = \frac{TP}{TP = FN} \tag{16}$$

Figure 12.6 compares the specificity of the existing SAB-UAS, MSCryptoNet, PPDP, and proposed DQ-NNPP method, where the number of epochs used for analysis is given on the X-axis, and specificity values obtained in percentage are on the Y-axis. The existing SAB-UAS, MSCryptoNet, and PPDP methods achieved a specificity of 90.7%, 91.44%, and 91.58%, respectively. In comparison, the proposed DQ-NNPP method achieved

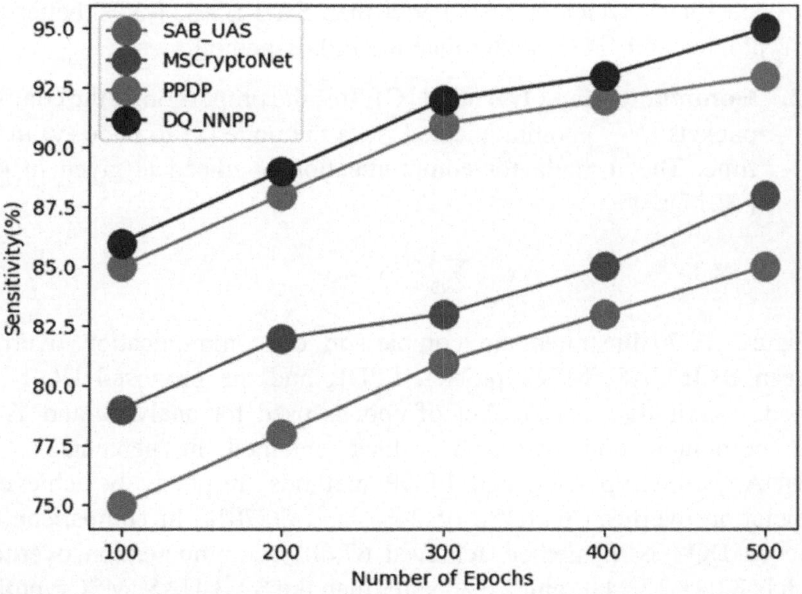

FIGURE 12.5 Comparison of sensitivity.

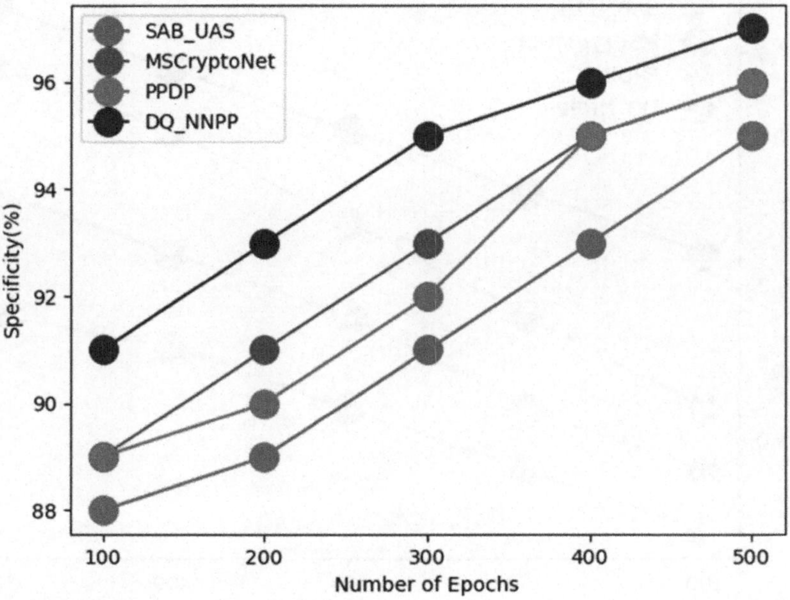

FIGURE 12.6 Comparison of specificity.

92.1% specificity, which is 2.6% better than SAB-UAS, 1.34% better than MSCryptoNet, and 1.48% better than the PPDP method.

2. **Communication Overhead (C):** It is the proportion of the complete packets (N_{pack}) communicated from the node (x) to node (y) in less time. The formula for communication overhead is given in Eqn. (12.17):

$$C = \sum_{0}^{N\,pack} x \rightarrow y \tag{17}$$

Figure 12.7 illustrates the comparison of communication overhead between SAB-UAS, MSCryptoNet, PPDP, and the proposed DQ-NNPP method. X-axis displays number of epochs used for analysis, and Y-axis gives communication overhead values obtained in percentage. The SAB-UAS, MSCryptoNet, and PPDP methods, respectively achieved a computation overhead 64.62%, 65.24%, and 66.76%. In comparison, the proposed DQ-NNPP method achieved 67.08% communication overhead, which is 3.04%, 2.24%, and 2.3% better than the SAB-UAS, MSCryptoNet, and PPDP methods, respectively.

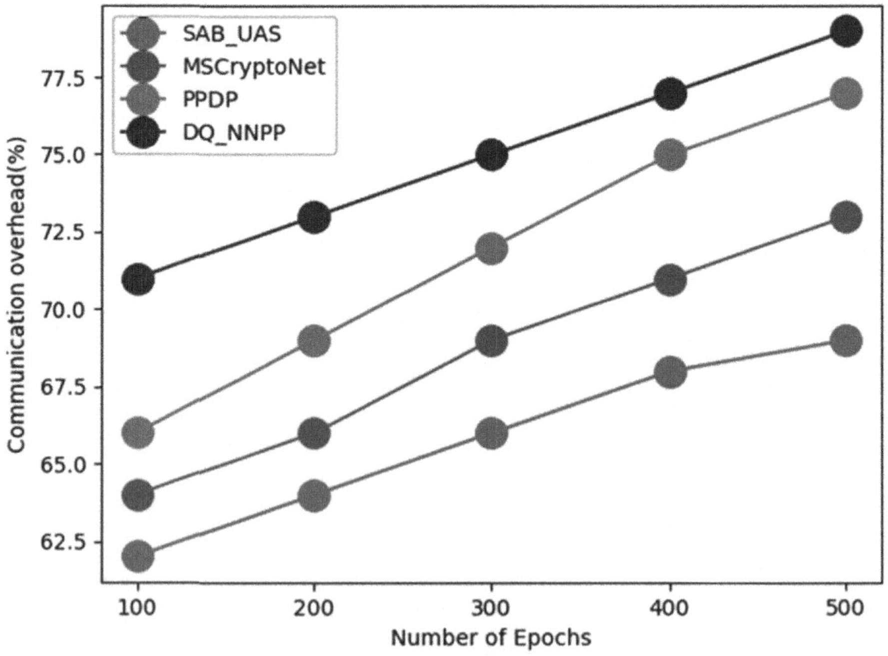

FIGURE 12.7 Comparison of communication overhead.

3. **Encryption Time (E):** It is the time taken by the algorithm to convert plain text (P) into cipher text (C) using the asymmetric or asymmetric keys. The formula for encryption time is defined in Eqn. (12.18):

$$E = Time(P \rightarrow C) \tag{18}$$

Figure 12.8 presents the evaluation of encryption time in the middle of existing techniques and the proposed technique, in which the number of epochs used for analysis is given on the X-axis and the encryption time values in milliseconds are on the Y-axis. When compared, existing SAB-UAS, MSCryptoNet, and PPDP methods achieved encryption times of 64, 62.2, and 60.52 ms, respectively. Comparatively, the proposed DQ-NNPP method achieved an encryption time of 58.72 ms, which is 6.72, 4.4, and 2.3 ms faster than the SAB-UAS, MSCryptoNet, and PPDP methods.

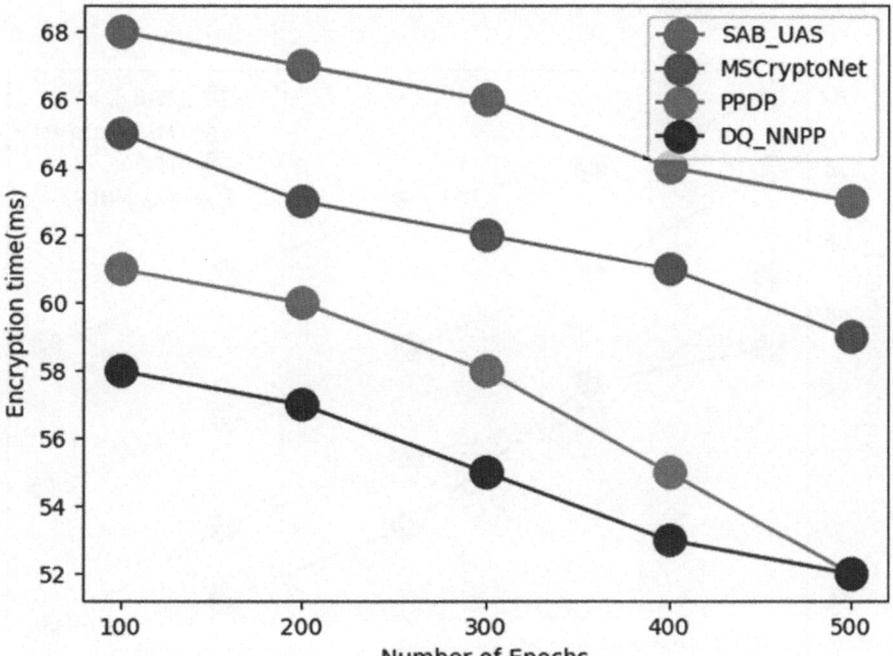

FIGURE 12.8 Comparison of encryption time.

4. **Decryption Time (D):** It is the time taken by an algorithm to convert cipher text (P) into plain text (C) using the asymmetric or asymmetric key. The formula for encryption time is provided in Eqn. (12.19):

$$D = Time(C \rightarrow P) \tag{19}$$

Figure 12.9 presents the comparison of decryption time between existing SAB-UAS, MSCryptoNet, and PPDP systems and the proposed DQ-NNPP method. X-axis displays number of epochs utilized for analysis, and Y-axis gives decryption time values obtained in milliseconds. The existing SAB-UAS, MSCryptoNet, and PPDP methods achieved decryption times of 67.48, 66.58, and 64.74, respectively. In comparison, the proposed DQ-NNPP method achieved a decryption time of 62.72 ms, which is 5.36 ms faster than SAB-UAS, 4.5 ms faster than MSCryptoNet, and 2.02 ms faster than the PPDP method. Table 12.1 provides the overall comparative analysis of all methods.

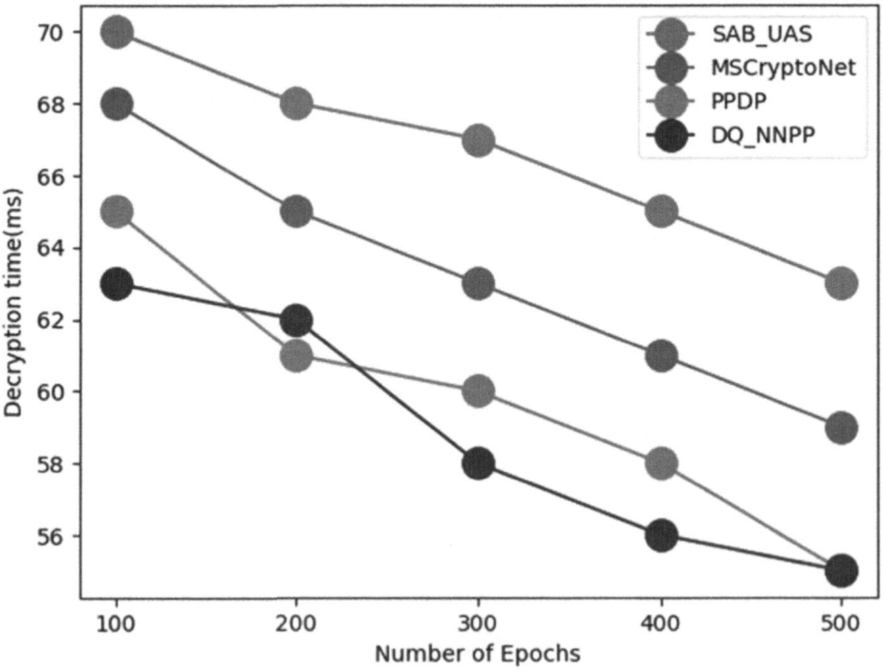

FIGURE 12.9 Comparison of decryption time.

TABLE 12.1 Overall Comparison between the Proposed and Existing Methods

Parameters	SAB-UAS [12]	MSCryptoNet [14]	PPDP [16]	DQ-NNPP [Proposed]
Accuracy (%)	92.02	94.3	93.04	93.74
Sensitivity (%)	79.4	84.72	86.42	92
Specificity (%)	90.7	91.44	91.58	92.1
Communication overhead (%)	64.62	65.24	66.76	67.08
Encryption time (ms)	64	62.2	60.52	58.72
Decryption time (ms)	67.48	66.58	64.74	62.72

12.5 CONCLUSION

Security and privacy are the most challenging issues in IoT healthcare applications. With limited resources in IoT, the existing security approaches are not appropriate. The proposed named DQ-NNPP architecture overcomes the challenges of security and privacy threats. This chapter introduces a novel Ciphertext-Policy Attribute-Based Privacy Preservation (Cip-PolAttPrivPre), which combines the benefits of the private key, public key, and master key to design a patient-centric access control approach used in electronic records in medical sectors, thereby ensuring security and privacy. The proposed method demonstrated superior results when compared with the existing SAB-UAS, MSCryptoNet, and PPDP methods, achieving 93.74% accuracy, 92% sensitivity, 92.1% specificity, 67.08% communication overhead, encryption time of 58.72 ms, and decryption time of 62.72 ms. Future works should also include anonymized data searching in a deep learning (DL) concept to improve security.

KEYWORDS

- **data transmission**
- **deep learning**
- **encryption**
- **healthcare**
- **internet of things**
- **performance analysis**
- **privacy**
- **Q-learning**

REFERENCES

1. Buttyan, L., & Hubaux, J. P., (2008). Privacy protection. In: *Security and Cooperation in Wireless Networks: Thwarting Malicious and Selfish Behavior in the Age of Ubiquitous Computing* (pp. 237–254). New York: Cambridge University Press.
2. Ramos, J. L. H., Bernabe, J. B., & Skarmeta, A. F., (2014). Towards privacy-preserving data sharing in smart environments. *IEEE 8th Int. Conf. on Innovative Mobile and Internet Services in Ubiquitous Computing, Birmingham* (pp. 334–339).
3. Gue, X., Duan, X., Gao, H., Huang, A., & Jiao, B., (2013). An ECG monitoring and alarming system based on android smart phone. *Communications and Networks, 5*, 584–589.
4. Sonar, K., & Upadhyay, H., (2014). A survey: DDOS attack on internet of things. *Int. J. of Engineering Research and Development, India* (pp. 58–63).
5. Miao, Y., Ma, J., Liu, X., Wei, F., Liu, Z., & Wang, X. A., (2016). m2-ABKS: Attribute-based multi-keyword search over encrypted personal health records in multi-owner setting. *Journal of Medical Systems*, *40*(11), article 246.
6. Huang, M., Liu, A., Wang, T., & Huang, C., (2018). Green data gathering under delay differentiated services constraint for internet of things. *Wireless Communications and Mobile Computing*. Article ID 9715428.
7. Rahim, Murugan, Mostafa, Dubey, Regin, Kulkarni, & Dhanalakshmi, (2020). Detecting the phishing attack using collaborative approach and secure login through dynamic virtual passwords. *Webology*, *17*(2).
8. Tang, J., Liu, A., Zhao, M., & TWang, T., (2018). An aggregate signature-based trust routing for data gathering in sensor networks. *Security and Communication Networks* (p. 30). Article ID 6328504.
9. Al-Qatf, M., Lasheng, Y., Al-Habib, M., & Al-Sabahi, K., (2018). Deep learning approach combining sparse autoencoder with SVM for network intrusion detection. In: *IEEE Access,* (pp. 52843–52856).
10. Otoum, S., Kantarci, B., & Mouftah, H. T., (2019). On the feasibility of deep learning in sensor network intrusion detection. *IEEE Networking Letters*, 68–71.
11. Ahamad, D., Shabi, A. H., & Mobin, A., (2020). A multi-objective privacy preservation model for cloud security using hybrid Jaya-based shark smell optimization. *Journal of King Saud University-Computer and Information Sciences*.
12. Deebak, B. D., et al., (2019). An authentic-based privacy preservation protocol for smart e-healthcare systems in IoT. *IEEE Access, 7*, 135632–135649.
13. Wang, K., et al., (2021). Forward privacy preservation in IoT-enabled healthcare systems. *IEEE Transactions on Industrial Informatics.*
14. Owusu-Agyemang, K., et al., (2019). MSCryptoNet: Multi-scheme privacy-preserving deep learning in cloud computing. *IEEE Access, 7*, 29344–29354.
15. Keshavarzian, A., Saeed, S., & Sanaz, S., (2019). Modified deep residual network architecture deployed on serverless framework of IoT platform based on human activity recognition application. *Future Generation Computer Systems, 101*, 14–28.
16. Zhang, C., et al., (2015). PPDP: An efficient and privacy-preserving disease prediction scheme in cloud-based e-Healthcare system. *Future Generation Computer Systems, 79*, 16–25.
17. Malviya, R., Ghinea, G., Dhanaraj, R. K., Balusamy, B., & Sundram, S., (2022). *Deep Learning for Targeted Treatment* (p. 436). Scrivener publishing.

18. Zhu, J., et al., (2017). A new deep-Q-learning-based transmission scheduling mechanism for the cognitive internet of things. *IEEE Internet of Things Journal, 5*, 2375–2385.
19. Guesmi, R., (2014). A novel design of chaos-based S-boxes using genetic algorithm techniques. In: *2014 IEEE/ACS 11th International Conference on Computer Systems and Applications (AICCSA).*
20. Qin, Q., Biyuan, J., & Yanqing, L., (2021). A secure storage and sharing scheme of stroke electronic medical records based on consortium blockchain. *BioMed Research International.*

CHAPTER 13

A Heterogeneous Graph-Based E-Health Solution in Cloud Computing with Semi-Supervision During Pandemic Periods

ANTONY XAVIER BRANSON,[1] SAI SHANMUGA RAJA,[1] SENDILVELAN SUBRAMANIA,[2] LARISSA R. SASSYKOVA,[3] FRANCIS JENCY,[4] GEETHA SOMAN,[1] KANYA NATARAJ,[5] and MOHANDOSS SUNDARAM[1]

[1]*Department of Computer Science and Engineering, Dr. M.G.R. Educational and Research Institute, Chennai, Tamil Nadu, India*

[2]*Department of Mechanical Engineering, Dr. M.G.R. Educational and Research Institute, Chennai, Tamil Nadu, India*

[3]*Faculty of Chemistry and Chemical Technology, Al-Farabi Kazakh National University, Almaty, Kazakhstan*

[4]*Department of Computer Science and Engineering, Kumaraguru College of Technology, Coimbatore, Tamil Nadu, India*

[5]*Department of Information Technology, Dr. M.G.R. Educational and Research Institute, Chennai, Tamil Nadu, India*

ABSTRACT

The unlabeled data that represents most of the acquired dataset poses the most difficult problem in the process of creating a classification model for risk prediction during COVID-19. Those unlabeled datasets characterize the individuals in health exams, for whom the health states can range from extremely healthy to severely ill, depending on the assessment. There is no objective way to distinguish between their varied states of health, surgical

Creating Smart Healthcare with Blockchain and Advanced Digital Technology.
Rishabha Malviya and Sonali Sundram (Eds.)

procedures, lab tests, observations, diagnostic reports, prescriptions, patient data, and allergies are all examples of information that can be found in an electronic health record (EHR). A personal health record (PHR), often known as a PHR, is a newly emerging patient-centered model for the interchange of health information. The storage of PHRs is typically outsourced to a third party, such as a cloud storage provider. Encrypting patients' health information before transferring them to a third party for processing is one technique that could help consumers retain control over who gets access to their own PHRs. This chapter introduces a novel paradigm called the patient-centric paradigm as well as a set of strategies for controlling data access to PHRs stored on semi-trusted servers. Achieve greater attention to data access control that is also scalable for PHRs, each patient's health record file is encrypted utilizing attribute-based encryption (ABE) technologies. Using the multi-authority technique protects a substantial degree of patient confidentiality at the same time. Furthermore, this system enables the dynamic change of access restrictions or file attributes, supports efficient user revocation, and gives access when required.

13.1 INTRODUCTION

In response to COVID-19, digital technologies are mostly utilized to aid public health efforts. These activities include population monitoring, contact tracing, case identification, and the evaluation of treatments are data based on communication and movement with the public. They are all part of population surveillance. Because of the large web datasets and linked devices, as well as breakthroughs in machine learning (ML), inexpensive computing resources, and natural language processing, many responses are possible [1]. For COVID-19, this review intends to examine all the digital innovations that have been implemented to date, their strengths and weaknesses, and the roadblocks that stand in the way of widespread adoption. Ethical, legal, and privacy problems, as well as workforce issues and organizations, are all examples of potential roadblocks. To improve and reinforce pandemic management and also be ready for the upcoming outbreaks of COVID-19 as well as other communicable diseases, a global strategy for the evaluation, regulation, and utilization of digital technologies is required. As time goes on, public health will become increasingly digital. Those who are vulnerable and disadvantaged are more at risk from this virus, and those in very low- and low-income nations with a weak system of health [2]. The World Health Organization (WHO) has declared a pandemic a respiratory infection caused by the coronavirus, COVID-19.

Finding clusters of illness, stopping community transmission of the disease, and preventing further spread are all key components in controlling the COVID-19 pandemic as they were during prior epidemics and outbreaks. When the plague struck Europe in the 14th century, sick people were isolated from the rest of the population, and mobility was prohibited to keep the disease from spreading. When dealing with an outbreak, public health approaches such as case detection on time, halting the spread of disease within the population, and widespread dissemination of information remain relevant today. It is critical to keep tabs on the effectiveness of these approaches and the impact they have on the number of cases and deaths they cause.

Each country must have the essential capabilities necessary to ensure that it is effectively equipped to cope with infectious risks that have the potential to spread to other countries to comply with the International Health Regulations [3]. As a result of an outbreak, innovative approaches and technologies are routinely researched and developed to strengthen these fundamental capacities. Ebola outbreaks happened in West Africa, and data from mobile phones were exploited to replicate travel patterns. It was also possible to do contact tracing more effectively and acquire a greater understanding of the outbreak dynamics thanks to handheld sequencing technology that was available. Like the COVID-19 pandemic, digital technology has been used to enhance public health measures.

The rise of digital technology has had an impact on many elements of modern life. Around 67% of the world's population is registered to mobile devices in 2019, with smartphones accounting for 66% of those subscriptions. The pace of Smartphone adoption is expanding the quickest in Sub-Saharan Africa. Downloads of mobile applications hit 204 billion in 2019, and the number of users actively using social media platforms worldwide reached 3.8 billion as of January 2020 [4]. In this section, an in-depth investigation is performed of how digital technologies are presently being exploited in the fight against COVID-19 all over the world. How many inventions are there, and how many limits are there for each? This approach, which focuses on the system, is vital for identifying digital tactics integrated into COVID-19 control plans and for assisting in the planning for future epidemics.

With a variety of digital technologies available, certain methods may also require internet and telecommunications infrastructure to be accessible. For simplicity, ML is treated as a separate topic from artificial intelligence (AI), despite its vital role in many other fields. Data dashboards use a significant percentage of the data generated by these technologies.

Information systems, including various automation, can hold precise information about the identifying and the sequence of events, which are the other two categories of the process model. Process This is the most essential task of the process model because it lays the groundwork that will lead to future studies, such as the application of the other two categories of the process model, compliance checking, and enhancement. Process discovery is a method in which event logs are used as inputs and a process model is constructed without the use of previous information. Many businesses may have difficulties when attempting to construct an actual process using event logs, owing to the disparity between theory and practice. Heuristic Miner, Alpha Miner, and Fuzzy Miner are some of the algorithms that are utilized for process discovery [5]. Event logs are examined by the process model and discovered flow, and it is confirmed that the carried-out process is in the way specified in its given model. The variations between the process that was performed, conformance checking, and the process model's specification are measured. The major purpose of this procedure would be to identify areas that need improvement based on the information gathered during the process. There are four viewpoints in the project model technique: organizational, control flow, time, and case. These viewpoints are not disjointed; rather, they are connected. When it comes to the activities and the development of the process model, the control viewpoint is concerned with finding the best definitions for all conceivable courses to take. As a result, the findings are represented in business process modeling notation (BPMN) format [6]. Categorize the roles of the process model and organizational contexts, the organizational viewpoint considers the actors (person, role, and system) and the actors' relationships that exist. The case viewpoint is concerned with the definition of cases as well as the factors that influence the facts. The time perspective is anxious with the frequency of events and occurrence time, and it aids in the identification of bottlenecks, the measurement of service levels, the tracking of resource use, and the prediction of the remaining time for ongoing events, among other things.

Because of these reasons, the application of this method in the medical field holds a lot of promise. Several types of automated information systems retain vast amounts of information regarding the identity and sequence of actual events. Process discovery is an essential activity of the project model because it provides future studies with a base for including the application of the other two types of the project model, which are checked, confirmed, and enhanced. Consequently, process discovery is the most critical activity in the project model. In the process model, both its flow and its discovery in the event logs are reviewed, and a check is made to determine if the process followed the model's parameters. The variations that exist between the actual process being conducted and the process model's specification are what are measured by conformance checking. Using the knowledge obtained during this process, the primary objective of this procedure is to establish which aspects of it require further development.

The institutional perspective considers the actors as well as the relationships between such actors to categorize the process model which is based on responsibilities and organization. The primary areas of focus for the case viewpoint are the definitions of scenarios and the elements that impact the actual data. The temporal perspective is focused on the times and frequency with which events occur. It also assists in detecting bottlenecks, monitoring levels of service, tracking resource utilization, and forecasting the overall amount of time remaining for currently happening activities.

13.2 SPARSE AREAS THAT ARE STABILIZED BY ORDINARY REGRESSION TO STRATIFY MEDICAL RISKS

Data mining is currently facing several significant difficulties and opportunities because of the recent widespread deployment of electronic medical records (EMR) [7]. The EMR data consists primarily of temporal information and is known to be noisy, irregular, and of high dimension. In this research, an innovative ordinal regression framework is constructed to predict the stratification of medical risk using EMR. First, a model representation of EMR is created in the form of a temporal image to extract a variety of different properties. Second, ordinal modeling is used for determining whether a risk is cumulative or progressive. One of the challenges is creating a transparent prediction model with a large number of features that are only mediocre predictors and stable against fluctuations while being like one another. The proposed approach makes use of sparsity approaches, which are then stabilized by domain-specific feature interaction networks. It assesses the stability of the model by comparing it to similar data using two indices that were developed. The use of feature networks (the Random Walk and Laplacian) results in the generation of two multivariate Gaussian priors having sparse precision matrices [8]. The applied framework to the problem of short-term prediction of a large suicide risk shows that the methods perform better than those of clinicians by a significant margin. It is also demonstrated that the methods discover the risk factors of suicide that are consistent with enhanced stability in mental health and produce models.

13.3 THE USE OF HOME TELEHEALTH MEASUREMENT DATA TO IDENTIFY THE PROBABILITY OF AN EXACERBATION IN INDIVIDUALS WHO HAVE COPD (CHRONIC OBSTRUCTIVE PULMONARY DISEASE)

Utilizing telehealth technologies to remotely monitor patients who are afflicted with chronic diseases may make it possible to provide preventative therapy for health conditions that are deteriorating before they cause a major change in the overall health status, which would otherwise require the subject to be admitted to the hospital. The goal of this study would have been to create and assess the algorithm classification of identifying persons having a history of COPD, who are at greater risk of suffering an impending exacerbation activity. The system attempts to forecast that patient's state one day ahead by comparing their current physiological effects measures to the range of those values gathered over the previous month. This analysis is based on the patient's previous medical records.

Telehealth measurement data were collected from the treatment of moderate to severe COPD living in the home to validate the proposed technique, which is based on a classification and regression tree (CART), commonly known as a CART. Telehealth home monitoring equipment was used during the data gathering process, which took place in February 2007 and January 2008 [9]. The CART algorithm, according to the findings, is capable of classifying home telehealth measurement data into "low level of risk" or "high level of risk" categories with an accuracy of 71.8%, specificity of 80.4%, and sensitivity of 61.1% [10]. The algorithm was able to identify a condition as having a "significant risk" a day before the patients were detected as having a worsening in their COPD condition. The records of symptoms and medications taken by the patients revealed a deterioration in the patient's COPD condition. According to the findings of the CART study, the sorts of indicators with the greatest predictive potential for stratifying a patient's health include forceful expiratory volume in one second, weight, and arterial oxygen saturation. This CART algorithm for early diagnosis could begin the onset of suitable medicine, which could, in turn, lower the severity of the exacerbation, minimize the time needed for recovery, and improve the patient's well-being. The above study emphasizes the significant advantage of automated classification of home telehealth data in detecting exacerbation occurrences in COPD patients [11].

13.4 ACQUIRING KNOWLEDGE OF CLASSIFICATION SCHEMES USING FUZZY LABELS

Objectives in the field of medicine, the learning of classification models frequently depend on data that has been tagged by a human specialist. Finding strategies to reduce the time and effort required for labeling clinical data is one of the most important things we can do to improve our capacity to study the new models automatically. In the above work, it is proposed an innovative approach to ML that is smart enough to learn improved binary classifier models in a more time and resource-efficient manner. This is accomplished during the training phases by modifying the binary class data with soft labels which reveal and identify how firmly the expert ends up feeling about the classic labels. The components and procedures are two distinct types of methodologies for learning enhanced binary classification models using soft labels. The very first employs probabilistic and numerical labels, whereas the second employs ordinal categorical labels. It is investigated and shows how these strategies can be beneficial for reading a notifying model for heparin-induced thrombocytopenia (HIT). Investigations are undertaken by employing data from 377 patient occurrences labeled by three different human professionals. The received operating characteristic curve score under the region would be used to compare the various techniques [12]. According to the results of our area underneath the receiver operating characteristic curve research, the novel method is more effective at studying classification models than more traditional learning approaches. When the number of cases from which to learn is small, the improvement in these areas of the receiver operating characteristic curve is noticeable. This method concludes that learning classification techniques by using expert labels to adopt a new framework of categorization studying that allows students to learn from supplemental soft-label data provided by a human expert. This would reduce the amount of effort and money spent labeling data [13].

13.5 DEVELOPING EXTENDED ASSOCIATION RULE SUMMARIZATION METHODS FOR EVALUATING THE DANGER OF DIABETES MELLITUS

By utilizing association rule mining (ARM), the primary objective of this is to provide a forecast for the patients of their heightened risk of developing diabetes and to provide a summary of their subpopulation. In the field of data mining, association rule learning is a method that has gained a lot of popularity and has been thoroughly investigated. This method is used to find interesting links between variables that are stored in huge databases. Use ARM on electronic medical data to identify groups of risk variables and the subpopulations that correspond to them to identify the high-risk individuals who are at an exceptionally high risk of developing diabetes. An EMR, often known as an EMR, is a notion that is still in the process of development. It is described as the systematic collection of electronic health data on a patient or community. The high dimensionality of EMRs generates ARM and a massive number of rules that must be summarized before they can be used in clinical settings. Applied four different strategies for the summary of association rule sets, and then conducted a comparative analysis to provide direction for the applicability, strengths, and shortcomings of each technique. It was discovered that each of the four methodologies created summaries that described the sub-populations getting diabetes who are at substantial risk. Each of the four methods had its distinct strengths. Considering our objectives, the bottom-up summarization (BuS) that has been developed represents the most effective use of the information presented in the initial summary.

13.6 BOOSTING FOR FAST AND COST-SENSITIVE GRAPH CLASSIFICATION WITH THE COG BOOST SYSTEM

The number of applications requiring items with intricate structural linkages has increased significantly in recent years, contributing to widespread interest in graph classification. To this day, all graph classification methods in use assume, either implicitly or explicitly, because improperly classifying occurrences results in an equivalent amount of expenditure. However, in real-world situations, that is not always the case. Even though there has been a lot of research done on cost-sensitive learning, all the methods are still predicated on data that has an instance-feature representation. The feature space of datasets is infinite and must be thoroughly investigated to choose classes with a greater cost. Graphs, on the other hand, do not contain any features that can be learned, and this feature space needs to be explored. In this research, it is proposed a method for the classification of graphs called Cog Boost [14]. It is a fast approach that is sensitive to costs and attempts to minimize the costs of misclassification rather than the errors themselves to achieve a large-scale graph dataset, a high learning speed is required. Cog Boost solves in each iteration a linear programming problem by utilizing the rule-based optimal loss function (Bayer decision) after iteratively picking one of the most discriminative sub-graphs by evaluating the costs of distinct classes. The goal of this process is to reduce the costs associated with misclassification as much as possible. Furthermore, cutting plane methods were developed to speed up solving linear programs, allowing for quick learning on large network databases. Tests and comparisons on big graph databases from the actual world demonstrate that the approach is both successful and efficient.

SHG-Health is a semi-supervised heterogeneous graph-based method for predicting health hazards based on health examination records. It was developed as a solution to the problem of health risk forecasting brought on by the presence of heterogeneity in health examination records as well as vast amounts of unlabeled data. A method of learning that is semi-supervised for the data that was generated. To tackle the one-of-a-kind problem posed by the proof-based risk prediction derived from medical examination records, the HeteroHER graph technique was utilized [15]. To solve the problem, the technique combines the benefits of class discovery with the benefits of dealing with heterogeneity. To begin to solve the learning problem, we create an objective function for it and show that it is convex. Then we use an optimization procedure to find a solution. Afterwards, we construct an efficient iterative algorithm and demonstrate that it is convergence-proof. Finally, the topic of time complexity is addressed.

13.7 ELECTRONIC HEALTH RECORD (EHR) SYSTEM CURRENTLY IN USE

Most currently available classification algorithms for healthcare data do not take unlabeled data into account. They have either expertly established reduced risk or control groups, or they simply regard non-positive cases as negative. The binary classification challenge is only addressed by the healthcare applications that are now available. Nguyen and colleagues presented mPUL, a multiclass extension. Nevertheless, this method used a mixed range of negative and unlabeled examples, whereas a negative example is not always accessible [16]. Both present and historical EHRs are required for early detection and prevention. When talking about "risk," also talks about unfavorable outcomes like death and disease. The disadvantage of the currently used SHG-Health method is a solution to the difficult problem of multi-class categorization that involves substantial unlabeled instances which may or may not be associated with the classifiers. The study pioneers risk prediction by utilizing medical assessment data in the context of vast amounts of unlabeled data.

13.8 ELECTRONIC HEALTH RECORD (EHR) SYSTEM UNDER CONSIDERATION

The SHG on health is a graph-based method that is offered as a proof-based risk prediction strategy to mine longitudinal health examination data. This method is founded on the idea that distinct types of people have distinct types of health histories. The algorithm is called the "semi-supervised heterogeneous graph on health," and its name describes its function. It investigates a heterogeneous graph termed the HeteroHER graph, which is built on Health Examination Records, to manage heterogeneity [17]. Examinable things are represented by separate sorts of nodes in this graph, and their historical relationships are represented as links. Overcoming the challenge of massive volumes of data that is unlabeled, SHG-Health employs a technique that employs both labeled and unlabeled samples.

The SHG-health algorithm is a solution to a difficult multi-class classification problem that contains a sizable number of unlabeled examples. A unique graph extraction mechanism is proposed to deal with the heterogeneity that can be noticed in the records of longitudinal health examinations. The suggested semi-supervised graph-based learning system health achieves considerable performance gains on a comprehensive and large real health examination dataset. The benefits of heterogeneous graph studying, and class identification are combined in this technique.

The suggested graph-based learning algorithm SHG-Health can handle a complex multi-class classification task with numerous unlabeled examples. Furthermore, coping with the heterogeneity seen in longitudinal health examination data necessitates the development of a novel graph extraction mechanism. Furthermore, the proposed learning method SHG-Health, which provides a combination of class discovery with heterogeneous graph learning, achieves considerable performance gains on a large number of unlabeled examples [18].

13.9 SOFTWARE AND HARDWARE REQUIREMENTS

Detailed system specification, including hardware requirements:

- Pentium III processor with a clock speed of 733 MHz.
- RAM: 128 megabytes

- 10 GB of storage space on a hard drive
- The monitor is a 14-inch VGA color monitor.
- Logitech Serial Mouse is the device in question.
- 1 GB of available disc space

Requirements for software:

- Platform: Java Development Kit (JDK) 1.8
- Microsoft Windows and NT 4.0 as the operating system
- JAVA – the programming language used in the program.
- MySql 5.5 is the database system.
- NETBEANS 8.0, SQLYog, and JDK 1.8 are the tools used.

13.10 METHODOLOGY

13.10.1 PATIENT AND DOCTOR

If a patient wishes to gain access to the information that is kept in a database during this module, he or she must first register their details to do so. These particulars are always kept in a database. After the patient has registered, they can request the database with their query. In this section, the patient can examine the list of available files and can retrieve the data in an encrypted format. Within the context of this module, the doctor will upload patient data via encryption. In this section, the doctor can view patient details and can upload a patient report with all the required information. The data will be encrypted in a time-effective manner by our SHG algorithm at this phase [19]. These particulars are stored in a database using a case diagram as shown in Figure 13.1.

13.10.2 A FEW RESULTS FOR THE HOSPITAL SEARCH

The patient will be able to look for hospital information that is local to him as well as hospitality services that are provided through this module. This module provides the patient with assistance in retrieving information about the hospital, including information on available doctors, operating hours, and so on, and the patient has already been entered into the database.

13.10.3 INFORMATION RELATING TO THE DISEASE

The module presents the general knowledge about the disease in the form of a frequently asked questions section, which generates information for patients regarding how they may protect themselves from disease and how they can

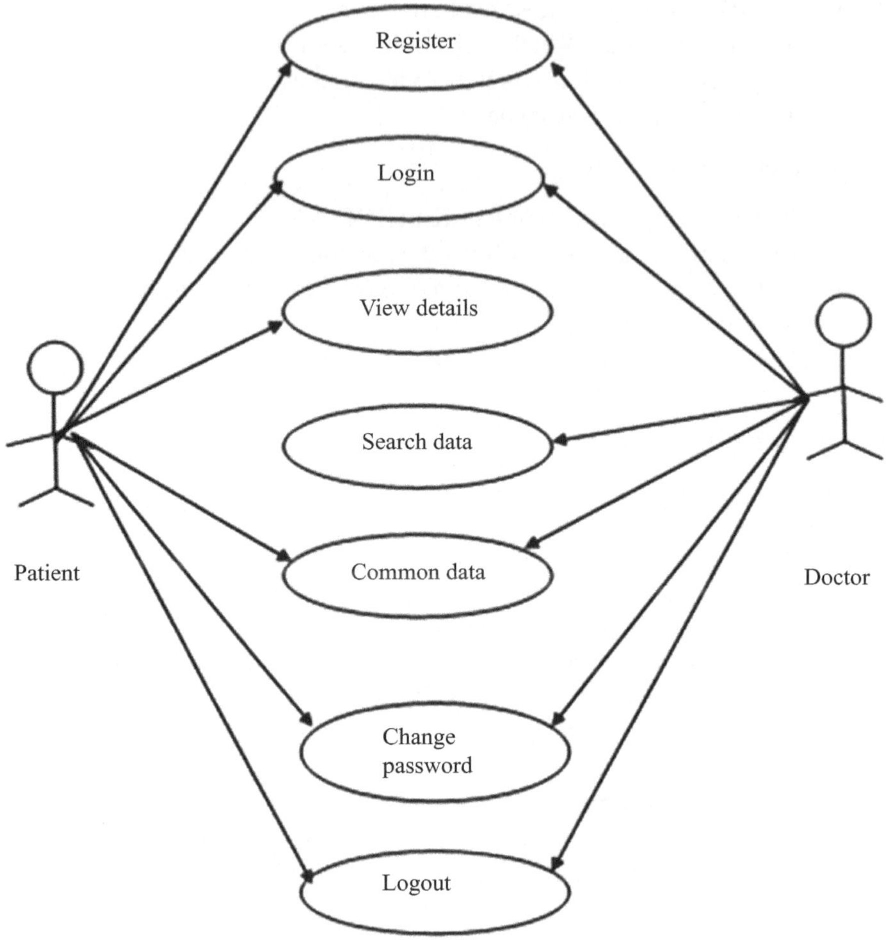

FIGURE 13.1 Case diagram between the patient and doctor.

best care for other patients who have a specific disease. This module is helpful for regular users to submit information, and they can do so by using it. The sequence diagram shows the information for the doctor, which gives the flow of activities during the process and the results as shown in Figure 13.2.

13.10.4 EXPLANATION OF THE SHG ALGORITHM

The challenge of predicting health risk based on health examination data, which contains heterogeneity difficulties as well as massive amounts of unlabeled data, is addressed by the SHG-Health solution, which is shown

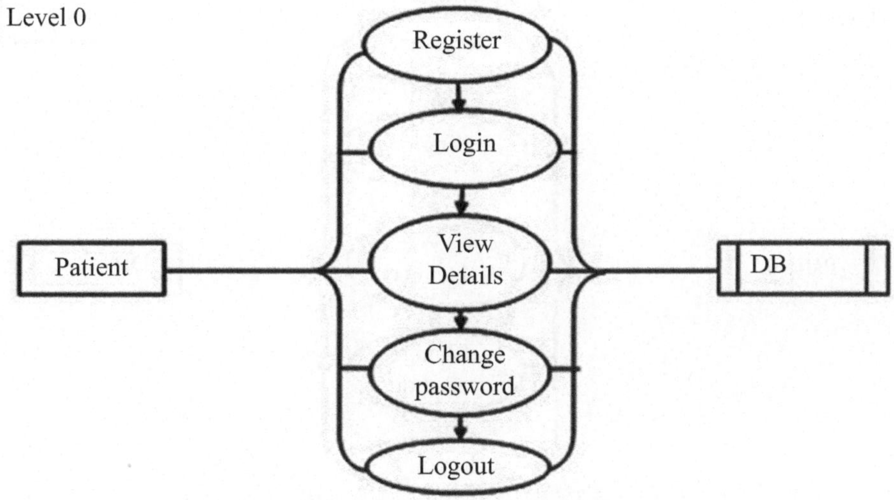

FIGURE 13.2 Sequence diagram for the patient and the activities.

here. Semi-supervised studying strategy for the HeteroHER network [20]. This approach combines the benefits of heterogeneity handling and class discovery to address a specific difficulty posed by evidence-based risk prediction using health examination records. The inability to effectively forecast dangers based on past medical history produced the dilemma. The convexity of the learning problems is an objective function that is proven first. The problem is then solved using an optimization approach. Then, demonstrate the convergence of the solution by deriving an effective iterative algorithm.

13.11 OPEN DATABASE CONNECTIVITY (ODBC)

Microsoft's ODBC standard is a programming interface that is widely utilized by app developers and database system manufacturers. Before ODBC became the de facto standard for Windows programs to use when interacting with database management systems, developers would have to connect to various databases using separate proprietary languages. From a coding point of view, the decision of which database system to use is unimportant now thanks to ODBC, exactly as it should be. There is a need for business to be changed abruptly, and app developers have thought a lot to consider about the syntax required in migrating their program from one database to another [21]. The data flow diagram shows how the process goes on and is digitized as shown in Figures 13.3–13.5. Figure 13.6 is the architecture diagram.

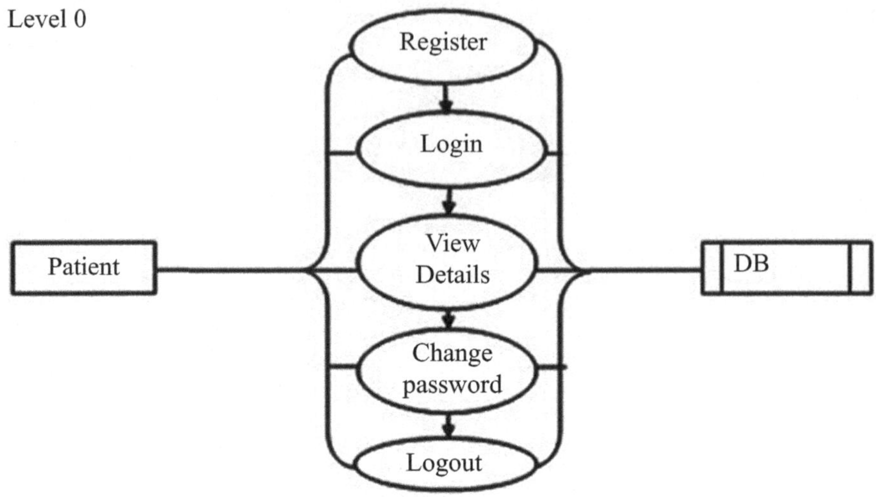

FIGURE 13.3 Flow diagram Level 0 data.

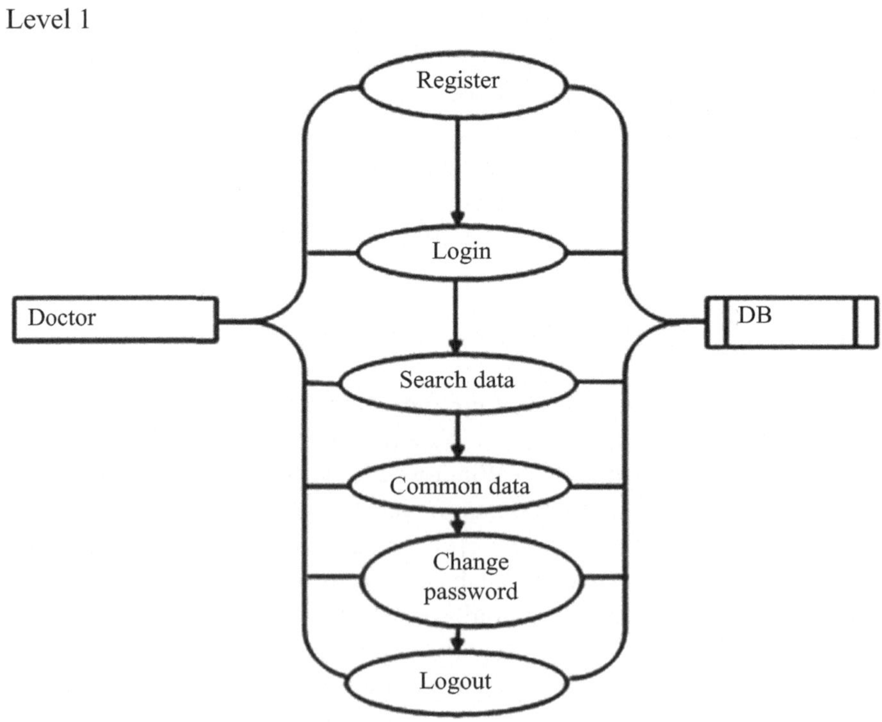

FIGURE 13.4 Flow diagram Level 1 data.

Level Context

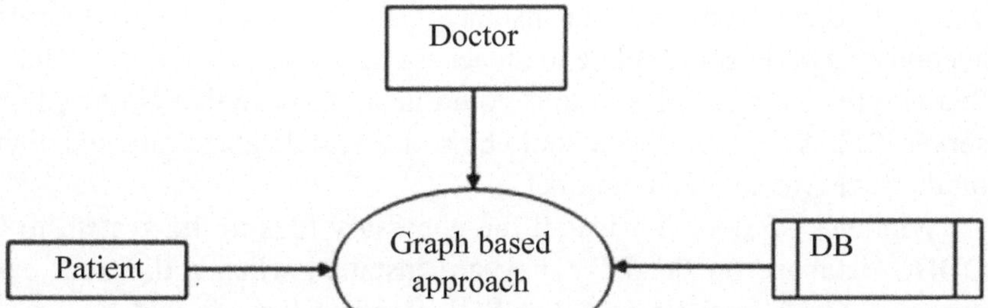

FIGURE 13.5 Level context flow diagram (data).

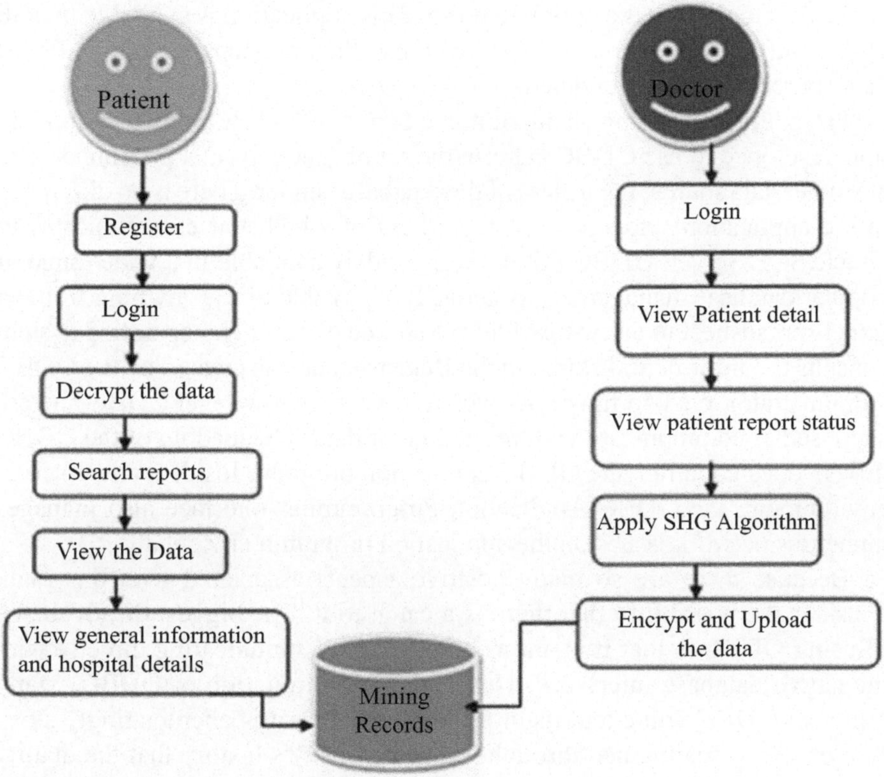

FIGURE 13.6 Architecture diagram.

The database given is linked to a data source that is used by an ODBC program that is designed to be used through the control panel's ODBC Administrator. Think of an open database connectivity (ODBC) data source as a door with a nameplate. It will eventually get to a different database if you go through each door. For instance, the data source that is referred to as accounts payable could relate to an access database, whereas the data source that is referred to as sales figures could be a database that is hosted on SQL server [22]. A source of data could be a physical database situated anywhere on the LAN (local area network).

Windows 95 does not install the necessary files in the system to use an ODBC database on the PC. They are installed when a different database program, like Visual Basic 4.0 or SQL Server Client, is installed and made available for usage. A file known as ODBCINST.DLL is utilized throughout the process of installing the ODBC icon in the control panel. You can also manage ODBC sources of data with a stand-alone tool called ODBCADM. EXE. This tool gives the option to do so. This application is available in both 16-bit and 32-bit flavors, and each of those flavors keeps its unique list of data sources of ODBC updated.

From a programming standpoint, the benefit of ODBC is that an application developed to use ODBC can use the set of function calls to connect with any other data source, regardless of the database vendor. There is no difference in the application's source code regardless of whether it communicates to Oracle/SQL Server. ODBC drivers were widely available in a wide range of popular database management systems. It is possible to use anything from an Excel spreadsheet to a raw text file as a source of data. The operating system consults the information stored in the Registry that was created by the ODBC Administrator to try to figure out which drivers are low-level ODBC and are supposed to communicate with the source of data. The loading of the ODBC drivers does not affect the ODBC application program. Inside a client-server environment, the ODBC Application Programming Interface also manages numerous network issues on the application programmer's behalf.

Because there are so many positive aspects associated with this plan, consider the possibility that there is a catch to it. The biggest disadvantage of using ODBC is that it is not as efficient as communicating directly with the native database interfaces. This is the only limitation of ODBC. Many critics of ODBC argue that its biggest issue is that it is excruciatingly slow. Microsoft has maintained throughout the company's history that the quality of the driver software that is employed is the single most key component in determining overall performance. Recently, there has been a significant increase in the number of good ODBC drivers that are available. And in any case, the complaints concerning performance are like those voiced by individuals who said that compilers would never be able to compete with the speed of assembly language written in its purest form. Perhaps not, but using the compiler (or ODBC) will allow developing programs that are cleaner, which will speed up the process and let you complete it sooner. Meanwhile, the speed of computers continues to increase annually.

13.12 JAVA DATABASE CONNECTIVITY (JDBC)

Java database connectivity, known as JDBC, was created by Sun Microsystems to offer an independent database standard application programming interface (API) for Java. JDBC is a standardized database access technology that offers a uniform front interface to a variety of RDBMSs. It supports the generic SQL database query language. The utilization of "plug-in" database connectivity modules, also known as drivers, is what enables this consistently functioning interface to be realized. He or she must provide the driver when a database provider wants JDBC support, for any platform that can run both Java and the database. Because Sun wanted JDBC to be used by more people, the JDBC framework was modeled after ODBC. You already know from earlier in just this chapter that ODBC offers comprehensive support across a large range of platforms; this fact was previously brought to your attention. When JDBC is built on ODBC, it can bring JDBC drivers to market considerably faster than if they had to create a whole new connectivity solution. The final version of the JDBC specification, version 1.0, was made available for user feedback not long after that [23]. The remaining content of this part will provide sufficient knowledge about JDBC to enable us to understand what it is all about and how to make efficient use of it. This is in no way intended to be a comprehensive summary of JDBC. There are not many instances of software products being built without any aims in mind. JDBC is responsible for driving the development of the API because of the many aims that it has. With the achievement of these goals and the incorporation of early reviewer feedback, the JDBC class libraries have been transformed into a robust platform for developing Java database applications. These goals that were established for JDBC were crucial. It might provide insight into the rationale for specific classes and functionalities' behavior in the system.

13.13 SQI LEVEL API

The designers considered the most critical stage in the process to be designing a SQL interface for Java. Although a database interface is not the lowest possible level, it enables the development of higher-level tools and APIs. It has developed to the point that application developers feel at ease using it. If this goal is realized, future tool manufacturers will be able to "generate" JDBC code and shield the end user from many of the complexity of JDBC.

13.13.1 CONFORMITY WITH SQL

From database vendor to database provider, SQL syntax varies. Support as many different suppliers as feasible, any query statement allowed by the JDBC will be sent to it to the underlying database driver. The connectivity module, as a result, can suitably manage non-standard functionality for the individuals who use it. Implementation of JDBC needs to be possible on top of standard database interfaces. It is required for the JDBC SQL API to "sit" atop other common APIs for the SQL level. This goal, by employing a software interface, allows JDBC to make use of current ODBC-level drivers. JDBC calls this interface will be translated to ODBC and likewise. Java user interface can be if matches the rest of the Java operating system. With the favorable reception that Java has received from the user community up to this point, the developers of Java believe that it should not depart from the core Java system design [24].

13.13.2 SIMPLE IS BEST

This goal is presumably included in every listing of software design goals. Even JDBC is not an exception. Sun stated that JDBC's design should be simple, with just one way to carry out each mechanism's responsibilities. The sole purpose served by allowing duplicate functionality is to confuse API users. Always opt for the robust and static method of typing wherever possible. Strong type enables more error checking to be done during compilation, which in turn results in fewer errors occurring during runtime. Keep the most typical scenarios as simple as possible [25]. These queries need to be easy to execute using JDBC because the typical SQL commands used by the programmer are direct INSERT's, SELECT's, UPDATE's, and DELETE's. This is the case most of the time. It should, however, be enabled to perform more complex SQL commands. Java is both a programming language and an operating system for computers. Simple architecture, neutral objects, distributed, high performance, multi-threaded, interpreted, dynamic, robust, and secure, are the characteristics that may be found in Java, which is a high-level programming language. Furthermore, Java is unique in that each Java code is developed and processed simultaneously [20]. Convert a Java program into an intermediate language known as Java byte codes while compiling it. The compilation occurs only once; after the program is executed, the interpretation occurs each time, as shown in Figure 13.7.

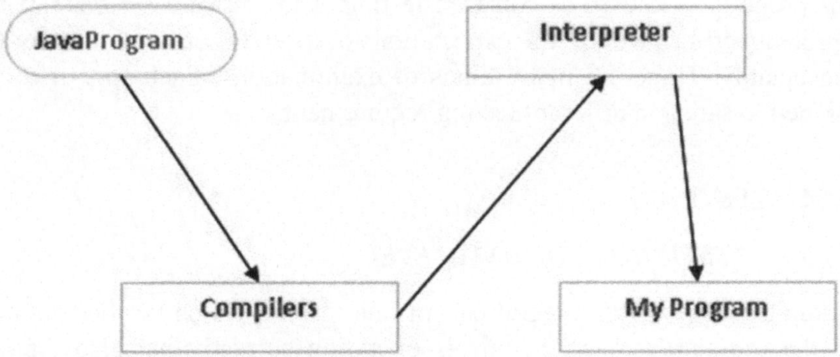

FIGURE 13.7 Java program compiled and interpreted.

This language contains platform-independent code instructions, which are then delivered to the computer and run there. Java byte codes can be thought of as machine code instructions that are executed by the Java Virtual Machine. Every Java interpreter, whether a dynamic or Java development tool that can run Java applets, must have an implementation of the Java Virtual Machine [27]. It is also possible to implement the Java Virtual Machine using hardware as shown in Figure 13.8. Java's "write once, execute anywhere" functionality is made feasible using byte codes.

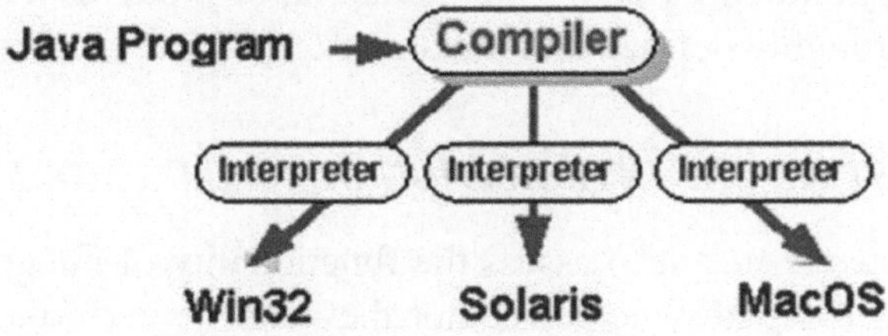

FIGURE 13.8 Java virtual machine.

Java programs can be compiled on a platform that includes a Java compiler by converting it to byte codes. The byte codes can then be run on any Java Virtual Machine implementation. The Java application, for example, can run on Macintosh, Windows NT, and Solaris computers.

Errors are to be found and eliminated through the testing process. The process of testing is searching for flaws or vulnerabilities in a work product in as many ways as possible. It makes it possible to test the functionality of individual components, subassemblies, assemblies, and even final products. The practice of putting the software through its paces to ensure that it functions properly is known as software testing. The software system satisfies its prerequisites as well as the expectations of its end users and does not fail unacceptably. There are many kinds of examinations. Each sort of test is designed to satisfy a different testing requirement.

13.14 TESTING

13.14.1 TESTING AT THE UNIT LEVEL

Writing test cases is an integral part of unit testing, which verifies not only that the program's internal logic is operating correctly but also that the program's inputs lead to legitimate outputs. The following is an explanation of what is meant by the term "unit testing": Validation needs to be performed on every decision branch and every internal code flow. It is the process of evaluating separate pieces of software that are included in a larger program. After each unit has been done, but before the units have been merged into a whole, it is finished. This is a destructive test of the structure's integrity, which is predicated on prior knowledge about the structure's construction. Unit tests are used to check a particular business process, application, or system configuration. They are also used to conduct straightforward component-level tests. In some circles, they are also known as component examinations. Unit tests guarantee that each branch of a business process adheres to the outlined guidelines and consists of inputs and outcomes that have been thoroughly defined and documented [28].

13.14.2 TESTING THE INTEGRATION OF TWO OR MORE SYSTEMS

Integration tests are meant to assess the functionality of integrated software components to evaluate whether or not they can be performed as a single program. The purpose of these tests is to determine whether or not the integrated software can be used. The general outcome of screens or fields is more significant than the minutiae of the testing procedure, and events are used to drive testing. Integration tests, when completed, establish that, even though the components were good when evaluated individually (as demonstrated by successful unit testing), the components, when merged, are accurate and consistent. This is true even if the individual component tests were successful. Integration testing is a type of testing that is specifically designed to reveal issues that develop because of the integration of components. The goal of this type of testing is to ensure that the final product functions as intended.

13.14.3 THE TEST IS FUNCTIONAL

Functional testing methods and processes demonstrate in practice that the capabilities under examination are available following the system documentation, user manuals, and business and technical requirements. These demonstrations can be seen in action. The following aspects are what the functional testing is mostly focused on:

1. **Valid Input:** It is necessary to acknowledge the various classes of valid input that have been found.
2. **Invalid Input:** It is necessary to get rid of any classes of invalid input that have been found.
3. **Functions:** To conduct the functions that have been outlined; it is important to have this.
4. **Output:** It is essential to practice the many sorts of application outputs that have been specified.
5. **Systems/Procedures:** It is essential to make use of the corresponding interface systems or procedures.

Functional tests are planned and prepared in such a way that they are centered on requirements, major functions, or particular test scenarios. This ensures that the tests accurately reflect the intended behavior of the application. Thorough coverage of data fields, business process flows, scheduled procedures, and following actions are some of the other considerations that should be made during testing [29]. More tests are identified before the completion of functional testing, and the effective value of the tests that are already being used is determined, among other things.

13.14.4 TEST OF THE SYSTEM

The purpose of system testing is to verify that the complete integrated software system satisfies all prerequisite conditions. It verifies a setup to make certain that the results are known and predictable. System testing can be illustrated with the use of an example such as a configuration-oriented system integration test. System testing is based on process descriptions and flows, with a focus on pre-driven process connections and integration points, as should be pointed out below. Testing that is carried out in an uncontrolled setting is referred to as white-box testing. White box testers are software testers who are familiar with the inner workings, structure, and language of the software, or at the very least, the purpose of the software. White box testers also have an understanding of the overall purpose of the software. It serves a certain function. It is utilized for testing areas that are inaccessible from the black box level of the test.

13.14.5 TESTING IN A BLACK BOX

The process of testing software without prior knowledge of the software's internal workings, structure, or language of the module under test is known as black-box testing. Black-box tests, like many other types of testing, must be developed using a definitive source document, such as a specification or requirements document [31]. The term "black box testing" refers to testing that treats the program under test as if it were a black box. You can't "see" within it. The exam creates inputs and responds to outputs without regard for how the software on the computer works.

13.14.6 TESTING CODING AND UNIT

It is normal practice to execute unit testing as part of the combined code and unit test phase of the software development lifecycle; nevertheless, it is not unheard of for coding and unit testing to be performed as separate stages of the software development lifecycle. Both the strategy and the method are put to the test:

- Hands-on testing in the field is going to be done, and careful planning is going to go into functional testing to ensure correctness.
- Test objectives have been specified.
- No duplicate entries are allowed, and all field entries must work properly.
- The pages must be triggered by the recognized link.
- There should be no latency between the entry screen, the messages, and the responses.

The following features will be subjected to testing:

- Examine the entries to ensure that they are in the correct format.
- All links must route users to the appropriate page.
- Integration testing is the process of combining two or more parts of the software to make them work as a whole.

Software integration testing is characterized by the progressive integration testing of two or more integrated software components that are all executed on the same platform. The goal of this testing is to identify and duplicate defects caused by interface difficulties. Integration testing is performed to ensure that individual software components and applications, such as those found in a software system or a higher-level software application at the corporate level, work properly in conjunction with one another.

13.14.7 RESULTS OF THE TESTS

All of the above-mentioned test cases passed with flying colors. There were no flaws found. Acceptance Testing is a form of test that assesses whether or not a product is acceptable. Acceptance by the user Testing is a critical component of every project, and it requires considerable feedback from the end-user throughout. It ensures that the system meets all functional specifications. Test results: All the above-mentioned test scenarios passed with flying colors. There were no flaws discovered. The output is shown in Figures 13.9 and 13.10.

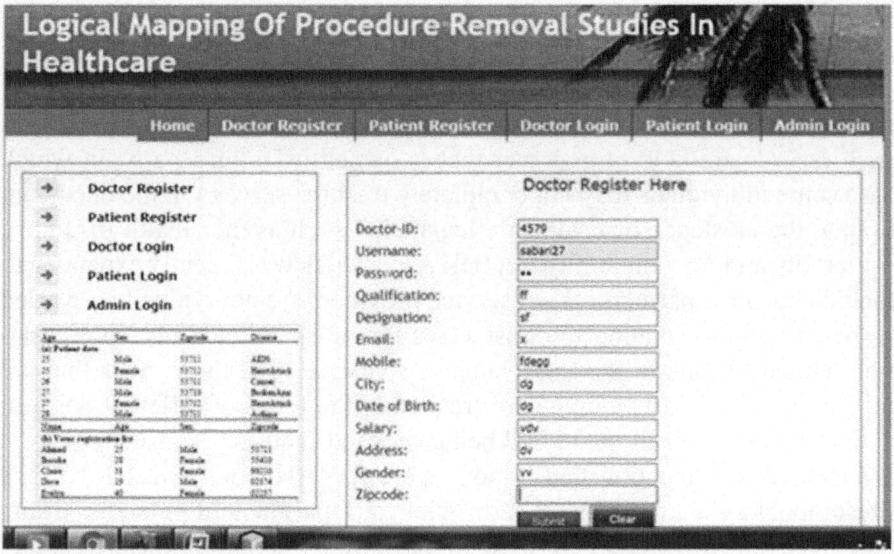

FIGURE 13.9 Portal of doctor registration.

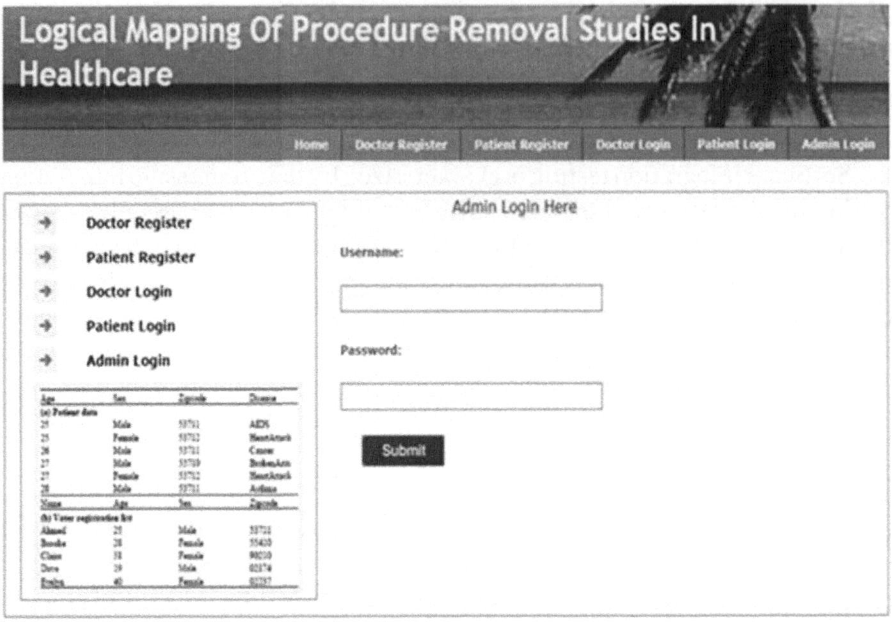

FIGURE 13.10 Portal of admin.

13.15 PERSONAL HEALTH INFORMATION (PHI) EXISTING SYSTEM

The availability of simple PHR services for everyone is highly exciting; nevertheless, widespread use of this technology may be hampered by the significant security and privacy dangers associated with it [32]. The most important question is whether or not patients will be able to restrict the sharing of their sensitive personal health information (PHI), particularly if such records are held on a server that is owned by a third party, in which case some individuals may not completely trust the server. On the one hand, despite the existence of healthcare legislation such as the Health Insurance Portability and Accountability Act (HIPAA), which was recently expanded to include business partners, cloud service providers are not typically regarded as being included among the businesses that are protected by this legislation. However, due to the high value of sensitive PHI, the servers that are utilized for third-party storage are frequently the focus of different harmful actions that may result in the PHI being exposed. This is because the servers are located in a location that is not secure [33]. This is because of PHI's great monetary worth. Without permission, a Department of Veterans Affairs employee took the secret PHI of 26.5 million war veterans' homes with them and stole the database, which contained information such as the veterans' social security numbers and health issues [34]. This is a well-known occurrence. To ensure that patients have total control over the privacy of their PHRs, fine-grained data access control approaches that are compatible with semi-trusted servers are required.

13.16 PERSONAL HEALTH INFORMATION (PHI) PROPOSED SYSTEM

With the participation of a large number of PHR owners, an ABE-based architecture has been developed to facilitate the secure and patient-centric sharing of PHRs in cloud computing settings. The users of the system should be conceptually divided into two distinct kinds of domains—public domains (PUD) and personal domains (PSD) to handle the core management concerns. In particular, attribute authorities in the latter handle a distributive way the large number of professional users, whereas, in the former, each owner simply needs to be responsible for handling the keys for a restricted number of users in her domain. Our architecture is built in this manner to suit the requirements of several diverse PHR sharing applications while imposing a minimal amount of key management overhead on both system owners and users [35]. In addition, the framework supports write access control, handles dynamic policy updates, and provides emergency break-glass access to protected health records (PHRs). To avoid key escrow, increase the level of security in the public domain by implementing multi-authority ABE (MA-ABE). Each attribute authority (AA) inside it is responsible for supervising a specific subset of user role characteristics, but none of those authorities is capable of regulating the overall system's safety on their own. We provide key distribution and encryption approaches during the encryption process so that PHR owners can implement configurable fine-grained role-based access controls. Under the data attributes of a PHR file in the personal domain, owners can encrypt it and directly assign access privileges to personal users. Furthermore, it improves MA-ABE by presenting an effective and on-demand user/attribute revocation mechanism and demonstrating that this technique is secure under standard security assumptions. In this manner, patients will have complete discretion over the level of privacy connected with their PHRs [36].

13.17 REGISTRATION

The sign-up of new users into the websites is included in the registration process. Personal information, a medical history, and a physical examination are all possible components of the registration. Email address, password, phone number, username, gender, height, and age are the components that make up personal information. The medical history includes the status of the owner, as well as any allergies and medications they use. The examination includes taking your pulse, your heart rate, and a blood sample. The acronym PHR stands for "personal health record," and it refers to records that contain information on their owners, such as their details, medical histories and examinations, information about insurance policies, and other sensitive data as shown in Figure 13.11.

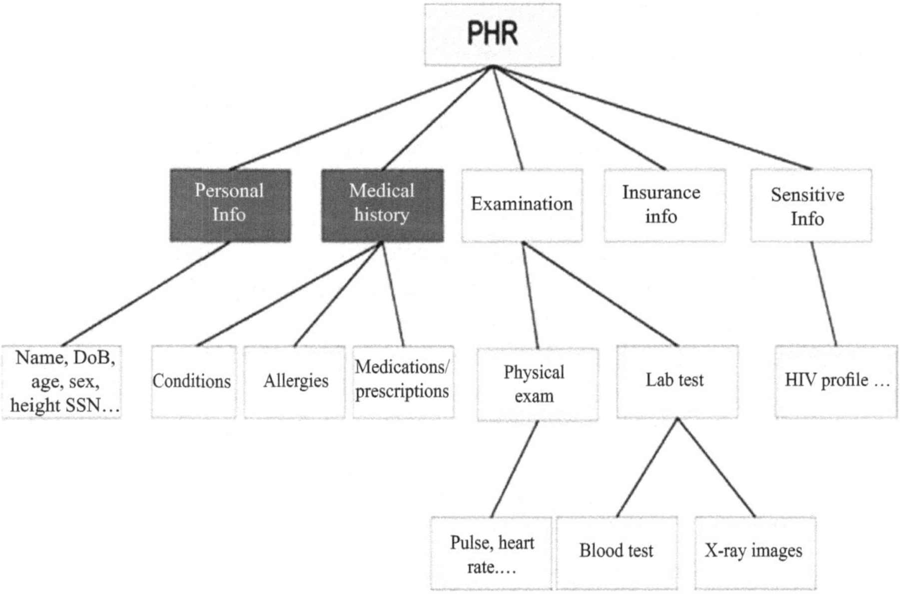

FIGURE 13.11 Personal health records.

13.18 PHR ENCRYPTION

The owners upload PHR files to the server that are encrypted using attribute-based encryption (ABE). Each owner's health record file is encrypted using both a specific fine-grained and role-based access policy that allows users from the PUD to access it, as well as a selected set of data attributes that allows access from users in the PSD [32, 36]. Both policies are enforced by the PSD. The PHR files can only be decrypted by authorized users; the server itself cannot do it. To achieve a higher level of productivity, the data attributes will incorporate every file type that lies between the root and the leaf nodes. For instance, the attributes of an "allergy" file are "PHR, medical history, allergy" in the figure that was just presented. The data readers get PHR files from the server, and the only way they can decrypt the files is if they have the appropriate attribute-based keys. If data contributors submit the necessary write keys, they will be granted write access to the PHR of the person whose data they contributed [37].

13.18.1 PHR ACCESS

Restriction of User Access. With the possibility of canceling a data reader's properties or access permissions, numerous scenarios are possible: (i) removal of one or more role attributes from a public domain user; (ii) removal of a public domain user, which has the same impact as removing all of that person's attributes. Both of these actions have the same effect. However, for the sake of enhanced efficiency, the actual computations may be delegated to the server rather than being done by the AA to which the user belongs; (iii) removal of access credentials associated with a personal domain user; and (iv) the deletion of an account associated with a personal user domain. These can also be triggered by utilizing the client application that is connected to the individual who owns the PHR. Changes to the Policies. By making changes to the characteristics (or access policy) in the cipher text, a PHR document's owner can modify the sharing policy that is associated with an existing PHR document [38]. Add, remove, and modify are some of the operations that are supported and that can be performed by the server on the user's behalf.

13.18.2 REGISTRATION OF PHYSICIANS

The registration process also involves signing new doctors up for accounts on the relevant websites. Personal information about the doctor, in addition to information about their practice, could be included in the registration. The individual's name, password, email address, and phone number make up his or her personal information, whereas the individual's profession, area of expertise, and the name of his or her hospital make up his or her professional information [39].

13.18.3 DOCTOR REMARKS

In this module, according to owner PHR records (personal information, medical history, Examination), the doctor provides the prescriptions [40].

Within cypher text-policy attribute-based encryption (CP-ABE), one of the primary overheads that contributes to the decline in scalability and efficiency is the process of updating policies. An owner of the data must do an update on the policy to bring it up to date. This involves adding, modifying, or removing attributes or logical gates (AND, OR, or M of N) from the policies. In this situation, the data owner is responsible for retrieving the policies, which have traditionally been stored at the location of the data owner, and then carrying out the update. After the policy has been modified, it will be necessary to re-encrypt any cipher texts that were previously encrypted using the policy that is being revised. Following the completion of the re-encryption process, the cipher texts will be stored in the cloud [40]. These kinds of activities are often carried out by the owners of the data, which results in an increase in the amount of processing and communication overhead on the owners' end. In the case of the management of PHRs, patients may need to update the access policy that is used to encrypt their medical data. This is necessary to grant access to their medical treatments to other physicians working in various hospitals. For the most part, providing policy updates in a CP-ABE scenario can be accomplished through either cipher text update or proxy re-encryption (PRE), both of which are two different ways.

13.19 CONCLUSION

In the context of cloud computing, an innovative new framework for the safe exchange of PHRs has been developed. To fully actualize the patient-centric approach and take into account the reality that cloud servers are only partially trustworthy, we believe that patients should have complete control over their privacy and be able to encrypt their health record data for granular access. The approach solves the specific issues that are brought up by a wide variety of PHR owners and users by drastically simplifying the process of key management while simultaneously increasing the number of privacy assurances that are provided in comparison to previous research. Encrypting patient health record data with an algorithm known as ABE so that patients can provide access to personal users but to users from PUD who hold a variety of professional positions, certifications, and affiliations. Because of this, patients can share the information included in their PHRs with a higher number of users. In addition to this, we improve an existing MA-ABE scheme by making it capable of managing user revocation in an effective and on-demand manner, and we demonstrate the system's security. Using both simulation and actual implementation, we demonstrate that our technique is both scalable and efficient.

COVID-19's extraordinary humanitarian and economic issues are prompting rapid and widespread use of cutting-edge digital technologies. Online databases can help epidemiological intelligence by identifying cases and clusters of diseases, easily tracing contacts, and monitoring movement patterns during lockdowns. Public health messages can also be sent out on a large scale using these digital technologies. There are still hurdles to overcome before digital solutions become commonplace. As the COVID-19 pandemic is ongoing, it is too early to accurately assess the contribution of digital technology to the fight against the pandemic. When it comes to dealing with a pandemic, digital tools can be helpful, but they are not a cure-all. In addition to standard public-health therapies, it is becoming increasingly apparent that it plays a comprehensive response to the outbreaks and pandemics, and as a result, they contribute to mitigating the effects of COVID-19 on individuals and the economy. It will be necessary to conduct rapid and widespread testing with digital symptom checkers and contact tracking, epidemiological information, and long-term clinical follow-up to develop digital online care pathways that link these talents with cost-effectiveness and sustainability. Although data sharing and community interaction are crucial in the expanding mobile and digital healthcare sector, the COVID-19 epidemic has emphasized the need for even more stringent evaluation and ethical frameworks that incorporate community engagement. COVID-19 is a highly contagious virus, as confirmed by the pandemic. The public's trust must be earned by establishing strategies for communication across all digital platforms and explaining a proper commitment to privacy protection. Public health and pandemic planning must acknowledge the significance of digital technologies, the public health future is anticipated to become digital. Similar to viruses, data and digital technologies do not appear to care where they originate. Urgently required is a global framework for the regulation, evaluation, and use of digital technology to improve pandemic management and future preparedness for COVID-19 and other infectious diseases. This alignment must be completed immediately.

13.20 FUTURE ENHANCEMENT

The application of the Apriori method to the data to be used in the proposed system will be used to prepare datasets, which will then be used to extract hidden knowledge. Predicting a person's smart health is only possible if the system behaves in the desired manner. ARM will be used to construct the final report, which will involve comparing these datasets with the queries that are being submitted. Patients will be able to receive an immediate diagnosis with the assistance of this proposed methodology because it will be based on actual historical data and will produce precise and effective findings. In the future, more work can be done to improve the classification by making use of additional datasets that are related to cardiovascular diseases and by making use of various methods of data reduction. The datasets that will be used must be quality-focused and free from outliers, inconsistencies, and missing values to achieve a higher level of accuracy in the diagnosis and prediction of cardiac illnesses. The functionality of this online application may be improved by developing it as an Android app. Users will be able to access this on their mobile devices, and there is potential for its use to expand even further. Also, the functionality makes the doctor available online via chat, so that patients can have a direct conversation with the concerned physicians. The modules that do cancer analysis can be combined to determine the relative proximity of the person connected with cancer. Because of this, the behavior of this web application will become more predictable.

ACKNOWLEDGMENT

The authors thank the management of Dr. M.G.R. Educational and Research Institute, Chennai, for the continuous encouragement to do the research work inside the campus. The authors also thank Mrs. J. Vijayalakshmi, Technical Assistant (Joint Registrar), Dr. M.G.R. Educational and Research Institute, Chennai for her work in editing and proofreading.

FUNDING

This research received no specific grant from any funding agency in the public, commercial, or not-for-profit sectors.

CONFLICT OF INTEREST

The authors declare that they do not have any conflicts of interest.

KEYWORDS

- **attributed-based encryption**
- **COVID-19**
- **digital technology**
- **e-health solution**
- **electronic health record**
- **personal health information**
- **personal health record**
- **PHR encryption**

REFERENCES

1. Khorsand, R., Ghobaei-Arani, M., & Ramezanpour, M., (2019). A self-learning fuzzy approach for proactive resource provisioning in cloud environment. *Softw: Pract. Exper., 49*(11), 1618–1642.
2. Jula, A., Sundararajan, E. A., Othman, Z., & Naseri, N. K., (2021). Color revolution: A novel operator for imperialist competitive algorithm in solving cloud computing service composition problem. *Symmetry, 13*(2), 177. doi: https://doi.org/10.3390/sym13020177.
3. Alboaneen, D., Tianfield, H., Zhang, Y., & Pranggono, B., (2020). A metaheuristic method for joint task scheduling and virtual machine placement in cloud data centers. *Future Generation Computer Systems, 115*, 201–212. doi: https://doi.org/10.1016/j.future.2020.08.036.
4. Otsetova, A., & Otsetova-Dudin, E., (2019). Growth and opportunities in mobile internet market in Bulgaria. *Transport and Communications, 7*(2), 21–27. doi: 10.26552/tac.C.2019.2.5.
5. Pang, J., Xu, H., Ren, J., et al., (2021). Process mining framework with time perspective for understanding acute care: A case study of AIS in hospitals. *BMC Med. Inform. Decis. Mak., 21*, 354. https://doi.org/10.1186/s12911-021-01725-1.
6. Jonnro, E., Irene, V., Konstantinos, T., & Paul, G., (2020). Using business process models for the specification of manufacturing operations. *Computers in Industry, 123*, 103297, ISSN 0166-3615, https://doi.org/10.1016/j.compind.2020.103297.
7. Ehrenstein, V., Kharrazi, H., Lehmann, H., et al., (2019). Obtaining data from electronic health records. In: Gliklich, R. E., Leavy, M. B., & Dreyer, N. A., (eds.), *Tools and Technologies for Registry Interoperability, Registries for Evaluating Patient Outcomes: A User's Guide* (3rd edn.). Addendum 2 [Internet]. Rockville (MD): Agency for Healthcare Research and Quality (US); Chapter 4. Available from: https://www.ncbi.nlm.nih.gov/books/NBK551878/ (accessed on 4 December 2023).
8. Tugnait, J. K., (2021). Sparse graph learning under Laplacian-related constraints. In: *IEEE Access* (vol. 9, pp. 151067–151079). doi: 10.1109/ACCESS.2021.3126675.

9. Pei, Z., Sun, Y., Wang, S., et al., (2020). Estimating mortality among inpatients with acute exacerbation of chronic obstructive pulmonary disease using registry data. *NPJ Prim. Care Respir. Med. 30*, 28. https://doi.org/10.1038/s41533-020-0186-y.
10. Celli, B. R., & Wedzicha, J. A., (2019). Update on clinical aspects of chronic obstructive pulmonary disease. *N. Engl. J. Med., 381*, 1257–1266.
11. Mathioudakis, A. G., Janssens, W., Sivapalan, P., et al., (2020). Acute exacerbations of chronic obstructive pulmonary disease: In search of diagnostic biomarkers and treatable traits. *Thorax., 75*, 520–527.
12. Lauritsen, S. M., Kristensen, M., Olsen, M. V., et al., (2020). Explainable artificial intelligence model to predict acute critical illness from electronic health records. *Nat. Commun., 11*, 3852. https://doi.org/10.1038/s41467-020-17431-x.
13. Juvé-Udina, M. E., Adamuz, J., López-Jimenez, M. M., et al., (2019). Predicting patient acuity according to their main problem. *J. Nurs. Manag., 27*, 1845–1858. https://doi.org/10.1111/jonm.12885
14. Bhuiyan, M., & Mohammad Al, H., (2018). Representing graphs as bag of vertices and partitions for graph classification. *Data Science and Engineering, 3*(2), 150. Gale Academic OneFile, link.gale.com/apps/doc/A550913925/AONE?u=googlescholar&sid=bookmark-AONE&xid=281d4ab9 (accessed on 4 December 2023).
15. Jones, A., Whyley, H., Doyle, J., & Bevan, L., (2018). Development of approaches and legislation to optimize nurse staffing levels. *Nursing Standard, 33*(5), 27–31. https://doi.org/10.7748/ns.2018.e11202.
16. Rosenberg, K., (2019). RN shortages negatively impact patient safety. *AJN American Journal of Nursing, 119*(3), 51. doi: 10.1097/01.NAJ.0000554040.98991.23.
17. Hawkins, M., Messier, A., Myers, K., Nihsen, A., & Kniewel, M., (2019). Using an acuity tool that interfaces with the electronic health record to balance nursing workload. *I-Manager's Journal on Nursing, 9*(2), 36–42. https://doi.org/10.26634/jnur.9.2.16250.
18. Rajkomar, A., Oren, E., Chen, K., et al., (2018). Scalable and accurate deep learning with electronic health records. *NPJ. Digit. Med., 1*, 18. doi: 10.1038/s41746-018-0029-1.
19. Gulmezoglu, B., Inci, M. S., Irazoqui, G., Eisenbarth, T., & Sunar, B., (2016). "Cross-VM cache attacks on AES. *IEEE Transactions on Multi-Scale Computing Systems* (Vol. 2, No. 3, pp. 211–222). doi: 10.1109/TMSCS.2016.2550438.
20. Mani, A., Reihaneh, K., & Mohammadreza, R., (2021). An adaptive fault detector strategy for scientific workflow scheduling based on improved differential evolution algorithm in cloud. *Applied Soft Computing, 99*, 106895. ISSN 1568-4946. https://doi.org/10.1016/j.asoc.2020.106895.
21. Wu, H., Wang, C., Lu, K., Fu, Y., & Zhu, L., (2018). One size does not fit all: The case for chunking configuration in backup deduplication. *Proceedings – 18th IEEE/ACM International Symposium on Cluster, Cloud and Grid Computing, CCGRID* (pp. 213–222). doi: 10.1109/CCGRID.2018.00036.
22. Maria, C. C., Marco, L. D. V., & Daniele, T., (2019). A methodological framework for cloud resource provisioning and scheduling of data-parallel applications under uncertainty. *Future Generation Computer Systems, 93*, 212–223. ISSN 0167-739X, https://doi.org/10.1016/j.future.2018.10.037.
23. Goshgar, I., & Haluk, R. T., (2020). Neural network-based multi-objective evolutionary algorithm for dynamic workflow scheduling in cloud computing. *Future Generation Computer Systems, 102*, 307–322. ISSN 0167-739X, https://doi.org/10.1016/j.future.2019.08.012.

24. Hadeer, A. H., Sameh, A. S., & Elsayed, M. S., (2020). A smart energy and reliability aware scheduling algorithm for workflow execution in DVFS-enabled cloud environment. *Future Generation Computer Systems, 112*, 431–448. ISSN 0167-739X, https://doi.org/10.1016/j.future.2020.05.040.
25. Tamilvizhi, T., & Parvathavarthini, B., (2019). A novel method for adaptive fault tolerance during load balancing in cloud computing. *Cluster Comput., 22*, 10425–10438. https://doi.org/10.1007/s10586-017-1038-6.
26. Shen, J., Deng, X., & Xu, Z., (2019). Multi-security-level cloud storage system based on improved proxy re-encryption. *J. Wireless Com Network, 2019*, 277. https://doi.org/10.1186/s13638-019-1614-y.
27. Kok, K. J., John, M., & Liam, M., (2022). Energy-efficient virtual-machine mapping algorithm (EViMA) for workflow tasks with deadlines in a cloud environment. *Journal of Network and Computer Applications, 203*, 103400. ISSN 1084-8045. https://doi.org/10.1016/j.jnca.2022.
28. Lin, C., Cao, Q., Huang, J., Yao, J., Li, X., & Xie, C., (2018). HPDV: A highly parallel deduplication cluster for virtual machine images. In: *Proceedings of the 18th IEEE/ACM International Symposium on Cluster, Cloud and Grid Computing* (pp. 472–481). doi: 10.1109/CCGRID.2018.00074.
29. Zuo, C., Shao, J., Liu, J. K., Wei, G., & Ling, Y., (2018). Fine-grained two-factor protection mechanism for data sharing in cloud storage. *IEEE Transactions on Information Forensics and Security* (Vol. 13, No. 1, pp. 186–196).
30. Mohan, E., Anandan, R., & Shakthibalan, S., (2021). The data de-duplication in cloud storage management. *Natural Volatiles & Essential Oils Journal, 8*(2), 118–124.
31. Hölbl, M., Kompara, M., Kamišalić, A., & Nemec, Z. L., (2018). A systematic review of the use of blockchain in healthcare. *Symmetry, 10*(10), 470. doi: 10.3390/sym10100470. C.
32. Li, M., Yu, S., Zheng, Y., Ren, K., & Lou, W., (2013). Scalable and secure sharing of personal health records in cloud computing using attribute-based encryption. In: *IEEE Transactions on Parallel and Distributed Systems* (Vol. 24, No. 1, pp. 131–143). doi: 10.1109/TPDS.2012.97.
33. Andrikopoulou, E., Scott, P., Herrera, H., & Good, A., (2019). What are the important design features of personal health records to improve medication adherence for patients with long-term conditions? A systematic literature review. *BMJ Open, 9*(9), e028628. doi: 10.1136/bmjopen-2018-028628. PMID: 31558449; PMCID: PMC6773318.
34. Fang, H., Tan, T. H., Tan, Y., & Tan, C., (2021). Blockchain personal health records: Systematic review. *Journal of Medical Internet Research, 23*(4), e25094. https://doi.org/10.2196/25094.
35. Miyachi, C., (2018). What is "Cloud"? It is time to update the NIST definition? In: *IEEE Cloud Computing* (Vol. 5, No. 3, pp. 6–11). doi: 10.1109/MCC.2018.032591611.
36. Li, M., (2012). *On the Confidentiality of Information Dispersal Algorithms and Their Erasure Codes* (pp. 1–4). [Online]. Available: http://arxiv.org/abs/1206.4123.
37. Zhe, L., Fuqun, W., Kefei, C., & Fei, T., (2020). A new user revocable ciphertext-policy attribute-based encryption with ciphertext update. *Security and Communication Networks, 2020*, 11. Article ID 8856592. https://doi.org/10.1155/2020/885659.2.
38. Chang, S. C., Lu, M. T., Pan, T. H., & Chen, C. S., (2021). Evaluating the e-health cloud computing systems adoption in Taiwan's healthcare industry. *Life, 11*(4), 310. https://doi.org/10.3390/life11040310.

39. Divya, P. A., & Pradeep, K. T. S., (2019). MLPPT-MHS: Multi-layered privacy-preserving and traceable mobile health system. *Procedia Computer Science, 165*, 598–614. ISSN 1877-0509. https://doi.org/10.1016/j.procs.2020.01.054.
40. Ismail, K., & Ammar, O., (2021). Security and privacy of electronic health records: Concerns and challenges, *Egyptian Informatics Journal, 22*(2), 177–183. ISSN 1110-8665, https://doi.org/10.1016/j.eij.2020.07.003.

CHAPTER 14

Autonomous Robots: A Disruptive Technology in the Health Sector

BIKASH RANJAN JENA,[1] G. S. N. KOTESWARA RAO,[2] NAGA JOGAYYA KOTHAKOTA,[1] ROJA RANI BUDHA,[3] L. SRINIVAS,[4] J. RAJKUMAR,[5] and SURYA KOVVASU[6]

[1]*School of Pharmacy and Life Sciences, Centurion University of Technology and Management, Jatni, Odisha, India*

[2]*Department of Pharmacy, School of Medical and Allied Sciences, Galgotias University, Greater Noida, Uttar Pradesh, India*

[3]*Department of Pharmacology, Institute of Pharmaceutical Technology, Sri Padmavati Mahila Visvavidyalayam, Tirupati, Andhra Pradesh, India*

[4]*Department Pharmaceutics, Gitam Institute of Pharmacy, Gitam University, Visakhapatnam, Andhra Pradesh, India*

[5]*Department of Pharmaceutics, Vaageswari College of Pharmacy, Karimnagar, Telangana, India*

[6]*Ambiopharm Inc., Beech Island, North Augusta, South Carolina, USA*

ABSTRACT

Upcoming healthcare systems design might result in more convenient, economical, and primary and specialty care. It might also minimize individual interference in challenging tasks. For example, the ability of artificial intelligence could revolutionize medical education, illness analysis, and popular drugs. In the twenty-first century, learning robots driven by artificial intelligence systems will be a new and inventive technology in healthcare. Professionals will be prepared to provide the finest care possible

Creating Smart Healthcare with Blockchain and Advanced Digital Technology.
Rishabha Malviya and Sonali Sundram (Eds.)

by integrating medical databases and their experience. The degree to which robots are self-sufficient is governed by the work at hand, the environment in which the robot is deployed, and the amount of interaction necessary between people and robots. Autonomous healthcare robots include delivery, nursing, and surgical robots. The capacity of robots to undertake automatic actions and sophisticated jobs is expanding responsibilities in various application industries. Autonomous robots may contribute to the advancement of therapeutic practice in the pharmaceutical, healthcare, and biotech sectors by delivering a safer, more dependable, and cost-effective form of improved therapies and diverse research methodologies. In addition, several enhancements will be necessary to integrate these new-fangled automated technologies fully. Furthermore, the ethical consequences of these technologies are unknown. This chapter emphasizes recent advances in artificial intelligence, case studies, current status, and future directions of autonomous robots in targeted medication therapy in healthcare systems, Pathogen identification using genetics and genomics, and other molecular-based investigations in the biotech industry.

14.1 INTRODUCTION

As technology progresses, autonomous robots (ARs) will eventually command future supply chains due to the increased human-like capabilities that will be available to them. Robots are revolutionizing surgical procedures in the healthcare industry. They are also helping to speed up the delivery of supplies and the cleaning process, which frees up more time for doctors to focus on patient care. Intel provides various technologies for developing medical robots, such as mobile surgical robots, modular components, and autonomous operations. These are only some of the options available. As advanced machine learning (ML), computational statistics (data analytics), computers, and other relevant technologies continue to grow, medical robotics will develop to the point where they can do jobs more independently and precisely. Intel is working with other companies that sell technology and academic institutions to investigate potential solutions for the next generation of robotics. Through financing investigation and technology, Intel contributes to developing innovative applications for AI and Internet of Things (IoT) technologies in medical robotics systems. These system contributions assist in funding ongoing technologies that upsurge automation, boost efficiency, and address several significant concerns that are vital to the healthcare industry. The development of health robots will continue in tandem with the evolution of other technologies above statistical data and computational analytics— ML, etc. Robots of every imaginable variety will continue to advance to carry out jobs independently, efficiently, and accurately. Intel is working with other companies that sell technology and academic institutions to investigate potential solutions for robotics for the next generation. Intel is providing research and technical assistance to aid in the process of determining new applications for artificial intelligence (AI) and IoT technologies in the arena of medical robotics. These contributions assist in funding technologies that can boost automation and efficiency and address several significant concerns vital to the healthcare industry. ARs and drone aircraft (aerial robots) are two new categories of technology that can be developed to perform activities with little to no involvement or input from humans. These robots can also be referred to as "aerial robots." They can range from flying vehicles to robotic process automation with significant data and picture-collecting capabilities in terms of stability, mobility power, and AI; they can cost; from a few dollars to millions of dollars.

An ever-increasing number of self-sufficient robots are currently going through the process of having AI installed in them so that they may recognize their surroundings, gain knowledge from them, and form their own opinions. This shift, which is having significant repercussions for the healthcare system, is being driven by the rapid development of analytics tools and the explosion in available healthcare data. In the field of medicine, some of the most common uses of AI include research on cancer, neurological disorders, and cardiovascular disease. After that, we will discuss how AI has been utilized to improve stroke care in the three critical areas of diacritical, rehabilitation, and prevention. Our discussion will come to a close with a look at some early examples of AI, such as IBM Watson, and then explore wider adoption of AI [10]. Similarly, today, there is a more significant demand to deliver high-quality healthcare worldwide, and this need has encouraged the creation of a wide variety of computerized and robotic healthcare tools that are assisted by AI. As a result, the next generation of digital diagnostic tools and healthcare robotics can benefit from an appropriate version of the Turing test to offer total diagnostic scores for AI [8–10].

14.2 CATEGORIES OF AUTONOMOUS ROBOTS (ARS)

14.2.1 SURGICAL-BASED ROBOTS

As motion-control technology has evolved, so have surgical robots. AI and computer vision help surgeons perform complex surgeries faster and more precisely. For example, some surgical robots may be able to work modifiers while surgeons monitor from a console [11].

14.2.2 *CRITICAL SURGERIES PERFORMED WITH ROBOTICS*

Modern robotics and AI can be beneficial for managing critical surgeries in medical centers, diagnostic centers, and the various robotics systems that help perform surgeries in other sectors. Significant examples are outlined in succeeding sections [11].

14.2.3 *MINIMALLY INVASIVE THORACIC SURGERY*

Procedures like robotic hysterectomy, prostatectomy, and weight loss surgeries mainly target soft tissues. These robots provide a secure foundation for remote surgical treatments and can be placed using minimally invasive techniques. Open surgery with huge incisions was the only option for doing most internal aesthetic operations in the past. In addition to a longer recovery time, the risk of infection and other complications was also higher. Manually operating via an incision, the size of a button, is challenging for even the most experienced surgeons. Surgical robots simplify procedures, increase accuracy, and decrease risks of infection and other complications [12].

14.2.4 *ORTHOPEDIC-DRIVEN SURGERIES*

Robots can perform common orthopedic surgeries, including total knee and hip replacements, using data analytics, 3D imaging, and intelligent robotic arms; these robots help surgeons with preoperative planning by more accurately outlining spaces. A robot can be taught to conduct a range of orthopedic treatments by using instructions derived from an AI-generated model. By transmitting a live video stream from the operating room to a nearby or faraway location, doctors can consult with each other. The top surgeons can now treat patients thanks to this. Now more than ever, AI is the backbone of today's surgical robots. The development of computer vision has enabled surgical robots to identify and distinguish between numerous tissue types. In robotic surgery, for instance, less damage to the patient's muscles and nerves is possible. High-definition Surgeons can benefit from 3D computer vision because it gives them a complete picture of their patients and a deeper comprehension of their conditions. Robots will soon be able to do suturing and other minor surgical procedures under the supervision of a surgeon. Now more than ever, robotic surgery training is required in medical school. Simulation systems for training surgical robots blend augmented reality with AI. By manipulating virtual surgical instruments with robotic arms, surgical trainees can gain experience in a safe, realistic environment [11–13].

14.2.5 ROBOTS BUILT-IN MODULES

Modular robots have more extraordinary adaptability and versatility than conventional systems. Robots with prosthetic limbs and exoskeletons are among them. Therapeutic robots can help people recover from injuries such as stroke, paralysis, or traumatic brain injury. They are also beneficial for people who have trouble moving around, such as individuals with MS. Intel and Accenture are working on a robotic arm that can be mounted to a wheelchair to aid individuals with spinal cord injuries. Equipped with AI, robots and profundity cameras can evaluate patients' mobility in several environments and track their progress more accurately than a human observer. It's also possible for them to communicate with patients and offer guidance and emotional support [10, 14].

14.2.6 AUTONOMOUS MOBILE ROBOTS (AMR)

Since autonomous mobile robots (AMRs) may help with various crucial activities in healthcare, including disinfection, telepresence, and the delivery of drugs and medical supplies, they have frequently used its boost security and frees up employees to dedicate more time to patient care. Light detection and ranging technology (LiDAR), Visual Computing, and capabilities mapping enable medical robots to navigate patients towards examination or hospital rooms without human intervention [15–17]. Professionals can now have remote interaction with patients. If AMRs can be controlled remotely by experts or other hospital employees, doctors may feel comfortable carrying them around the facility as they see fit. An expert may offer real-time advice on a patient's diagnosis and treatment from the safety behind a computer screen. Robots can help with pre-admission activities before a patient is ever admitted. Using a robot created by the Mexican business Roomie, doctors in Mexico can treat high-risk patients with COVID-19. Roomie Bot records a patient's vitals and medical history as soon as they check-in. Intel® Movidius

TM vision processing units (VPUs), 8th Generation Intel® NUCs, and Intel® RealSense TM cameras are some of the Intel technologies that power Roomie Bot. The terms "service" and "social" robots collectively make up another category of AMRs with potential medical applications [16, 17].

14.2.7 SOCIAL-BASED ROBOTS

In the medical field, service robots can relieve some of the everyday strain on human workers by performing menial duties. Machines that can hold authentic conversations with humans are called "social robots." In elderly facilities, these "warm and fluffy" robots can act as friends and guard dogs. Cognitive engagement and treatment adherence strategies can help patients stay attentive and cheerful. They can also serve as wayfinding aids for visitors and patients alike. Overall, using social robots has been shown to improve the well-being of patients and caregivers [15, 16].

14.2.8 SERVICES ENABLED ROBOTS

Service robots are meant to perform repetitive tasks, which can help alleviate some of the monotony experienced by human healthcare professionals regularly. "Social robots" refer to machines that can hold natural conversations with humans. These "warm and fuzzy" robots can serve as friends and guardians for the elderly and disabled in nursing homes. Patients might be encouraged to stay optimistic and alert through cognitive engagement and interventions that improve treatment adherence. Additionally, they can help patients and visitors find their way around the entire facility. The employment of social robots has been shown to improve both the patients' and their caregivers' psychological and physiological well-being [10, 16, 17].

14.2.9 DENTAL ROBOTICS

The earliest robots required a human to control them. Still, automated systems have traveled a long way in the past 10 years, and the most recent medical robots are capable of performing patient intervention or remote monitoring on their own. Dental replanting, oral and maxillofacial operations, prosthetic and restorative dentistry, root canal therapy, orthodontics, oral radiographs, and dentistry education are some disciplines that have successfully implemented robot systems [4–6, 16].

14.3 NANOROBOTS: A MODERN APPROACH TO SYSTEMIZED ROBOTICS

In the present scenario, the Nanorobots are used in various sophisticated handling of human care like ophthalmology or ophthalmic treatments, Hematology, treating cancer cells, antiviral therapies, tissue engineering, cellular assistance in the inflammatory response, early monitoring of microbes, etc. However, some of the practical applications of Nanorobot's and its reliable applicability in healthcare diagnosis, mitigation, and eradication of all critical health diseases are specified below. The modern era of Nanorobots is designed to counteract tumors of chronic stages and is known as "Nanobots." Nanobots refer to engineered nanomachines or simply tiny robots at the nanoscale level.

14.3.1 TINY ENGINE-BASED NANOROBOTS

German physicists created the smallest engine in the world from a single atom. Like other engines, it transfers heat into motion, albeit on a smaller scale. Atoms are trapped within a cone of electromagnetic radiation, and lasers heat and cool them, causing them to oscillate like a piston [10, 17].

14.3.2 DNA-ENABLED 3D-MOTION NANOMACHINES

By expanding on the complex nanoscale mechanical components using 'the DNA origami,' a team of mechanical engineers and experts from Ohio State University have shown the basic design for applying the same principles that apply to normal machine fragments can now be functional to DNA to configurable machinery and strategy complex towards upcoming nanorobotics [17–19].

14.3.3 ADVANCED NANOSWIMMERS

Researchers from Technion and ETH Zurich developed an elastic "nano-swimmers" polypyrrole (Ppy) nanowire that can fly over biological fluid surroundings at about 15 micrometers per second. This nanowire is around 200 nanometers thick and 15 micrometers long. The ability to distribute pharmaceuticals and target cancer cells using magnetic targeting might be added to the functionality of the nano-swimmers [17].

14.3.4 A NANO-ENGINE LOOKS LIKE AN ANT

Scientists at Cambridge have developed an ant-like nano-engine having 100 times the force/unit weight. New nano-engines have the potential to pave the way for disease-fighting nanorobots that can enter living cells, according to the study's authors. The study director was Professor Jeremy Baumberg of the Cavendish Laboratory (ANTs). In the same way, real ants can produce disproportionately strong forces for their size [17, 18].

14.3.5 SPERM-INSPIRED MICROROBOTS

Microrobots relied on the sperm morphologies created by researchers at the German University in Cairo and the University of Twente in the Netherlands and were programmed to move in response to fluctuating moderate magnetic fields. Complex micro-manipulation and focused therapy will also incorporate them [17–19].

14.3.6 BACTERIA-POWERED ROBOTS

Robots powered by bacteria can use electric fields to sense their surroundings and navigate around obstacles, according to researchers at Drexel University. Medications may be delivered, stem cells can be manipulated to affect growth, and microstructures can be built [17–19].

14.3.7 NANOROCKETS

Researchers have created high-speed, remote-controlled nanoscale rockets by mixing nanoparticles with biological molecules. Researchers seek to construct a rocket that may be used in any setting, such as to deliver medications [18, 19]. The outline of various categories of Nanorobots is represented below for systematic understanding [20]. A glimpse of different nanorobots and their categories are drawn in Figure 14.1.

14.4 MICROROBOTS AND THEIR APPLICATIONS

Medical and biological tasks are just two examples of the many new uses for microrobots and microscopic robots. Several unique designs have

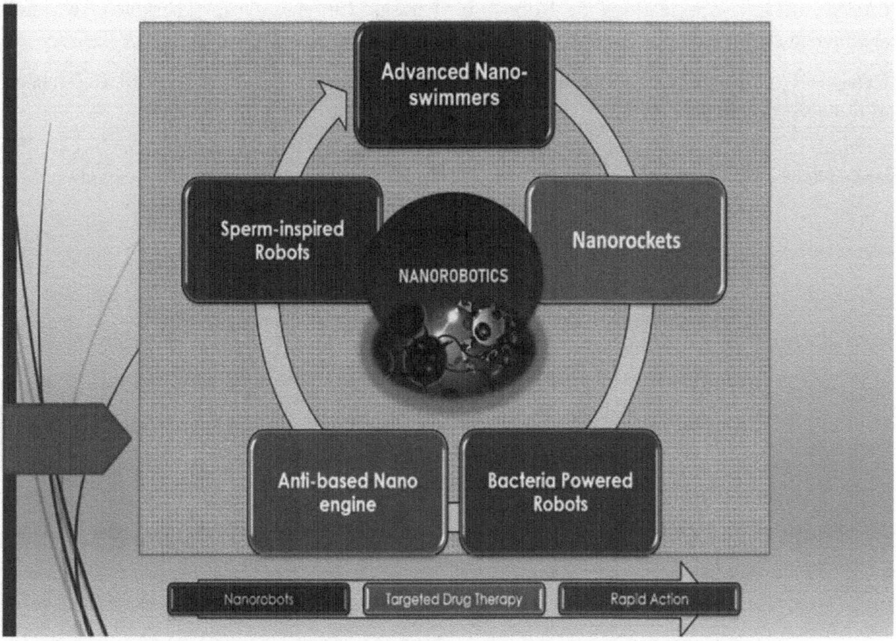

FIGURE 14.1 Diagram indicating categories of nanorobots in diverse fields.

been presented for microrobots; Microrobots (particularly bacterium-empowered robots) have demonstrated outstanding potential to undertake microscale activities, including drug delivery, cell manipulation, micro-assembly, and biosensing [19–21] via manual control. Recently, medical micro-/nanorobotic platforms incorporating magnetic resonance imaging (MRI) have been researched to reach deep regions in the human body while boosting targeting efficacy. Recent advances have been made in the field of microrobotics. For example, biological microrobots may directly leverage the power of pathogens for propulsion and sensing, while synthetic micro-robots can duplicate the motions of microorganisms to achieve mobility successfully. Systemic chemotherapy remains the backbone of many cancer treatments [19–26]. Engineering microrobots are rapidly garnering this attention, particularly their mobility, allowing the microrobots to penetrate tissues and access malignancies cell lines more efficiently [12, 27–29]. The applications of different categories of Robots and their applications in targeted drug therapies in medicine and healthcare systems are illustrated in Table 14.1.

TABLE 14.1 Applications of Robots in Various Targeted Drug Therapies and their Mechanisms

Categories of Robots	Targeted Drug Therapies/Site of Action	Applications	References
Surgical-based robots	The applications of robotics are vast, and they have helped to enrich surgical subspecialties by providing benefits such as improved three-dimensional visualization and wristed articulation. Robotics applications have helped to enrich surgical subspecialties by providing benefits such as improved three-dimensional visualization, wristed articulation, enhanced surgeon autonomy and control, enhanced instrument dexterity, and enhanced tissue management.	Despite general trending surgery, the count includes the surgical subspecialties of colorectal surgery, cardiac surgery, biliary and pancreatic systems, gastric oncology, bariatric surgery, surgery of the anterior digestive tract, pediatric surgery, and endocrine surgery. The large area of expertise has generated a plethora of first-rate randomized Meta-Analyzes, measured trials, and retrospective and prospective studies.	[11, 12, 29, 31]
Modular robots	Robotic systems capable of self-reconfiguration are called "modular" or "self-reconfigurable" robots and are autonomous kinematic machines of varying morphology.	Sensors, actuators, CPUs, power supplies, and so on are only some of the functionalities that can be bundled into small, portable modules in modular robots. These modules connect using reusable connectors that rearrange their configurations with various ranges for an extensive range of morphological studies. Examples of such devices include exoskeletons and artificial limbs.	[14]
Social robots	Service robots relieve some of the burden of mundane work traditionally performed by healthcare workers. Machines that can hold authentic conversations with humans are called "social robots."	Social robots can take over complete job duties in the workplace, such as welcoming people and providing basic customer service. Examples include. Social robots have the potential to perform a variety of tasks, including psychological treatment, cognitive instruction, social facilitation, companionship, and even physiological therapy.	[34]
Industrial robots	Drug discovery is used in the pharmaceutical and therapeutic device manufacturing industries for various targeted therapies, such as oncology remission.	The pick-and-place robotics pattern for syringe tray loader is used in pharmaceutical packaging.	[35]

TABLE 14.1 *(Continued)*

Categories of Robots	Targeted Drug Therapies/Site of Action	Applications	References
Nanorobots	Much hope rests on medical micro- and nanorobotics, which can improve passive diffusion approaches by delivering drugs more precisely and quickly. Because their delivery rate may be raised without sacrificing accuracy, this is the situation. For instance, magnetically guided nanorobots were utilized to deliver the drug fluorouracil to prevent tumors from developing in a mouse model. The study's goal was to find a way to slow or stop tumor development; therefore, this was done. However, biohybrid nanorobots have also been used to accurately implant payloads inside live living creatures. This was achieved by carefully inserting the nanorobots under the animal's skin.	• Applications of *in-vivo* micro- and nanorobotics include, among other things, propulsion through the eye, as well as improved capacities for medicine delivery to tissues and retinal cells, as well as the posterior section of the eye. • It is utilized in the therapy of cancer in order to eradicate malignant cells. Among the most critical applications of this technology are more efficient vaccines, the administration of DNA probes, materials for cell imaging, and delivery vehicles that are particular to individual cells.	[24, 37, 38]
Autonomous mobile robots (AMRs)	AMRs can be used to dispense medication, sterilize surfaces, or give the capability for mobile telepresence. Cobots can also assist medical professionals during rehabilitation or provide nurses with assistance to provide better patient care.	• Utilized in the medical field to improve the overall experience of the patient. • Utilized in the biopharmaceutical and biotech industries, which have stringently controlled production procedures.	[39, 40]

14.5 MODERN ROBOTICS IN THE COURSE OF SUPPLY CHAIN MANAGEMENT (SCM)

It is anticipated that ARs will skyrocket over the next five years, specifically in areas of the supply chain that perform low-value and high-risk operations. Production, assembly, and storage are just a few examples of the stories currently seeing widespread adoption of ARs. In the future, more ARs will be utilized in these industries, freeing humans to focus on more functional, less dangerous, and more strategic activities throughout the supply chain [19–24]. In the future supply chain, ARs will play an increasingly important role as technology advances. Increased haptic (touch) sensors, for instance, will allow robots to pick up everything from delicate eggshells to sophisticated metal assembly pieces without requiring further programming or hardware updates [25–28].

ARs are becoming increasingly sophisticated, reducing the time needed to set them up, reducing the amount of monitoring they need, and cooperating more closely with people. The benefits will increase when ARs evolve to the point where they can work autonomously around the clock with improved quality and productivity. As a result, these robots will be able to work autonomously. It is projected that as the market for ARs expands, the supply chain will have a more flexible end-to-end alignment [26–29]. As more companies adopt ARs for specialized operations in the supply chain, pilot programs are testing a variety of robots to ensure that productivity increases will occur due to this trend. In the future, forward-thinking corporations may employ more robots whose primary purpose is to put together other robots. The general applications of ARs for managing the healthcare system are enlisted in Figure 14.2.

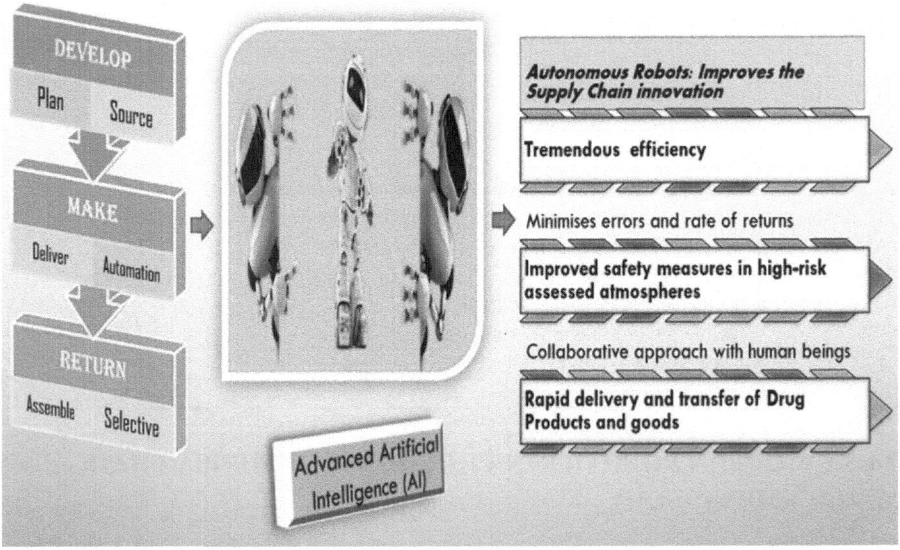

FIGURE 14.2 Autonomous robots driven supply chain management.

14.5.1 SYSTEMS OF ROBOTICS IN TREATING HOSPITALITY AND ECOSYSTEM

Traditionally, ARs have been employed for mundane, repetitive jobs. They were inflexible, requiring complicated programming both to set up and operate. Better AI means less programming time, less oversight, and the possibility of human-robot collaboration. Future supply chains will reap even more benefits from ARs as they improve their ability to work around the clock while maintaining high quality and productivity standards [12, 14, 31, 32, 34]. They can perform tasks that people cannot or choose not to. Supply chain innovation and value creation are propelled mainly by ARs' ability to reduce direct and indirect operating costs while simultaneously raising revenue. In particular, ARs can: Improve efficiency and productivity. Errors, repeating work, and taking unnecessary risks should be minimized [14, 34]. Help those who must operate in hazardous conditions by making such environments safer. Put forth the time and effort to complete the tedious, low-value activities so that people can collaborate on the more critical, strategic endeavors that robots can't handle. Sales growth through enhanced order accuracy, expedited shipping, and satisfied customers.

AI is being integrated into the design of increasingly complex ARs so that they can recognize objects, learn from their experiences, and act independently [14, 24, 31, 32, 34, 35, 37]. ARs are creating innovation and tremendous value in the supply chain because they can: raise the rapidity and correctness of consistent processes, specifically in warehousing and industries. Upsurge competence working along with humans decreases the possibility of manpower damage in the workplace hazardous. Self-driving robots may also boost human worth by freeing them to focus on higher-value activities such as strategy development rather than menial errands. Reduce the number of time workers spend in hazardous environments to protect them. The company's reputation was bolstered since its innovative methods and cutting-edge technology became more apparent [14, 24, 31, 32, 34, 35].

14.5.2 NEW TECHNOLOGIES TO IMPROVE THE HOSPITAL ECOSYSTEM

Recent advancements in digital healthcare technology can assist in enhancing healthcare delivery systems in terms of cost, accessibility, and quality. Additionally, it has the potential to make people safer when they are engaging in risky activities.

14.6 IMPLEMENTATION OF ARTIFICIAL INTELLIGENCE (AI) IN RESEARCH AND DEVELOPMENT

14.6.1 GENETICS-BASED SOLUTIONS

Within the next few decades, a significant portion of the world's population will undergo whole genome sequencing to identify and store their genetic data, either from birth or later in life. The whole genome sequencing will take between 100 and 150 gigabases of data, allowing for more precise therapy. Can interplay between genomics and phenotype is still ongoing. The existing clinical system requires a makeover so that it can make use of genetic data [13]. A new company in the health technology sector called Deep Genomics is attempting to establish a connection between genetic data and EMRs and other disease markers. This company performs correlation analysis to discover treatment targets, either existing targets or new ones, to manufacture individualized genetic drugs. AI is used for various tasks, including toxicity testing, lead optimization, target identification, and innovative trial design. It can be challenging to interpret data from an individual's whole genome for many hereditary conditions towards various types of genomic profiles. Whole genome sequencing and AI can expand the mutation of genomics for identification in precision medicine [13–15].

14.6.2 DRUG DISCOVERY AND DEVELOPMENT

It is conceivable that more than a decade will pass between the time that molecular targets are recognized and the time that an approved therapeutic product is introduced to the market throughout the drug discovery and development process. Most potential pharmacological treatments fail at some stage throughout development and are never brought to the consumer market. This can significantly influence the amount of money spent [12–14]. The ever-increasing regulatory roadblocks and the difficulties in continually locating medicine compounds that are substantial enhancements over those that are now available on the market both contribute to the complexity of the situation and make it more difficult to find a solution. Because of this, developing new pharmaceuticals is complex and inefficient, and the expense of bringing a novel treatment to market is a significant financial investment [14–16]. In recent years, a plethora of information regarding pharmacological compounds' activity and biology data has become accessible. This is because of advancements in automation and the development of novel experimental methods, such as the hidden Markov model (HMV) dependent speech-to-text synthesis and equivalent synthesis. These approaches are responsible for this development. Mining of large-scale chemical data is required, however, in order to resourcefully identify possible medicinal compounds. Contraption learning methods have revealed tremendous promise in this regard, one area in which they have been applied [15–17]. Since the 1990s, various approaches have been used to design models, which have helped to facilitate the discovery of new drugs. Vector machine supports, random forests, and neural systems are examples of these types of models. Because of the amount of data and the speed at which computers can handle it, data lakes have become increasingly applicable in recent years. Several new drug development stages can be made more straightforward by utilizing ML in various capacities. Predicting the properties and activities of medications, creating novel pharmaceuticals from the ground up, understanding how drugs interact with receptors, and estimating how drugs will react inside the body are all aspects of this [16, 17]. The drug molecules and attributes utilized by the in-silico models are transformed into a vector format before being presented to the learning systems. This enables the learning systems to comprehend the information. Examples of the kind of data utilized in this context include grids for convolutional neural networks (CNNs) [17] and strings of molecular input line entry systems that have been simplified (SMILES). More examples include molecular fingerprints and descriptors (such as physicochemical properties). Molecular descriptors are another example (molecular structure). Making educated guesses about the properties and behaviors of medications is essential to understand the properties and activity of a pharmaceutical molecule to accurately forecast how it will function inside the body of a human being. Methods that are based on ML have been used to evaluate the biological activity, ADME characteristics, and physicochemical aspects of pharmaceutical substances. In recent years, millions of compounds aimed at various disease targets have been recorded because of the availability of several chemical and biological data repositories such as ChEMBL and PubChem. Computers can read these libraries, which are then used to develop ML models that can be applied to the drug discovery process [15–18]. For instance, to develop molecular fingerprints, a vast collection of molecular graphs containing information on each atom in the molecule can be used in conjunction with CNN's. These fingerprints can be used to identify the molecule. It is possible to use a neural fingerprint developed for a specific chemical to generate predictions about the molecule that the fingerprint represents. This method can be used to evaluate molecular properties such as octanol, solubility, melting point, and biological activity, and then the results can be used to predict new characteristics of pharmacological compounds, as Coley et al. and others have demonstrated [18, 19]. Other researchers have also demonstrated this. Using these methodologies with a scoring function allows for selecting pharmaceutical compounds with the desired levels of biological activity and physiochemical characteristics.

The vast majority of recently developed pharmaceuticals are notoriously tricky to use due to their unfavorable properties, such as their insolubility, instability, poor absorption, and complicated molecular structures. It is especially true for older pharmaceuticals, which tend to have more superficial molecular structures [18, 20–22].

14.6.3 ROBOTS IN CLINICAL AND NEW PUBLIC HEALTH-DRIVEN TECHNOLOGIES

The use of robots in the medical industry makes it possible to provide patients with treatment of the highest possible standard, streamline clinical workflows, and create a safe environment for patients and members of the medical staff. These benefits are all made possible by using robots [32, 33].

14.6.3.1 PATIENT TREATMENT WITH NEW-DRIVEN TECHNOLOGIES

Medical robots make it possible to perform surgeries with a minimally invasive incision, monitor patients with chronic illnesses in a tailored manner, provide intelligent therapy, and provide social interaction for elderly patients. Other applications of medical robots include monitoring patients with chronic diseases in a tailored style and regularly [21, 22]. All these advantages are attainable by using medical robots in the appropriate settings. As a result of having less work to complete, nurses and other caregivers may be able to spend more time with patients, which would benefit both the patients and the staff. They will be able to establish relationships with patients, which are vital to the patient's long-term health, and will be made possible as a result of this [22, 23].

14.6.3.2 RATIONALIZED CLINICAL ROADMAPS

Autonomous mobile robots, also known as AMRs, may one day be utilized to improve therapeutic procedures in the workplace. This would be accomplished by reducing the physical strain placed on workers and ensuring a higher level of reproducibility. These robots can help alleviate concerns about staffing levels and guarantee that the necessary materials, equipment, and pharmaceuticals are constantly on hand by keeping track of inventories and making purchases at the appropriate times [22–24]. Automated medical robots (AMRs) make it simpler to sanitize and prepare patient rooms promptly, enabling medical personnel to devote more attention to providing patients with the highest possible level of care [23–25].

14.6.3.3 PACIFIC WORK-BASED ATMOSPHERE

To stop disease transmission, hospitals frequently use AMRs to convey soiled linens and other potentially infectious items. To prevent the spread of hospital-acquired illnesses, hundreds of medical facilities have already put robotic cleaning and disinfection systems in place (HAIs). A subgroup of AMR known as social robots can assist with labor-intensive tasks like moving patients or beds [14, 15, 26, 28].

14.6.3.4 AUTOMATED GUIDED VEHICLES (AGVS)

Real ARs can do their tasks without human guidance or intervention. For the past 15 to 20 years, robotics has primarily been used in teleoperated mobile robots equipped with cameras to monitor out-of-reach places or in basic industrial settings. Automated guided vehicles (AGVs) are used for transporting goods in workshops and granaries, unmanned aerial vehicles (UAVs) are utilized in emergencies, and underwater robots are used to locate sunken ships. While there is no denying the usefulness of robots in many applications, past uses do not indicate the future of fully ARs [40].

14.7 OTHER PROMISING APPLICATIONS OF AUTONOMOUS ROBOTS (ARS) FOR THERAPEUTIC ACTIVITIES

14.7.1 ARS IN MEDICINE AND HEALTHCARE

Because of the improvements in robot performance and usability brought forth by AMR, they are finding new applications. The medical field is making greater use of ARs. ARs have several applications in the healthcare industry, but one of the most important is the efficient management of the flow of materials and medications across the institution. This is especially vital in infectious disease units because it protects nurses from potentially harmful substances while allowing them to provide adequate patient care. Secondly, medical AMRs can be used to keep public places clean without putting people in danger by giving robots empowered with UV lights with virus-killing capacity or decontamination sprays. Some of the tremendous applications of ARs are supply of medicine, sanitizing exteriors, delivering MTF (mobile telepresence functionality), assisting public health professionals at the time of rehabilitation, affording operative support to the staff nurses and other paramedics for patient handling and acute care management diseases like cancer, stroke, life-threatening illness [38–40].

14.7.2 ARS FOR CLINICAL DATA MANAGEMENT (CDM)

This new application space for AMRs is secure autonomous mobility in the operations of data centers and research facilities. Protecting high-priced items during transport and keeping the chain of custody intact is possible with the help of independent robots equipped with cabinets and lock boxes. It paves the way for comprehensive procedure documentation that can be accessed quickly and accurately [38–40].

14.7.3 ARS IN BIOTECH RESEARCH ACTIVITIES

Despite the growing demand for biopharmaceuticals, producing biomedical products that align with the tight requirements established by the industry is a labor-intensive procedure for biotech companies. Monitoring must occur continuously and nonstop to carry out tasks such as sampling and maintaining protocols for cell culture. Mobile robots equipped with robotic arms have the potential to be used safely to remove waste from the production line, control vital process inputs, and carry out routine monitoring tasks. Because AMRs take care of the menial tasks, human workers are free to concentrate on the more essential parts of the manufacture of biopharmaceuticals. These aspects include monitoring growth parameters, running periodic testing, and adjusting the process as it moves forward [38–40].

14.7.4 ARS FOR ANALYTICAL AND TECHNOLOGY DEVELOPMENT

Research and development use AMRs to make the mundane task of delivering materials for experiments and other engineering tasks more bearable. The field of research is beginning to pay more and more attention to AMRs. One field that shows promise is engineering sensors and robots capable of transporting items. There is a constant demand for innovative uses of cutting-edge technologies, but many academic institutions lack the means to build the infrastructure necessary to take full advantage of the latest scientific breakthroughs. With the help of flexible, AMRs, sensors and manipulators for research can be simply incorporated into a portable platform not only facilitates financial and time savings but also gives these new technologies the freedom to move around independently [40, 41].

14.7.5 LOGISTICS, MANUFACTURING, WAREHOUSING

Even though AMRs are constantly developing new applications, transportation is still their most common and widely used function. While manufacturing pharmaceutical dosage forms, these robots are frequently used for additional tasks, such as sorting APIs, moving raw materials, and processing returns. Controlling stock and sorting packages, etc. [39–41].

The majority of the biotech and biopharma businesses around the globe are experiencing rapid expansion. As a result, the world is experiencing an increase in these industries while it is undergoing the production process following human needs. This process involves labor-intensive tasks such as the isolation of cells from various biological sources, the maintenance of cell culture, and the processing of cell cultures toward research and development, and additionally, it has necessitated constant monitoring by rigorous day-to-day labor 24 hours a day, seven days a week. ARs are becoming increasingly important in many industries today, particularly the biological and pharmaceutical industries, to shorten the most labor-intensive jobs and shift the focus to time management with the assistance of robots. Intelligent devices, such as ARs, can carry out activities in the real world without the direct intervention of a person [42]. Because of this self-sufficiency, the labor force can delegate the fascinating and valuable aspects of their employment to robots, allowing them to spend more time doing the parts of their professions for which they are uniquely equipped. In recent decades, roboticists have drawn much more inspiration from biology than computer science or electronics.

Moreover, around the middle of the previous century, attempts at artificial robotics or proto-robots borrowed significantly more from mathematics, mechanics, and electronics than from natural robotics. This tendency continues today. This technique, which utilizes robotics, invariably results in the high creation of successful items, particularly in the industrial sectors [42].

On the other hand, it was helpful in better grasping the chasm that still exists between a robot and an animal, at least when it comes to the need for autonomy and the ability to adapt to quality. In addition, the rates are required since the range of applications, from household to industrial, is expanding continuously. In modern robotics, there has been a startling shift in focus away from living organisms and toward artificially created ones. Without a doubt, the synergies of the new wave of robotics would not be feasible if it were not for the recent advancements in biology [41, 42]. ARs are a natural source of inspiration for the "new wave" of robotics.

14.8 AUTONOMOUS ROBOTS (ARS) FOR BIOTECHNOLOGICAL RESEARCH AND DEVELOPMENT

Automated robots can reduce the number of tiresome transport operations required for research and development. These jobs may include repetitive testing or other technical requirements. In addition, there has been a significant increase in research towards developing robotic manipulation technologies. An example of this would be the development of technology that allows for automated manipulation and innovation in sensors in one hot region [41]. The advanced studies for researchers looking at the ways to robotics and technology, the manipulator and sensors can be used for research and development can be integrated easily into the robotic platform provided that an easy-to-use autonomous mobile robotics expansion process towards skills, industries, companies saving and research and development institutions substantial money and time. In addition to the advanced studies for researchers looking at the ways of robotics and technology, the manipulator and sensors used for research studies can be simply combined into the robotic portfolio [42, 43].

14.8.1 AUTONOMOUS ROBOTICS IN HEMATOLOGY

Because blood testing is so commonplace in clinical practice, robotic systems like HaemoBot and VenousPro are increasingly used to draw blood automatically for diagnostic purposes. But that hinges on the technician's expertise and the patient's individual physiology. Automatic blood testing, for instance, protects healthcare workers against potential infection. HaemoBot [42] and VenousPro [43] are the results of recent advances in medical research. Ultrasound navigation and force sensing are used in both systems to detect and cannulate the vein in a person's forearm without human intervention.

More recently, a prototype of VenousPro was evaluated in human subjects [44-46]. In addition, the robot was developed for collecting blood from peripheral venous, i.e., hand-held robot catheterization for various health industrial and pediatric applications [47]. More advanced development towards these systems can find various applications for infectious disease-affected people with viral transferable across the world [48, 49].

14.8.2 AUTONOMOUS ROBOTICS IN DNA ANALYSIS

Researchers are working to build biochip devices that are based on microfluidics in order to simplify the analysis of DNA with biological sample solutions and complications. A single, fully automated device having an electron chip called a biochip with microfluidic valves, chambers, pumps, heaters, mixers, channels, and DNA microarray biosensors is utilized to perform based on magnetic beads rare cell apprehension, cell preconcentration, and decontamination, hybridization of DNA, PCR, and electrochemical detection. These procedures were carried out in a directive to accomplish the desired consequences. It is done to ensure that the device can perform every one of these functions. For the sole purpose of holding these components, a microfluidic chip is deployed [48–50].

14.8.3 AUTONOMOUS ROBOTICS IN MICROBIOLOGY

SteriMax smart thermal sterilizer, MALDI (matrix assisted laser desorption ionization) Biotyper mass Spectrometer, Panda robot manipulator MBT Biotarget 96, and disposable MALDI target plates. The end-effector tool consisted of the ZG2-WDS8T – a laser sensor position system of measurement, an RGB camera a2A3840-45ucPRO, a force sensor Nano17, Feedback 360° high-speed servo motor, and a stainless-steel needle depicted in Figure 14.4 [47–50].

The petri dish picture was taken from an RGB camera that operates to estimate the chosen bacterial colony location. Using 2D laser profile measurement equipment for calculating the surrounding area around the estimated place is then detected with a measurement of 2D laser profile equipment. In addition, it gave a detailed 3D representation of the room to the operator, site lauding the bacterial colony [47–49].

The colonies were selected and positioned with the help of a needle made of stainless steel. Before examining MALDI Biotyper Mass Spectrometer for the colony, selection needs to be plated out MBT Biotarget 96 plates [48–50].

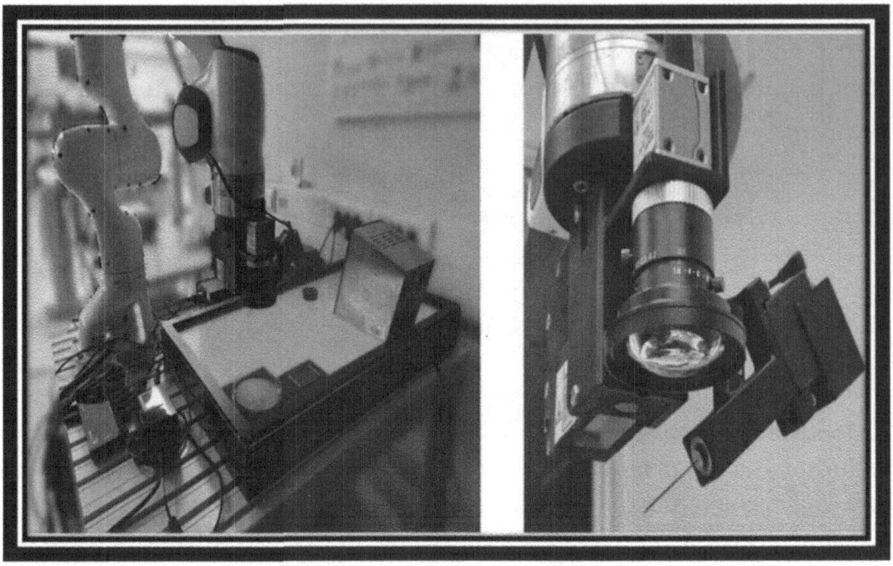

FIGURE 14.3 Schematic diagram representing feedback 360° high-speed servo motor, and a stainless-steel needle.

Source: Reprinted with permission from Ref. [52]. Copyright © 2022 by the authors. Licensee MDPI, Basel, Switzerland. https://creativecommons.org/licenses/by/4.0/

14.8.4 NOVEL AUTONOMOUS ROBOTS (ARS) FOR TREATING MEDICAL FIELDS

In research and development, laborious transport duties help reduce the need for additional engineering needs and involvement in repetitive testing. Additionally, autonomy is becoming an increasingly important aspect of research and the robots' development. Take, for instance, the rapidly expanding field of robotic sensor manipulation technology development as an example of a hot area of innovation. Studies at a more advanced level of research are looking into how technology may be mobilized. Incorporating sensors and manipulators into the mobile platform is simple, allowing these emerging technologies to be mobile and independent while saving companies and research institutions significant time and money. Despite this, many organizations lack the resources to establish their platforms. Mechanical biology produces chemical byproducts. The process of interconversion of mechanical, chemical, and electromagnetic energy that occurs in mitochondria is related to the phenomena known as mechanochemiemission. For individuals suffering from cancer, for instance, microbial robots might be employed as a treatment.

A biological brain created from cultured neurons that were first segregated could identify the neurological activities afterwards incorporated within a robot body as the neurological entity [53]. The brain is the robot's only component that generates motor signals, and it does so by processing information sent to it by sensors located on the robot's body. The artificial brain cannot compare to the complexity and versatility of the biological brain. Examples are Implants in the cochlea and bone-anchored hearing aids (also known as Baha). People who suffered from acute hearing loss were the ones who made use of these hearing aids. One of the ARs, known as Baha hearing aids, for instance, attaches itself to the bones in the middle ear to generate sound vibrations in the skull and then transmits those vibrations to the cochlea, artificial sensing skin. In its current iteration, artificial sensing skin can sense any pressure applied to it. People who have lost all sensation in some portions of their body, such as those with diabetes who suffer from peripheral neuropathy, are the intended recipients of this treatment. Bionic eye – the bionic eye is a bioelectronic device that can give those blind their sight back. And endoscopic robotics – these robots can remove a polyp from a colon while examining it with a colonoscope. Implantation of cochlear hearing aids, known as cochlear implants, is available for hard-of-hearing persons [49, 50]. In contrast to traditional hearing aids, which just direct the electrical signals to the ear canal, cochlear implants are surgically implanted in the skull and transmit them directly to the auditory nerve, which is the nerve responsible for processing sound information [48–50].

14.8.5 AUTONOMOUS ROBOTS (ARS) IN BATTLING COVID-19

The COVID-19 pandemic has developed into a severe problem on a global scale; as a result of increased economic interdependence and globalization, the majority of countries will be impacted by the epidemic. To stop the spread of viruses, everyone needs to work together on a global scale. Using various robots as appropriate resources to fight against COVID-19 is possible. ARs can perform various tasks, including measuring vital signs, providing food and medication, disinfecting an area, and assisting with border control. As the number of epidemics increases, the function of robotics is becoming more and more apparent. In the wake of the Ebola pandemic that broke out in 2015, the Science and Technology department located at the White House office and the National Science Foundation co-hosted a series of workshops that focused on how advances in autonomous robotics could improve clinical care (such as decontamination and telemedicine), surveillance (such as voluntary quarantines monitoring compliance), and logistics (e.g., handling and delivery of waste contaminants) [37, 55]. Even though it's limited to specific areas like the notion of evidence, China and other countries are actively researching the majority of autonomous applications. Most front-line personnel who are most frequently exposed to pathogens in direct contact with patients are those who work in the healthcare industry. The utilization of safety equipment in conjunction with Albeit led to introducing the fourth domain in socioeconomics' work continuity and maintenance duties [46–49]. Additional research into remote operations with various wide applications illustrates the numerous different kinds of occupations that entail dexterity manipulation. These jobs range from manufacturing to controlling waste treatment and power plants remotely. The fields of illness prevention, diagnosis and screening, disease management, and patient care can all benefit significantly from ARs. The application of noncontact ultraviolet (UV) robot-controlled surface disinfection is utilized because COVID-19 transmits from one to another via close contact with respiratory droplets and infected surfaces [55]. These areas are pervasive development opportunities in robotics that should be explored to avoid infection. It can cling to living surfaces for days, regardless of whether the surfaces are made of steel, acrylic, or polycarbonate. UV light systems that include the UV robot are used in most hospitals, which help to reduce the amount of contamination on high-touch surfaces. Manual disinfection necessitates workforce mobilization, and the exposure risk to cleaning personnel will increase as a result. In contrast, remote or controlled autonomous disinfection robots are efficient, quick, and inexpensive [47, 48].

Opportunities can be found in intelligent navigation, in which a high risk of detection is combined with preventive measures to continuously navigate the development of high-risk areas and sterilize all high-touch surface areas. Mobile ARs capable of sensing temperature in public gathering spaces and entry ports practically employ advanced techniques [54]. These robots are used for treatment and screening. It is normal practice to utilize highly developed and automated video systems to screen several people concurrently in huge spaces. For example, the effectiveness of autonomous or remotely controlled robots' thermal sensors and vision algorithms could be improved by adding coverage screening and reducing overlap. This movable robot could also be used to regularly check the temperatures of in and outpatients in diverse parts of the hospital. The information from these checks could be sent to the hospital's information systems [55]. Existing security systems networked with facial recognition software can retrace infected persons' links and warn others who may be at risk is made possible by networking existing security systems.

To protect people's privacy, however, establishing proper rules is essential. It is recommended that nasopharyngeal and oropharyngeal swabs are collected and tested as part of the initial diagnosis process for COVID-19 in most nations requires the collection of samples, their handling, their transfer, and their testing. The absence of skilled personnel to swab patients and process test samples is one of the most significant obstacles that must be overcome during a big outbreak. Swabbing the nasopharyngeal and oropharyngeal cavities using an automated system or one aided by a robot may lower the risk of infection, speed up the process, and free up employees for other work [47–50].

For example, some people may not have symptoms or may not have the virus when they are tested. For example, a blood test for antibodies may be necessary to find noiseless infections. In these cases, collecting blood for research or testing laboratory might be automated, relieving doctors of a potentially dangerous duty. For example, researchers are looking into automatic devices for venipuncture that use ultrasound imaging to find veins in the forearm. With real-time assays, it would be possible to quickly and accurately find infections in vitro. Autonomous ground vehicles and drones can move samples and give medications to diseased patients when they shouldn't pass. By using a variety of self-driving robots, COVID-19 could lead to the development of robotic systems that can be quickly set up and give specialists and essential service providers remote access without having to go to the battlefield (Table 14.2). When many people are quarantined, they may not be able to talk to others for a long time, which may be bad for their mental health [45–47]. Social robots could keep people connected and on their treatments without worrying about spreading diseases, making social interactions hard to grow because you have to keep track of a lot of information [55].

Teleoperation is an established method that is used for both telework and telemedicine. In the past few weeks, most universities, colleges, and businesses have started to use online learning. Large international exhibitions and conferences might not be canceled, but new ways to meet online might become more popular. For example, remote participants might get used to using robot avatars and controls. In the same way, fighting infectious diseases means making an environment that humans can't work in, but that autonomous robot can.

The COVID-19 pandemic has become a serious global problem as it has spread out to most countries; since the economies and globalization are becoming more and more linked, the whole world needs to work together. Could robots be used along with other tools to fight COVID-19? The self-driving robots might be able to deliver medicines, food, and cleaning supplies, measure vital signs and help control the border. As diseases spread, robots are becoming more important. During the Ebola outbreak in 2015, the WHOSTNF (National Science Foundations and the White House Office of Science and Technology) held workshops to produce how important ARs were in three areas: clinical care (like decontamination and telemedicine), surveillance (like monitoring compliance in voluntary quarantines), and logistics (e.g., transportation) [48, 49, 55].

TABLE 14.2 Various Advanced Autonomous Robots in the Field of Biology

Name of Autonomous Robots	Importance in the Biology Sector	References
Number 250, Sartorius	24 parallel 250 ml individually regulated bioreactors. Online, you can control and measure things like DO (dissolved oxygen), biomass aeration, FOAMING, pH, stirring, off-gases, temperature, sampling, and feeding.	[50]
	Regular computerized specimen for offline analysis. Cultivations in bioreactors with maximum throughput and good scalability.	
Screening Robot, Beckman Coulter	Custom setup using a variety of gadgets. Several tens of microtiter plates can be processed each second.	[50]
	An influential Biomek pipetting station for handling multiwell plates.	
	Different options, including a tower incubator, washer-dispenser, thermal cycler, multimode plate reader, and thermosphere, are available for automated cultivation and HT-scale experiments.	
FLUENT 780, Tecan	Station for handling liquids that may do multiple types of pipetting.	[50]
	Span-8 head versatile tube and reservoir pipetting.	
	Beneficial mainly in plasmid purification and molecular biology, protein assays.	
	Integral multimode SPARK plate reader, Agilent centrifuge, Thermo Scientific thermoshaker, and Tecan vacuum workstation.	
Biolector Pro and Biolector II, m2p-labs	On-the-fly, online optical testing of 48-well plates for pH, DO, biomass, and a wide range of fluorescence wavelengths.	[50]
	Controlling pH and operating in a fed-batch mode with microfluidics (PRO).	
	The bioreactor, used for anaerobic cultivations, will be plate-mounted.	
DXA 5000 Total Lab Automation System	The DXA 5000 whole laboratory automation system and its proprietary innovations enable you to improve high-volume laboratories while delivering high-quality results.	[51]
	Enjoy a quick turnaround time that is consistent, thorough pre-analytical sample quality detection, and less manual processing.	

14.8.6 CHALLENGES AND ADAPTATION OF AUTONOMOUS ROBOTS (ARS) FOR DISINFECTION AND PERSONALIZED MEDICINES

The next generation of start-up companies devoted to eliminating the coronavirus is focused on developing disinfection robots. The response is self-evident and unaffected by the specifics of the situation. Because of their sophisticated navigational technology, ARs are an excellent choice for delivering UV-C light disinfection equipment. The AMR system serves as the primary building block for the UV-C Disinfection Robot. This UV lamp emitter allows this robot to disinfect its surroundings and clean up after itself by removing bacteria and viruses from its immediate environment. The Autonomous Navigation Technology that AMR possesses grants it the ability to freely navigate, and the UVC Light that it possesses simultaneously cleans and illuminates surfaces. The antimicrobial peptide (AMP) manufacturers CASUN, SMART GUARD, OTSAW, and SESTROROBOTICS are among the most prominent worldwide [54–56]. In addition, Argos Therapeutics and Invetech, a business specializing in custom automation and contract manufacturing, have partnered to deliver automated production systems for customized immunotherapies as a component of the Arcelis technology platform.

According to Richard Grant, the Arcelis system, the chairman of cell therapy at Invetech, harvests mRNA from a patient's tumor using two five-axis robotic arms. After the mRNA is extracted, it is loaded into dendritic cells generated by the cellular processing machinery. The killer T-cells created using this technology will target metastatic cancers once administered to a patient. According to Grant, RNA robots operate closed disposables in the same cleanroom classified as a 100,000 class. The utilization of closed disposables helps cut down on the facility's initial and ongoing costs because so many patients' belongings may be managed simultaneously. For example, Argos's leading candidate is currently undergoing Phase III clinical tests, and those tests make use of a technology capable of being rapidly scaled up and entirely automated. According to Grant [30], commercializing therapeutic procedures on a broad scale is impractical and inefficient from a financial standpoint. Robots, on the other hand, make it easier to bring these processes into the commercial realm. Moreover, Grant demonstrates that a scale-out model makes it possible to replicate production processes in additional locations all over the world with minimal training required for establishing and validating these new locations and minimal variation in the production processes themselves.

TABLE 14.2 *(Continued)*

Because of robotics, it is now possible to fill vials at a more leisurely pace [30, 33]. "ESS Technologies' head of sales and marketing, Walt Langosch, says robotic vial manipulation moves components before and after filling and packing. "Both of these processes take place simultaneously." In addition, the company is in charge of the pre-processing, buffering, and initial and final packing of pre-filled syringes. One of the recommendations that Langosch provided was that "Robots can be engaged to put together syringes, verify them, and wrap them." Robotics, the real benefit of having sterile settings is that they have a decreased danger of being contaminated by both humans and the environment in which they are located is an advantage that can be considered mutually exclusive. In addition to the various benefits they offer, such as increased precision and productivity, robots also contribute to an increase in the overall output of industrial production. This is because they can finish their tasks in a shorter amount of time and with a lower amount of waste than humans. When using an automated inspection system, each component can be put through extensive testing before being utilized. However, with the assistance of vision-recognition technology, it is possible to verify the authenticity of the serial numbers that may be found printed on the packaging of drugs. According to Langosch, a fully automated system can be developed by utilizing serialization software in conjunction with current and future optical technologies that would allow for the system to function without human intervention. However, the findings of a trend study that PMMI carried out indicate that color imaging, a development in vision sensors, makes it possible for robots to differentiate between bottle caps of varied colors. The development of end-of-arm tooling that includes vision sensors has made it much easier for robots to recognize objects and place them in the correct area. As a result, robots now have access to more accurate data [30, 33].

14.8.7 APPLICATIONS OF ROBOTICS IN THE CLEANROOM AND THE LABORATORY PRACTICE

Robotic technology dramatically enhances the processes because it eliminates the risk of humanoid contamination, and cleanroom filling is aseptic. According to Langosch, robotics can create an ISO 5 microbe-proof environment. It's no secret that ESS Technologies and Fanuc Robotics work together to develop secondary packaging and palletizing solutions for the pharmaceutical industry. As a result, the Fanuc M-430iA/2PV is waterproof and sterilization-resistant when sterilized with hydrogen peroxide vapor. Cleanroom-designed robots must produce as few particles as possible to meet cleanroom criteria. Therefore, it is vital to minimize cracks and make the robot resistant to cleaning or sterilizing solutions, Grant argues. The robot needs to be contained or guarded for the operator's safety. In order to limit the influence on airflow and particle formation, Grant says the cleanroom's heating, ventilation, and air conditioning system must also be managed. According to Mike Ouren, Precise Automation's manager of Life Sciences, the use of robots in pharmaceutical laboratories has increased significantly during the last few years. For example, a robot can transport a microtiter plate in a laboratory. According to Ouren, "an automaton associated with a planning software program reduces error rates, preserves observation reliability, and allows organizations to concentrate on the purpose of the laboratory activity rather than the way it will be carried out." Even though instruments can be manually loaded, one of the main differences between laboratories and industrial applications is that in the laboratory, the results of repeated activities are less predictable and subject to change depending on the results of an experiment. New communicative robotic systems that don't demand safety precautions can meet the laboratory's necessity for easy access to nearby equipment and the robot's space limitations. Precise Automation's one-kilogram PreciseFlex 400 SCARA robot is safe for individuals to operate near and can lift less than one kilogram. The term was first utilized in 2012. The robot's small footprint is ideal for laboratory workstations, saving space and money [30, 56, 57].

The PF400's Precise Guidelines Control enables medical researchers to "practice" the robot with their hands. In this case, the operator does not need a remote-control necklace to tell the robot what to do. Lab robots can move vials. Fanuc robots, for example, are used in laboratory facilities to process vials in a single location. The robot has a tool attached to its end that can handle 10 vials simultaneously [30]. Robots are increasingly used in laboratories and manufacturing facilities to improve quality and output. It is only a matter of time before medical robots are routinely used to treat patients. AI, miniaturization, and computer power advancements make medical robots more common. An industrial robot and computed tomography (CT) navigation were used approximately 34 years ago to insert a probe into the brain to obtain a biopsy specimen [33]. Robots that could conduct urological treatments and complete hip arthroplasty were developed in the following years. As a result of doctors' disdain for these fully autonomous machines, future robots were designed to serve the surgeon rather than the other way around. For various types of surgery, medical robots are currently widely used to precisely manipulate surgical equipment through a single or several tiny incisions [33, 36]. Three-dimensional (3D) high-definition magnified views of the surgical field improve precision and control. Since 2000, the FDA-approved da Vinci surgical system has reportedly conducted more than 6 million procedures. In addition to the smaller incisions, less blood loss, and quicker recovery times of laparoscopic surgery, robot-assisted surgery also has numerous other advantages. Regular surgery appears to have the same long-term results as long-term surgery [30, 33, 36].

14.9 CONCLUSION

Integrating ARs in healthcare could one day enable safer, more reliable, and more easily reproducible medical procedures. Before these new technologies can be fully included, numerous changes must be made. First, the importance of AI and robots in our healthcare ecosystem is growing. Life-threatening diseases are already being diagnosed and treated using AI in their earliest, most treatable stages. AI is also being used to monitor early-stage cardiovascular disease, enabling physicians and other caretakers to monitor and diagnose potentially fatal incidents at previously untreatable stages. The proliferation of consumer wearables and other healthcare gadgets used to monitor heart disease is used in its early stages.

14.10 CURRENT STATUS AND FUTURE DIRECTIONS

Not only in the operating room but also in a wide variety of other clinical settings, robots are increasingly being used to assist medical professionals in their tasks more efficiently and in providing patients with care of higher quality, not only in the operating room but also in a wide variety of other clinical settings. For instance, hospitals and clinics are increasingly putting robots to work to battle the spread of disease during the present COVID-19 pandemic is being done to do a wider variety of tasks. Robotics and automation are also utilized in research facilities to expedite the discovery process. These technologies take over the repetitive, high-volume tasks that technicians and scientists previously carried out. Because of robotics' capacity to boost productivity while simultaneously lowering danger, the medical field is finding more and more uses for the technology. For example, robots can clean and arrange patient rooms independently, significantly lowering the amount of human interaction required in isolation units. The procedure of locating the appropriate medication and dispensing it to hospitalized patients can be sped up by robots outfitted with drug identifier software powered by AI. Robots will be able to assume an increasing amount of responsibility as technology continues to advance, and eventually, they will be able to take over entirely autonomous operations. There will be more time for doctors, nurses, and others working in the medical field to provide direct, hands-on patient treatment. So, robotics and its application in the healthcare field will be a driving force for our human civilization, for the existence, establishment, and combating of life-threatening diseases.

KEYWORDS

- **artificial intelligence**
- **biosensors**
- **biotechnology**
- **pathogen detection**
- **surgical robots**
- **targeted drug therapy**

REFERENCES

1. Bhandari, M., Zeffiro, T., & Reddiboina, M., (2020). Artificial intelligence and robotic surgery: Current perspective and future directions. *Curr Opin Urol.*, *1*, 48–54. doi: 10.1097/MOU.0000000000000692.
2. Bohr, A., & Memarzadeh, K., (2020). The rise of artificial intelligence in healthcare applications. In: *Artificial Intelligence in Healthcare* (pp. 25–60). Academic Press.
3. Gumbs, A. A., Frigerio, I., Spolverato, G., Croner, R., Illanes, A., Chouillard, E., & Elyan, E., (2021). Artificial intelligence surgery: How do we get to autonomous actions in surgery? *Sensors (Basel, Switzerland)*, *21*(16), 5526. https://doi.org/10.3390/s21165526.
4. Grischke, J., Johannsmeier, L., Eich, L., Griga, L., & Haddadin, S., (2020). Dentronics: Towards robotics and artificial intelligence in dentistry. *Dental Materials*, *36*, 765–778.
5. Shan, T., Tay, F. R., & Gu, L., (2021). Application of artificial intelligence in dentistry. *Journal of Dental Research*, *100*(3), 232–244.

6. Dzobo, K., Adotey, S., Thomford, N. E., & Dzobo, W., (2020). Integrating artificial and human intelligence: A partnership for responsible innovation in biomedical engineering and medicine. *Omics: A Journal of Integrative Biology, 24*(5), 247–263.
7. Howard, J., (2019). Artificial intelligence: Implications for the future of work. *American Journal of Industrial Medicine, 62*, 917–926.
8. Hamet, P., & Tremblay, J., (2017). Artificial intelligence in medicine. *Metabolism, 69*, S36–S40.
9. Ashrafian, H., Darzi, A., & Athanasiou, T., (2015). A novel modification of the Turing test for artificial intelligence and robotics in healthcare. *The International Journal of Medical Robotics and Computer Assisted Surgery, 11*, 38–43.
10. Jiang, F., Jiang, Y., Zhi, H., Dong, Y., Li, H., Ma, S., Wang, Y., et al., (2017). Artificial intelligence in healthcare: Past, present, and future. *Stroke and Vascular Neurology, 2*(4), 230–243. https://doi.org/10.1136/svn-2017-000101.
11. Küçük, S., (2018). *Surgical Robotics*. IntechOpen.; https://doi.org/10.5772/65524.
12. Morris, B., (2005). Robotic surgery: Applications, limitations, and impact on surgical education. *Medscape General Medicine, 7*, 72.
13. Panait, L., Doarn, C. R., & Merrell, R. C., (2002). Applications of robotics in surgery. *Chirurgia (Bucur), 97*(6), 549–555. PMID: 12731212.
14. Yao, M., Belke, C. H., Cui, H., & Paik, J., (2019). A reconfiguration strategy for modular robots using origami folding. *The International Journal of Robotics Research, 38*, 73–89.
15. Grabowski, R., Navarro-Serment, L. E., Paredis, C. J., et al., (2000). Heterogeneous teams of modular robots for mapping and exploration. *Autonomous Robots, 8*, 293–308 https://doi.org/10.1023/A:100893382641.
16. https://www.robotics.org/content-detail.cfm/Industrial-Robotics-IndustryInsights/Robotics-in-the-Pharmaceutical-andLife-Sciences-Industry/content_id/2867 (accessed on 4 December 2023).
17. https://advancedmaterials2018.wordpress.com/2018/10/08/different-types-of-nanorobots-and-applications-advanced-materials-2019/ (accessed on 4 December 2023).
18. Saadeh, Y., & Vyas, D., (2014). Nanorobotic applications in medicine: Current proposals and designs. *American Journal of Robotic Surgery, 1*, 4–11. doi: 10.1166/ajrs.2014.1010. PMID: 26361635; PMCID: PMC4562685.
19. Kim, M., Julius, A. A., & Cheang, U. K. (2017). *Microbiorobotics: Biologically Inspired Microscale Robotic Systems* (2nd edn. pp. 245–246). Elsevier Imprint.
20. https://www.theweek.in/news/sci-tech/2019/01/22/Nano-robots-swim-through-blood-vessels-to deliver-drugs.html (accessed on 4 December 2023).
21. Schmidt, C. K., Medina-Sánchez, M., Edmondson, R. J., *et al., (*2020*).* Engineering microrobots for targeted cancer therapies from a medical perspective. *Nat Commun., 11*, 5618. https://doi.org/10.1038/s41467-020-19322-7.
22. Aziz, A., et al., (2020). Medical imaging of microrobots: Toward in vivo applications. *ACS Nano*. https://doi.org/10.1021/acsnano.0c05530,.acsnano.0c05530.
23. Wang, S., et al., (2019). Biocompatibility of artificial micro/nanomotors for use in biomedicine. *Nanoscale, 11*, 14099–14112.
24. https://www.frontiersin.org/articles/10.3389/fbioe.2018.00170/full (accessed on 4 December 2023).

25. Salido, J., Paredis, C. J. J., & Khosla, P. K., (1999). Continuous probabilistic mapping by autonomous robots. In: *Proceedings of the International Symposium on Experimental Robotics. Sydney, Australia*.
26. http://loop-impact.frontiersin.org/impact/article/856727#totalviews/views (accessed on 4 December 2023).
27. McLurkin, J. D., (1996). *Using Cooperative Robots for Explosive Ordnance Disposal.* Technical Document, Massachusetts Institute of Technology, Artificial Intelligence Laboratory, Cambridge, MA: USA 02139.
28. Kleeman, L., (1992). Optimal estimation of position and heading for mobile robots using ultrasonic beacons and dead-reckoning. In: *Proceedings of the 1992 IEEE International Conference on Robotics and Automation, May, Nice, France* (pp. 2582–2587).
29. https://builtin.com/robotics/surgical-medical-healthcare-robotics-companies (accessed on 4 December 2023).
30. https://www.pharmtech.com/view/using-robotics-pharmaceutical-manufacturing (accessed on 4 December 2023).
31. https://bentork.com/stationary-robots-and-autonomous-robots/ (accessed on 4 December 2023).
32. Panait, L., Doarn, C. R., & Merrell, R. C., (2002). Applications of robotics in surgery. *Chirurgia (Bucur), 97*, 549–555.
33. *Robot-Assisted Surgery,* (2019). Available from: https://aabme.asme.org/posts/robot-assisted-surgery (accessed on 4 December 2023).
34. Hung, L., Liu, C., Woldum, E., et al., (2019). The benefits of and barriers to using a social robot PARO in care settings: A scoping review. *BMC. Geriatr.*, *19*, 232. doi.org/10.1186/s12877-019-1244-6.
35. https://www.robotics.org/content-detail.cfm/Industrial-Robotics-Industry-Insights/Robotiamrcs-in-the-Pharmaceutical-andLife-Sciences-Industry/content_id/2867 (accessed on 4 December 2023).
36. *Medical Robots That Are Changing the World*, (2019). Available from: https://www.flomedicalsales.com.au/15-medical-robots-that-are-changing-the-world/ (accessed on 4 December 2023).
37. Aggarwal, M., & Kumar, S. (2022). The Use of Nanorobotics in the Treatment Therapy of Cancer and Its Future Aspects: A Review. *Cureus 14*(9), e29366. doi:10.7759/cureus.29366.
38. Zhiguang, W., Jonas, T., Hyeon-Ho, J., Qiang, W., Marius, S., Focke, Z., Zegao, W., et al., (2018). A swarm of slippery micropropellers penetrates the vitreous body of the eye. *Science Advances, 4*(11), eaat4388. doi: 10.1126/sciadv.aat4388.
38. Wu, Z., Troll, J., Jeong, H. H., Wei, Q., Stang, M., Ziemssen, F., Wang, Z., et al., (2018). A swarm of slippery micro propellers penetrates the vitreous body of the eye. *Science Advances*, 4 eaat4388. https://doi.org/10.1126/sciadv.aat4388.
39. Gómez Rivas, J., Toribio-Vázquez, C., Taratkin, M., Marenco, J.L., Grossmann, R.(2021). Autonomous robots: a new reality in healthcare? A project by European Association of Urology-Young Academic Urologist group. *Curr Opin Urol. 1; 31*(2), 155–159..
40. https://www.intel.com/content/www/us/en/robotics/types-andapplications (accessed on 4 December 2023).
41. https://www.pwc.com/gx/en/industries/healthcare/publications/ai-robotics-new-health/transforming-healthcare.html (accessed on 4 December 2023).

42. Brewer, R. D., (2015). *Improving Peripheral IV Catheterization Through Robotics: From Simple Assistive Devices to a Fully-Autonomous System*. thesis, Stanford University, Stanford, CA. http://purl.stanford.edu/qh215qd3853 (accessed on 4 December 2023).
43. Chen, A., Nikitczuk, K., Nikitczuk, J., Maguire, T., & Yarmush, M., (2013). Portable robot for autonomous venipuncture using 3D near-infrared image guidance. *Dent. Tech., 1*, 72–87.
44. Balter, M. L., Chen, A. I., Maguire, T. J., & Yarmush, M. L., (2015). The system design and evaluation of a 7-of image-guided venipuncture robot. *IEEE Trans. Robot., 31*, 1044–1053.
45. Balter, M., Leipheimer, J. M., Chen, A. I., Shrirao, A., Maguire, T. J., & Yarmush, M. L., (2018). Automated end-to-end blood testing at the point-of-care: Integration of robotic phlebotomy with downstream sample processing. *Technology*, *6*, 59–66.
46. Leipheimer, J. M., Balter, M. L., Chen, A. I., Pantin, E. J., Davidovich, A. E., Labazzo, K. S., & Yarmush, M. L., (2019). First-in-human evaluation of a hand-held automated venipuncture device for rapid venous blood draws. *Technology, 7*, 98–107.
47. Cheng, Z., Davies, B.L., Caldwell, D.G., & De Mattos, L.S. (2019). A Hand-Held Robot for Precise and Safe PIVC. *IEEE Robotics and Automation Letters, 4,* 655–661.
48. Chen, A. I., Balter, M. L., Maguire, T. J., & Yarmush, M. L., (2020). Deep learning robotic guidance for autonomous vascular access. *Nat. Mach. Intel., 2*, 104–115.
49. Tsai, S. C., Samani, H., Kao, Y. W., Zhu, K., & Jalaian, B., (2018). Design and development of interactive intelligent medical agent. In: *Proceedings of the IEEE International Conference on Artificial Intelligence and Virtual Reality (AIVR)* (pp. 210–215).
50. *Automation and Robotics for Biotechnology – VTT's Research Information Portal*. https://cris.vtt.fi/en/equipments/automation-and-robotics-for-biotechnology. (accessed on 2 December 2023).
51. http://.www.BeckmanCoulter.com (accessed on 4 December 2023).
52. Baumkircher, A., Seme, K., Munih, M., & Mihelj, M., (2022). Collaborative robot precision task in medical microbiology laboratory. *Sensors, 22*, 2862. https://doi.org/10.3390/s22082862.
53. Kevin, W., et al., (2022). *The Future of Artificial Intelligence and Cybernetics a Test Book of Artificial Intelligent*. https:www.bbvaopenmind.com/en/articles/the-future-of-artificial-intelligence-and-cybernetics/.
54. Kovach, C. R., Taneli, Y., Neiman, T., Dyer, E. M., Arzaga, A. J. A., & Kelber, S. T., (2017). Evaluation of an ultraviolet room disinfection protocol to decrease nursing home microbial burden, infection, and hospitalization rates. *BMC Infect. Dis.*, *17*, 186.
55. *Centers for Disease Control and Prevention, Interim Guidelines for Collecting, Handling, and Testing Clinical Specimens from Persons Under Investigation (PUIs) for Coronavirus Disease (2019). (COVID-19),* 9 March (2020). www.cdc.gov/coronavirus/2019-ncov/lab/guidelines-clinical-specimens.html (accessed on 4 December 2023).
56. *Medical Device Technologies: A Systems Based Overview Using Engineering Standards Book* (2nd edn., 2020).
57. PMMI Packaging Intelligence Brief, (2014). *Trends in Robotics: Market Assessment*. https://docplayer.net/11692206-Packaging-intelligence-brief-trends-in-robotics-market-assessment-april-2014.html (accessed on 4 December 2023).

CHAPTER 15

Challenges to Digital Transformation in the Healthcare Industry

PRACHI PACHUARY,[1] YASHRAJ SHARMA,[1] SHARDA SHAMBHAKAR,[2] SUDHANSHU MISHRA,[2] and PALAK GUPTA[3]

[1]*Department of Management Studies, Kanya Gurukula, Haridwar, Uttarakhand, India*

[2]*Department of Pharmacy, Banasthali Vidyapith, Vanasthali, Rajasthan, India*

[3]*Department of Chemistry, University of Florida, Florida, USA*

ABSTRACT

The digital revolution is increasing its significance for scholars and practitioners in the field of healthcare. The healthcare system's focus is shifting from disease-centered to patient-centered services. The digital healthcare system is an interdisciplinary domain that aims to enrich the efficiency of monitoring patients, their diagnosis, rehabilitation, prevention, and lasting with their care delivery. The digital revolution has changed the world in every aspect of human life involving human health, the medical industry, and the health economy. A digital change in the healthcare industry has enlarged the medical field with major improvements in the quality of healthcare, lowering the cost of clinical research, patients, the healthcare system, and its effectiveness as well. Adopting the digital healthcare revolution has rapidly accelerated after welcoming our newest guest, "The coronavirus" or "COVID-19" pandemic. It started in China and spread all over the world, affecting millions of people's lifestyles. Starting from physical distancing to wearing a mask and also quarantine. The abrupt increase of patients gave

Creating Smart Healthcare with Blockchain and Advanced Digital Technology.
Rishabha Malviya and Sonali Sundram (Eds.)

a serious challenge to the healthcare system to maintain and keep a proper record of the patients in a "no-touch" emergency state. Accessing healthcare data, consistency of data with providers, security regarding technology, and budgetary restrictions are found to be a few issues for the healthcare industry. Keeping the information of the patients and their records in safe mode is also a big concern, as the problem of re-identification hacking occurs because of merging old data with new data. The key challenges faced by the healthcare industry which are affecting the growth of this industry are as follows: data privacy, data governance, ethical challenges, and evidence-based digital health standards. Out of the aforementioned problems, privacy emerged as one of the main key challenges for this industry. As in today's era, the role of the consumer is changing, few apps and companies are there such as Apple, Facebook, Amazon, Google, Samsung, etc., are recording the medical data of the person and all the health-related information, which indirectly affects the privacy of the user. Coming to the core concern accessibility, consistency, and privacy are considered to be the main key challenges that need to be focused upon to bring a perfect digital revolution to the healthcare system. Besides this, the digital growth of the healthcare industry and the revolution will be helpful for researchers, scientists, technologists, and clinical payers to help patients live their lives longer and feel better.

15.1 INTRODUCTION

The digital revolution has changed our lives in both aspects, or we can say personally and professionally. It has been observed that technology is changing very rapidly. Earlier, the things which we have seen in science and fiction are now we are seeing in reality. Even the diagnoses of a doctor have changed from clinical to precise digital diagnoses, nowadays doctors are checking their patients completely online. From booking an appointment to prescribing them their medicine, everything is going online and digitally. The outbreak of COVID-19 or coronavirus also introduced digital solutions to each and everything, this virus created unforeseen situations in everybody's life. By default, all the people or families are becoming digital, from paperless to contact the world has witnessed a change in every phase of lifestyle. A few concerns which arise from using the healthcare industry are Accessibility, Consistency, and Privacy. Out of these three Privacy stands as one of the most important concerns which need to be looked upon. A report by OECD in 2016 gave an alert on data privacy, the report explains the difference between Legal and Ethical. The report explains the European Commission's tracking and growth towards the usage of the Internet in context with digitalization [1]. The member of the EU ensures the need for the digitization because the usage of the Internet is increasing. As far as privacy is concerned it is a risk and also a worsening of digital barring which needs to be avoided to make the system fully digitalized.

A report by Internet word stats in the year 2020 explains the usage of the internet in India and the European Union (EU). There is a massive difference in both the countries, the report states that there is only 58% of the world population estimated who are using the internet and when it comes to the EU 90% of the population are internet users. Studies also revealed that the pandemic has given a positive future for the country; it gave a digital divide among the people of the world. When we discuss our newest guest, COVID-19 or Coronavirus, it gave us a very positive impact on the healthcare industry it turned the healthcare industry into a digital healthcare society. With only one click patients can get themselves diagnosed from anywhere in the world and from whatever doctor they want to get the check. With the help of Digitalization India has offered various apps which can deliver medicines to your doorsteps. Online pharmaceuticals gave a great option to buy your medicines online with huge discounts and authenticity rather than visiting your local medical shop [2, 3]. Here are a few applications which are offering medicines at your doorsteps with no time:

1. **Netmeds:** It is a leading online pharmacy which is based in Pan-India. It delivers life-saving drugs to every state, also ensuring no-hassle delivery. One can set up a subscription and medicines will be delivered automatically every month. This application also provides a subscription to their customers to save some amount from your bill.
2. **Practo:** It offers an extensive catalog of medicines and healthcare products and provides hassle-free service across 100+ cities in India. It has an automated prescription refill option which allows checking the medicine order history and reordering.
3. **1 mg:** This app is considered to be one of the best apps where you can buy medicines online. On this platform, we can also check and order alternative medicine consisting of a different compound of the same medicine. Based on the medicines that we have ordered, this app provides health tips from well-known doctors.

4. **PharmEasy:** It offers more than 1 lakh products to choose from the app which fulfills healthcare needs with quality service. It also offers delivery in 24-48 hours across 1.2k cities in India. It also contains one of the unique features of giving a gentle reminder of your medicine and also provides cash-on-delivery services.
5. **Apollo Pharmacy:** It got accreditation of International Quality Certification and offers more than 5,000 products in various categories. Also having more than 3,000 outlets in key locations, it offers round-the-clock service.
6. **Medlife:** If you are purchasing medicine from this app then you must simply need to upload a prescription and get it confirmed on call before ordering the medicines. If the customer does not have a valid prescription, they can even consult a 'Medlife doctor.' Moreover, one can also book a Lab Test with them.

With the growing business of technology and the world becoming digitalized, the above graph shows how the popularity of these apps is increasing in the market. In today's era, online medicine delivery apps are capturing the market around the whole world, all this is happening because of digitalization and technology [4].

Technology is capturing the market very fast, from supermarkets to hypermarkets, from car manufacturing to selling cars online. Buying and selling goods and services online became a global trend in this era. Considering the popularity of online business, healthcare products and medicines also came into this market. People have started using mobile health applications these days, and their trust and promise toward online health prescriptions and consultation show their interest in digital healthcare. It is very important to analyze and check all challenges the healthcare industry is facing or is going to face shortly. This chapter will also help us to analyze how digitalization is taking place or capturing the healthcare market shortly [5].

15.2 BEGINNING OF DIGITAL MOVEMENT

The starting internet came into force in the year 1960, it was initially invented for the military and then expanded for communication with researchers and scientists. During the cold war, it was very necessary to have proper communication between military people, and those computers which are placed in the universities. Internet is one of the compound and complex revolutions which changes the whole world. Its revolutionary invention came into force in the year 1965 and gave global communication to the entire society, industry, and also to the whole world. It is considered to be one of the broadcasting capabilities worldwide. It can also be explained as the network of networks that has connected government, private computers, and universities with each other. Internet provided many services for people to be in touch properly. Services like E-mail, fax, documents, instant messages, and exchanging of data help the users to communicate properly. From 1965 to 2022 internet shows massive growth in the technology factor from email messages to WhatsApp messages, from normal calls to video calls which created the telephone network very strong. The internet network transformed nationwide infrastructure into an international network. In the year 1990 one of the most important inventions happened was the invention of WWW (world wide web). With this invention people can do around about everything whatever they want to do things like shopping, learning, chatting, listening to music even buying and selling goods and services. With this technology, you can buy anything from anywhere from whole around the world. With an increment in technology, there is a massive increment in the speed of the internet also. From 2G, 3G, 4G, and now it is 5G. Section 15.3 explains the evolution of communication [6].

15.3 EVOLUTION OF CONNECTION

1. **1G:** In 1G, G stands for "GENERATION," it is a term that was not used earlier until 2G came into force or 2G was available for common people.
2. **2G:** This is after the first generation of cell phone transmission.
3. **3G:** This is the generation that came into force in the year 2008 and set the benchmark for most of the wireless technology which we are using even today.
4. **4G:** This generation is also having the standards which a network needs to pass to get available to society. They need 100 megabits per second and also up to 1 Gigabit per second to pass as a 4G network.
5. **5G:** Till now we are only listening to the rumors about this 5G network, everyone is waiting for the launch of the 5G network. According to DOT (Department of Telecommunication), this network will go to be launched by the 15th of August.

As is already explained in the earlier paragraph that each and everything has a positive and negative impact. The things which give you a positive impact will also have some negative consequences [7]. Here are some of the advantages and disadvantages of technology or we can give a different word to technology which is "Digitalization." The cons and pros that cannot be neglected while using technology are given in succeeding sections.

15.4 ADVANTAGES OF THE DIGITAL INDUSTRY

15.4.1 QUICK SERVICE

Nowadays, everyone is so busy that they want things immediately without moving out of their houses. Items such as groceries, vegetables, medicines, food, and electronic appliances are delivered to their doorstep. Also, after COVID-19, it has rapidly increased as most people found it convenient as the required materials were delivered to them at their doorstep without much hassle and within the limited time. The latest development was done in the digital industry as per the citizens' requirements, such as a few apps taking orders in the early morning to deliver items such as fresh juices, slices of bread, milk, and eggs as these were during breakfast time. A few of the applications have also started delivering within 15 minutes after the order, even for the order of items having a value of 100 Rs was getting delivered to the doorstep in less than 15 minutes. Many platforms were started such as doc online, Practo, Lybrate, M-fine, and Tata health where one can log in and consult the doctors online on video or audio chat. These apps helped the doctors as well as their patients as during COVID, it was very difficult to move out and many of the citizens faced problems related to the medical facilities, so these apps worked well as they provided good consultations to citizens and doctors. It was helpful for doctors as well as during COVID, few doctors were unable to visit their clinics and hospitals, so they opted to use these platforms and give their consultations via calls. It helped them to earn some income while doing their duty during the difficult days [8]. The consultations seemed to be easy and hassle-free, as there was direct contact between the patient and the doctor, and it was much easier for everyone to showcase their issues and get the desired resolution. These apps are working fine on these normal days as well, as many of the patients are unable to go to doctors' clinics and hospitals due to their ill health, so they can consult with doctors and doctors can treat them online and give the required treatment or prescription [9].

15.4.2 RELIABILITY

The products listed on online platforms are much more reliable and trustworthy as most of the items are covered under services such as a 30-day return policy, no hassle exchange, instant refunds, and warranty clarity of products. The products sold at e-commerce websites have reliable bills and authenticity certifications. The same goes for the healthcare societies where the digital world has played an important role, such as medical tests, prescribed medicines, and doctor's consultations provided through online methods. Nowadays, many applications such as Healthians, Apollo 24×7, Lal Pathlabs, Flebo, etc., are in the market which give full body check-ups or required test samples being collected at doorsteps without much hassle. Samples are collected by trained professionals holding certifications related to the medical fields. The samples are collected and kept without any contamination, and the laboratory that performs the test on the collected samples is certified with the given government standards. The results are quick and clear to understand [10]. Few apps also provide a free consultation with doctors based on the reports, and the diet to be followed is also provided upon request.

15.4.3 EASE OF FACILITY

The digital world has opened a new way of life for those who are unable to go out due to their health conditions and disabilities. Before the digital awareness, mostly elderly people or couples with multiple health issues used to be dependent on others for their needs and requirements. However, as digitalization has increased day by day, especially after the COVID waves, it has opened new ways to solve the problems faced by citizens who were unable to leave their homes. Now, they can access fresh vegetables, groceries, fruits, medicines, and medical tests right at their doorstep. This only requires them to click on the application from their smartphones to get the desired product or service. If they are unable to do so, they can also ask other family members or distant relatives to order or book for them at their specific address [11].

15.5 DISADVANTAGES OF THE DIGITAL INDUSTRY

15.5.1 HEARING LOSS

Nowadays in our society, we can see people with headphones in their ears all the time as they are convenient. But on the other hand, they are even dangerous for us. This can harshly affect our hearing ability. This is how the technology is destroying our health.

15.5.2 POOR POSTURE

Continued use of technology such as laptops, mobiles, and digital devices can cause back pain, neck pain, and cervical pain. This is due to the head-down position and incorrect postures. If we do these things more than our routine, it will become more of a curse and critical situation for the person.

15.5.3 DIGITAL EYE STRAIN

Excessive use of screens causes a syndrome called digital eye strain. This syndrome leads to reduced eyesight and vision problems, which are most common in kids as well. The symptoms of digital eye strain syndrome are dry eyes, severe headache, blurred vision, and shoulder pain. The main reason for this is screen light at an inappropriate distance from the screen.

15.5.4 EMOTIONAL PROBLEMS

When patients get physically treated by the doctor, they become emotionally connected to the doctor's prescriptions and counseling. However, during digital consultation, the patient does not receive any physical or emotional support. It feels like an imaginary consultation. Research shows that digitally consulted patients do not experience psychological and mental satisfaction.

Digitalization is the process of converting data and information into digital forms through various methods. Digitalization relies on the usage of the internet. As the number of internet users increases, things become more digitalized [12]. The digital revolution came to India with the introduction of the internet in 1995. However, it had a slow and steady growth at that time.

After the government's vision of digital India in 2015, many changes have been made in policies and many new technologies have been introduced to bring about major reform in digitalization. This is the point from which many digital advancements have started in all sectors, including healthcare.

15.6 THE FUTURE OF HEALTHCARE

In the decades ahead, healthcare has undergone many dramatic transformations. The medicines will become more precise and valuable, patients will become empowered consumers and digitalization will transform every area of healthcare. Patients will have digital twins, a customized computerized model of themselves, and predict the outcome of procedures. Patients will get artificial intelligence (AI)-powered diagnoses and decisions. Healthcare will become organized and anticipatory in all medical conditions around the clock and around the world with real-time delivery [13]. The highly productive and multidisciplinary team will be able to work at the same time in each cycle. All interactions with patients will become more convenient and patients will get digital reports in easy-to-understand formats where no medical expertise will be required to treat patients. It will also be beneficial for patient attendants. Through this digitalization, patients will become more accessible to real-time doctors and experts monitoring through virtual meetings, so in these ways digitalization is helping and shaping future healthcare [14].

15.7 DATA HANDLING AND ANALYSIS

This digitization process has made the patient record, history, information, and data handling in a systematic order. Once the data is recorded and stored in a prescribed format, then its analysis becomes effective, efficient, and easy to understand. This practice is helpful for both the patients and medical practitioners. Through this practice, doctors can access all the information about their patients from any part of the world and can easily prescribe patient treatment [15].

Data handling and record maintenance are mostly required for lifelong diseases such as Alzheimer's, cancer, diabetes, heart disease, etc. In these types of diseases, it requires more and continuous monitoring of patient reports and clinical records. With the help of these, doctors and medical practitioners can easily study the nature of the disease, and these available data will further help in medical research as well.

15.8 SMART CITIES AND DIGITALIZATION

There is a direct relation between smart cities and digitalization as smart cities are based on digitalization. Healthcare sector development is an important part of smart city development. The vision of smart cities is to provide medical support as soon as possible without any hindrance. With the help of this digitalization, hospitals can send an ambulance to the patient on time and smart cities will be helpful in traffic management. In each case, patients will get good and required treatment from the best specialized medical practitioners across the world [16].

15.9 CHALLENGES FACED BY USING DIGITALIZATION IN THE HEALTHCARE INDUSTRY

Digitalization has both pros and cons. Despite many advantages, it also has many disadvantages and challenges. As India is a developing country, we have not completely adopted the digitalization model. We are facing shortages in many areas such as internet, power cuts, infrastructure, and skilled and trained personnel. Digitalization is growing rapidly in India at a very high growth rate, but it will take many years to achieve 100% digitalization in every sector, especially in the healthcare sector. In rural India, we have not even provided basic healthcare facilities such as first aid. It is unfortunate that after so many years of Independence, we have not been able to spread basic healthcare facilities all over India. However, the government's vision of digitalization in the healthcare sector gives hope for growth at a very high rate [17, 18].

15.9.1 LACK OF INTERNET AND ELECTRICITY

Digitalization depends on electrification and access to the internet. Without the internet, we cannot go digitalized. In India, we do not have internet connection everywhere. Currently, we have internet access in metro cities only. But after the entry of the 4G network in India, it has increased at a rapid growth rate. Currently, there are 47% of internet users in India, and the government is expecting that the percentage will increase to 80% by 2030. To increase digitalization in every sector, especially in the healthcare sector, we first need to provide internet and electricity access. It is one of the biggest challenges in adopting digitalization in the healthcare sector [19].

15.9.2 HABITS OF EMPLOYEE

Digitalization is easy to understand, but it requires specific training and special skills to use in the healthcare sector. We have old, untrained, and unaware staff in digitalization, making it very difficult for them to adopt new technologies and adapt to digitalization. To make the healthcare sector digitalized, we need to produce more trained and skilled workers and medical practitioners to achieve our digitalization target. This is the biggest manpower challenge for the healthcare industry in achieving digitalized healthcare. Nowadays, the government has made many computer certification courses mandatory to obtain a job. Without completing these types of computer certification courses, individuals cannot get a job. This type of step will help us to have trained and active staff, which will assist us in achieving our digitalization target [20].

15.9.3 NEED FOR DESIGNING A NEW PROCESS

The most important thing is to design a new process according to the needs and requirements. So, let's assume that you are carefully analyzing your medical business leaves and preparing an upgraded digital transformation strategy. You choose the best software for the market and invested in additional business solutions like interactive websites, mobile apps for patients, chatbot for voice assistant. Extra, you have all modern digital products (MDP) [21].

15.9.4 LACK OF SOFTWARE AWARENESS

To exchange information between two or more systems is a very desirable feature in business software, especially in the healthcare sector. If we want to give our patients access to their medical records stored in the database of your patient management system software or quickly gain information about patient insurance integrations with medical suppliers' software and laboratory software, it also increases the efficiency of our medical sector.

The absence of standards for interoperability and a rather complex path for digital health software integration makes communication between your company and third parties less efficient because you cannot fully realize the potential of your organization. Fortunately, the healthcare industry is evolving quite fast and there are already some software houses with considerable experience in developing a healthcare system that focuses on making the system more user-friendly and efficient [22].

15.9.5 COST OF DIGITALIZATION

Adopting digitalization is expensive as it requires a lot of money, time, and effort, etc. Digitalization is an expensive process because it requires new tech devices, we should get updated from time to time as per the requirement of digitalization, it is costly, and it makes a direct impact on the patients' expenses because at last the final consumer is the patient, so he has to bear the cost [23]. Digitalization will become cheaper only when it will be accepted at a very large scale in every system of healthcare.

15.10 LITERATURE REVIEW RELATED TO HEALTHCARE AND DIGITALIZATION

1. **Hantrais et al. [24]:** This research is based on "COVID-19 and the Digital Revolution" in 2020. It explains the digital revolution in the context of COVID-19. In this chapter, the researchers accumulated different evidence from various areas of social science and explained the impact of COVID-19 on a digital society. The authors show how COVID-19 changed the way data on patients is collected online and how e-health treatment will largely overcome traditional methods. This chapter also explains how families have become "digital by default." The spike in COVID-19 cases and the spread of the pandemic also created a breeding ground for crime and cybercrime. It explains the challenges faced by ordinary people, such as the fast-tracking of digital supplies, the construction of online platforms, the development of video-conferencing products, and the creation of different platforms for teaching and learning. All these things are not possible without cost, so there is a revolution in the healthcare

industry and other industries as well. Therefore, it is crucial to keep an eye on these revolutionary changes [24].

2. **Sriram & Subrahmanian [25]:** This research is based on "Transforming healthcare through the digital revolution." This researcher gave an example of recurring work at the National Institute of Standards and Technology (NIST). It explains the IoT and also about the devices of IoT are mobile devices, smart medical devices, smartphones, and personal computing devices. As far as a network is concerned, the Internet has widespread the areas network-wise, and also shows a paradigm shift in symbiotic networks. A researcher explains that the new generation will surely take the benefit of these devices more properly and appropriately. There will be proper and optimum utilization of the resources of these devices and also helpful in multimodal information from "biological," "cognitive," "semantic," and "social networks." This chapter not only explains the IoT revolution but also explains the Omics revolution, which is a combination of social networks and socio-omics. The researcher says that these things are directly and significantly giving implications to healthcare delivered in the United States [25]. The researcher also introduces a P9 healthcare concept which is shown in Table 15.1.

3. **Hasselberg [26]:** This research is based on "The Digital Revolution in Behavioral Health." This chapter analyzes the pros and consequences of technology-enabled healthcare providers, from more than 50 years ago. It also helps us to examine the movement which took place in psychiatry. Digital Revolution also helps the industry to include the opportunity of Video Conferencing, online consultation, Online education, and online healthcare providers. In this research, the researcher uses secondary data analysis, uses recent reports based on innovation and Behavioral health and also on the Digital revolution. This research also reviews the model of the University of Rochester to examine the current status of digital behavioral healthcare. As far as research results were concerned not giving enough attention to mental healthcare professionals specifically in rural areas, who did not know the proper usage of the internet became a hurdle for the Digital revolution in Behavioral health. Apart from attention, there are many challenges and issues which were faced to adopt Digital Revolution these are Knowledge gap, usage of internet gap and digital healthcare

TABLE 15.1 Details About the P9 Healthcare Concept

Sl. No.	P9 Healthcare Concept	Conception
1.	Personalized	This concept includes personalized medicines, or we can say customized treatment for every single individual.
2.	Predictive	The provided information by EHR (electronic health records), also defines individual susceptibility with the help of genomic data.
3.	Preventive	Decision analytics tools were used to check the disease of an individual rather than treating a disease when it infects a person.
4.	Participatory	Proper participation is necessary for an individual in the treatment and diagnosis of his/her medical condition.
5.	Pervasive	The basic meaning of pervasive is to present anywhere and everywhere. So, the healthcare industry should provide treatment anytime and anywhere.
6.	Precise	To get appropriate therapeutic action proper collection of data and information is very much necessary. Once the information is gathered all the tools can be used precisely for taking necessary actions for the treatment of the disease.
7.	Privacy-preserving	For minimizing the problems of patients processing the data of the patients is appropriate.
8.	Protective	For ensuring the protection of the patients, security of patients' information is required, and appropriate measures should be taken to avoid any harm to them.
9.	Priced reasonably	This is one of the most important factors of all the P9 factors is Price. Price plays a very important role in the healthcare industry as well. It is very essential to keep the rates affordable.

as well. Concluding it has been understood that it is very much important for behavioral health to bring digital healthcare into revolution [26].

4. **Bucci et al. [27]:** This research is based on "The digital revolution and its impact on mental health." The researcher explains the digital revolution and how it impacted mental healthcare. As the whole world is emphasizing big data, the technology of mobile, computing power, and information network. The mental healthcare industry came under high pressure than ever before. The author states that the development of the digital revolution is very much necessary for a theory-driven approach and also for a data-driven approach. Also, the need for co-production of digital health devices is important for minimizing chronic and mental health difficulties [27].

5. **Keesara et al. [28]:** This study is based on "COVID-19 and Healthcare's Digital Revolution." In this study, the researcher explains the digital revolution in the healthcare industry. This study is based on the American people. It shows that there came an emergency where the COVID-19 virus spread in the whole world and created an emergency for the healthcare industry. There comes the need arise where no-touch situation arose. It became clear to everyone that there is and will be an immediate need for the digital revolution. COVID-19 clearly explains the delivery of urgent action that needs to be taken for checking the patients and getting them diagnosed. Hospital at home policy also started, and patients can treat themselves online. Even they can order their food, medicine, and other miscellaneous items online. This is possible only because of digitalization. It is very important to make use of technology in practice as we are living in the 21st century, not in the old era where we do not have technology [28].
6. **Dionisio & Paula [29]:** This research is based on "Innovation and digital transformation in healthcare: A systematic review," in this study researchers created a systematic literature review to examine the evolution of digital transformation in healthcare concerning four factors: applications, benefits, opportunities, and threats, and explain how it is impacting the market. This study covers the Scopus database from the year 2015-2022. It covered 77 peer-reviewed articles in the study. This research is based on a systematic literature review of healthcare in the context of digital transformation. A bibliometric and content analysis is used to identify the latest trends with the most discussed topics related to healthcare and digital transformation [29]. In this study, the researchers find relevant keywords for healthcare, Digital Transformation, and also about the Nine Pillars of Industry 4.0. These keywords are shown in Figure 15.1.

Using these keywords, researchers used 1,578 articles and then filtered out the papers using the following filters: document type, language, year, and subject area as well. In this research, the researchers only focus on "Articles" which are from the English language. The subject areas in which they focus are Medicine, Computer Science, Engineering, Social Sciences, Business Management, Accounting, Nursing, Health Profession, Finance, Economics, and Econometrics. After this, the researchers came up with 505 articles, and

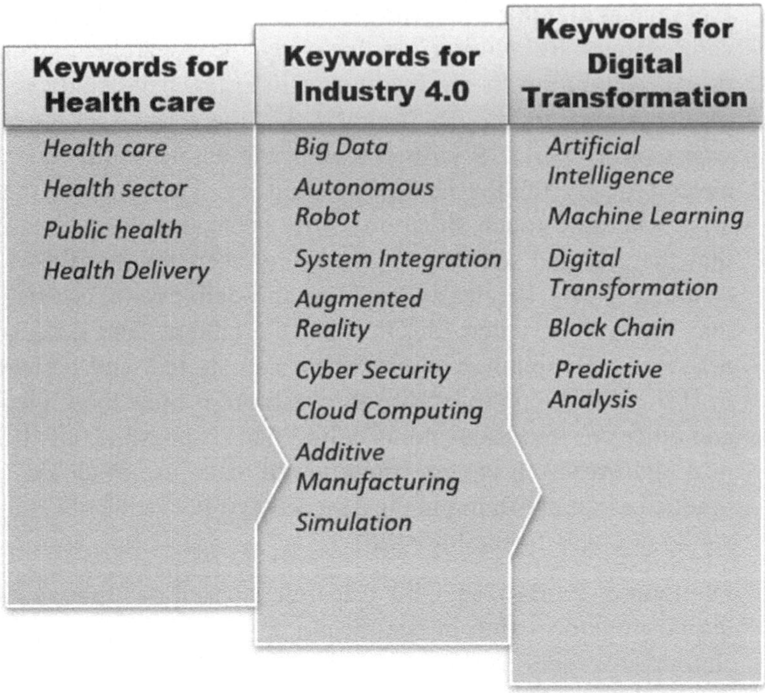

FIGURE 15.1 Various keywords are used in different fields.

then they searched for those articles which have only one citation. After applying all the filters, the graph of the article systematic review comes to 77 articles. After analyzing all the 77 articles, the researchers explain that there is a massive growth in the research of the healthcare industry and digitalization after 2014. With the help of content analysis, the researchers explain that the world needs to adopt a few things, especially "artificial intelligence," "internet of things," "blockchain," "big data," and "cloud computing solutions." As far as security is concerned, a few factors examined by the researchers are as follows: privacy, ethics, and data security. These factors need to be worked upon for the proper development of healthcare and digital technology.

7. **Compaoré et al. [30]:** This research is based on the title "The head issue of the digital revolution: an emergent challenge for the future of jobs." The study focuses on the difference between the two countries, and these countries are Burkina and Africa. Are these countries ready enough to go for digital transformation?

The main objective of this study is to suggest some guidelines to help managers while facing challenges because of the digital revolution at the local and international levels. Another objective is to have a good comprehension of "Human Resource Management" at local and international levels. The researcher also explains the challenges which occurred in Human Resource Management due to the emergence of the digital revolution. So, in this research, the researcher tries to explain the problems and challenges that the Human Resource of any organization is facing. The challenges this study explains are innovation and ICT (information technology) [30]. ICT comprises some of the factors which are helpful for the development of IT, as shown in Figure 15.2.

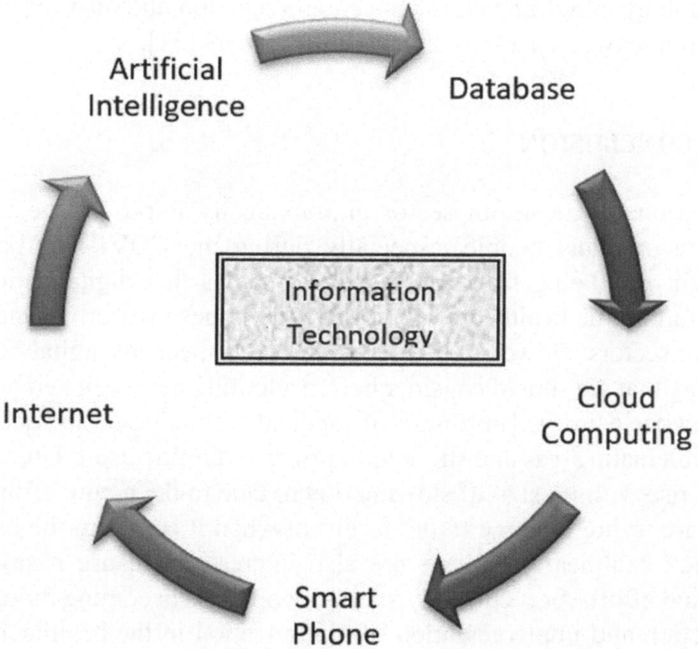

FIGURE 15.2 Some factors related to the development of information technology.

In this study, the researcher used secondary data based on an empirical and conceptual literature review. As far as Digital Transformation was concerned, researchers used "UNESCO (United Nations Educational, Scientific, and Cultural Organization)," "OECD," and also "France Government" reports for analyzing the future of Digital Transformation.

8. **Attaran [31]:** This study is based on "Blockchain technology in healthcare: Challenges and opportunities." The researcher explains blockchain technology and also analyzes the challenges and opportunities that patients are facing while using digital technology. The main aim of this study is to analyze practical implications and find out the benefits and negative aspects of the healthcare industry by the use of blockchain technology. This study shared that patients are facing the challenge of "accessing," "integrating," "data sharing," and "managing." As far as opportunities are concerned, the study examines the pros of the technology. Data can be easily managed, everything is visible with a single click, and all the reports can be recorded online. This study concluded that the proper use of technology could be helpful for communication and also for coordination between patients and health providers [31].

15.11 CONCLUSION

Digitalization in the health sector grammatically improves the lives and well-being of many people, especially during the COVID-19 pandemic. The tough time being faced by the world shows that digitalization has a bright future in the healthcare sector and high hopes to improve and change healthcare sectors. However, there are multiple aspects of digital healthcare technology that we should consider before adopting new digitized processes, such as cybersecurity. The future of medical technology must account for these problematic areas and strive to improve and refine itself. Digitalization is on the rise with no sign of slowing down. Due to the nature of industries, patients are trying to come to the forefront when it comes to the expansion into digital healthcare. Patients are also interested because it saves time, money, and effort. As it currently stands, people are becoming more open to the detection and implementation of digitalization in the healthcare sector. However, there is still a large number of people against it because they are not aware or knowledgeable enough to use digitalized software. Becoming more and more technology-centric makes patients feel that their needs are not being met. It's up to those within the industry to provide a humanistic touch to this ever-growing industry.

But we can say that digitalization is the need of this time and era. Specifically in India, we have to make drastic changes in our healthcare sector as we are a developing country. We are not fully equipped with basic amenities and facilities at our hospitals. In rural India, there are still places without any medical hospitals in 2022. The government of India is still working on it, but in my opinion, digitalization would help us achieve this target very shortly and make it accessible. With the help of digitalization, we can reduce costs and increase expansion.

The main drawback of digitalization in the healthcare sector is that only technically skilled people can use it. It is not beneficial for unskilled people, both for doctors and patients. This digitalization in the healthcare sector also lacks the physical checkup and psychological satisfaction of patients towards the disease. In a few studies, we have found that some parts of the disease get treated psychologically after consulting a specific doctor. However, in the digital healthcare system, this aspect is missing. Here, a patient can only see a doctor virtually and does not get any physical satisfaction or physical checkup. This is true for developed countries as well, and it will take time to get settled in developing countries. In conclusion, digitalization is needed in the healthcare sector, but it should be tailored to the requirements of patients, doctors, and health institutions.

15.12 FUTURE PERSPECTIVE

From the above study, one can easily find out the challenges which were faced by the country's people and healthcare industry because of the digital revolution. But there is not much research that was based on the Indian context. So, there is a need to research that as well. Few factors or challenges were examined by this study with the help of secondary data that needs to be looked upon and some challenges can be minimized by using digital technology properly. Digital revolution is necessary and is going to be helpful in upcoming years, but the knowledge and its proper use have to be conveyed so it can be used in better directions. It will surely help to have great sustainability and availability with good credibility. Sooner or later, the healthcare industry will surely rely on digitalization processes as they are quick, accurate, and reliable.

CONFLICT OF INTEREST

Authors have no conflict of interest.

FUNDING

Authors have received no funding from any government or non-government organization.

KEYWORDS

- **coronavirus**
- **data privacy**
- **digital healthcare**
- **digital industry**
- **digital revolution**
- **digitalization**
- **healthcare industry**

REFERENCES

1. Joshi, A., Mishra, S., Jain, D., Ludhiani, S., & Rajput, A. (2023). Artificial intelligence: An emerging technique in pharmaceutical and healthcare systems. In: *Bioinformatics Tools and Big Data Analytics for Patient Care* (pp. 71–90). Chapman and Hall/CRC.
2. Mahor, S., Chadha, H., Prajapati, S., Mishra, S., & Ojha, S., (2022). An update on COVID-19 outbreak: The longest pandemic. *Biological Sciences, 2*(1), 114–126.
3. Sharma, P., Srivastava, P., & Singh, A., (2010). Rishabha Malviya. *Education.*
4. Sharma, K., Singh, H., Sharma, D. K., Kumar, A., Nayyar, A., & Krishnamurthi, R., (2021). Dynamic models and control techniques for drone delivery of medications and other healthcare items in COVID-19 hotspots. In: *Emerging Technologies for Battling COVID-19* (pp. 1–34). Springer, Cham.
5. Singh, H., Majumdar, A., & Malviya, N., (2020). E-pharmacy impacts on society and pharma sector in economical pandemic situation: A review. *Journal of Drug Delivery and Therapeutics., 10*(3-s), 335–340.
6. Andrews, G. J., & Duff, C., (2019). Matter beginning to matter: On posthumanist understandings of the vital emergence of health. *Social Science & Medicine, 226*, 123–134.
7. Davis, D. Z., & Calitz, W., (2016). Finding healthcare support in online communities: An exploration of the evolution and efficacy of virtual support groups. *Handbook on 3D3C Platforms.*, 475–486.
8. Dash, S., Shakyawar, S. K., Sharma, M., & Kaushik, S., (2019). Big data in healthcare: Management, analysis, and future prospects. *Journal of Big Data, 6*(1), 1–25.

9. Mettler, M., (2016). Blockchain technology in healthcare: The revolution starts here. In: *2016 IEEE 18th International Conference on e-Health Networking, Applications, and Services (Healthcom)* (pp. 1–3). IEEE.
10. Sujan, M. A., Embrey, D., & Huang, H., (2020). On the application of human reliability analysis in healthcare: Opportunities and challenges. *Reliability Engineering & System Safety., 194*, 106189.
11. Stadler, J. G., Donlon, K., Siewert, J. D., Franken, T., & Lewis, N. E., (2016). Improving the efficiency and ease of healthcare analysis through use of data visualization dashboards. *Big Data, 4*(2), 129–135.
12. Meirte, J., Hellemans, N., Anthonissen, M., Denteneer, L., Maertens, K., Moortgat, P., & Van, D. U., (2020). Benefits and disadvantages of electronic patient-reported outcome measures: Systematic review. *JMIR Perioperative Medicine, 3*(1), e15588.
13. Qadri, Y. A., Nauman, A., Zikria, Y. B., Vasilakos, A. V., & Kim, S. W., (2020). The future of healthcare internet of things: A survey of emerging technologies. *IEEE Communications Surveys & Tutorials, 22*(2), 1121–1167.
14. Venkatesh, D. A., (2019). Reimagining the future of healthcare industry through internet of medical things (IoMT), artificial intelligence (AI), machine learning (ML), big data, mobile apps and advanced sensors. *Artificial Intelligence (AI), Machine Learning (ML), Big Data, Mobile Apps and Advanced Sensors.*
15. Deepa, N., Prabadevi, B., Maddikunta, P. K., Gadekallu, T. R., Baker, T., Khan, M. A., & Tariq, U., (2021). An AI-based intelligent system for healthcare analysis using ridge-Adaline stochastic gradient descent classifier. *The Journal of Supercomputing, 77*(2), 1998–2017.
16. Ghazal, T. M., Hasan, M. K., Alshurideh, M. T., Alzoubi, H. M., Ahmad, M., Akbar, S. S., Al Kurdi, B., & Akour, I. A., (2021). IoT for smart cities: Machine learning approaches in smart healthcare—A review. *Future Internet, 13*(8), 218.
17. Laurenza, E., Quintano, M., Schiavone, F., & Vrontis, D., (2018). The effect of digital technologies adoption in healthcare industry: A case-based analysis. *Business Process Management Journal.*
18. Agarwal, R., Gao, G., DesRoches, C., & Jha, A. K., (2010). Research commentary—The digital transformation of healthcare: Current status and the road ahead. *Information Systems Research, 21*(4):796–809.
19. Kakhi, K., Alizadehsani, R., Khosravi, A., Nahavandi, S., & Islam, S. M., (2021). Challenges of internet of medical things for electronic healthcare. In: *2021 IEEE 4th International Conference and Workshop Óbuda on Electrical and Power Engineering (CANDO-EPE)* (pp. 19–24). IEEE.
20. Abu, D. A. M., Gorty, A., Jenkins, S. M., Murad, M. H., & Hensrud, D. D., (2016). Health habits of employees in a large medical center: Time trends and impact of a worksite wellness facility. *Scientific Reports, 6*(1), 1–7.
21. Aronsson, H., Abrahamsson, M., & Spens, K., (2011). Developing lean and agile health care supply chains. *Supply Chain Management: An International Journal, 16*(3), 176–183.
22. Ghazvini, A., & Shukur, Z., (2016). Awareness training transfer and information security content development for healthcare industry. *International Journal of Advanced Computer Science and Applications, 7*(5).

23. Moro, V. R., & Morea, D., (2020). Healthcare digitalization and pay-for-performance incentives in smart hospital project financing. *International Journal of Environmental Research and Public Health, 17*(7), 2318.
24. Hantrais, L., & Lenihan, A. T., (2021). Social dimensions of evidence-based policy in a digital society. *Contemporary Social Science, 16*(2), 141–155.
25. Sriram, R. D., & Subrahmanian, E., (2020). Transforming health care through digital revolutions. *Journal of the Indian Institute of Science, 100*(4), 753–772.
26. Hasselberg, M. J., (2020). The digital revolution in behavioral health. *Journal of the American Psychiatric Nurses Association, 26*(1), 102–111.
27. Bucci, S., Schwannauer, M., & Berry, N., (2019). The digital revolution and its impact on mental health care. *Psychology and Psychotherapy: Theory, Research and Practice, 92*(2), 277–297.
28. Keesara, S., Jonas, A., & Schulman, K., (2020). COVID-19 and health care's digital revolution. *New England Journal of Medicine, 382*(23), e82.
29. Dionisio, M., Paula, F., & De Souza, Jr. S. J. (2022). *Innovation and Digital Transformation in Healthcare: A Systematic Review.* This paper was presented at The XXXIII ISPIM Innovation Conference "Innovating in a Digital World," held in Copenhagen, Denmark on 05 June to 08 June 2022. Event Proceedings: LUT Scientific and Expertise Publications: ISBN 978-952-335-694-8. Year: 2022.
30. Compaoré, I., Ouedraogo, H., Nassè, T. B., & Salakpi, A., (2022). The headic issue of digital revolution: An emergent challenge for the future of jobs. *International Journal of Management & Entrepreneurship Research, 3*(1), 1–10.
31. Attaran, M., (2022). Blockchain technology in healthcare: Challenges and opportunities. *International Journal of Healthcare Management, 15*(1), 70–83.

Index

A

Academic institutions, 20, 366, 367, 383
Acceptance testing, 353
Accountability, 221, 230, 295, 354
Acoer, 82, 106
Activated partial thromboplastin time, 168
Active
  community involvement, 174
  pharmaceutical ingredient (API), 81, 146, 153, 154, 251, 252, 273, 291, 292, 347, 348, 383
Adaptability, 9, 81, 109, 369
Adhere, 69, 263
Adherence, 15, 269, 370
Administrative
  officer (AO), 251
  safeguards, 263
Administrator, 9, 67, 70–72, 101, 135, 345, 346
Adoption, 12, 14–16, 23, 47, 108, 163, 196, 201, 222, 225–227, 232, 234, 236, 243, 249, 284, 297, 303, 332, 333, 367, 375
  rates, 227
Advanced digital technology, 1, 41, 53, 91, 115, 145, 163, 181, 213, 241, 279, 311, 331, 365, 399
Affordable care act (ACA), 227
Africa, 76, 109, 128, 223, 333, 414
Aggregation, 99, 103, 169, 226
  datasets aggregation, 171
Aging systems, 14
Algorithm, 3, 23, 45, 70, 71, 98, 103, 105, 151, 159, 165, 166, 170, 184, 234, 261, 284, 318, 319, 325, 326, 336, 339–341, 343, 358
Algorithmic contact tracing, 103
Alliance-based referral medical systems, 288
Alpha miner, 334
American healthcare system, 43, 47
Announcement system, 67
Anomaly identification (ADSs), 135
Anonymity, 3, 19, 21, 42, 63, 71, 77, 80, 124, 130, 219, 221, 262, 302
Anticipate factors, 166
Antimicrobial peptide (AMP), 391
Anxiety, 200
Apollo pharmacy, 402
App vendors, 42
Application
  program, 116, 119, 153, 227, 251, 291, 346, 347
  programming interface (API), 153, 227, 251, 291, 346, 347
Apriori method, 359
Area under curve (AUC), 168
Arthritis, 190
Artificial
  intelligence (AI), 1, 7, 10, 11, 14, 15, 31, 49, 55, 67, 81, 85, 94, 95, 98–100, 106, 109, 120, 130, 132, 133, 136, 145, 150, 159, 160, 163, 176–178, 181–203, 213, 225, 242, 260, 275, 276, 287, 288, 304, 311, 333, 365–369, 376–378, 393–395, 407, 414
    adoption, 163
    algorithms, 190, 197
    imaging technologies, 195
    programming, 184
    systems, 11, 159, 187–189, 191, 195, 196
    techniques, 197
    technology, 182, 188, 190, 192, 198, 201, 311
    tools, 11, 194
  neural networks, 185
Assets, 13, 24, 62, 118–120, 150, 154, 178
Assistive devices, 183, 200, 202, 203
Association rule mining (ARM), 337
Attribute
  authority (AA), 355
  based encryption (ABE), 332, 355, 356, 358, 361
Audit trail, 254
Authentic conversations, 370, 374

Automated
guided vehicles (AGVs), 381
robots, 384
Automatic payments, 7
Automation, 7, 189, 390, 393
Automobiles, 83
Autonomous
healthcare robots, 366
mobile robot (AMRs), 369, 375, 380, 384
navigation technology, 391
robots (ARs), 201, 365–367, 375–377, 381–384, 387, 388, 390, 391, 394
systems, 7
Autonomy, 173
Avatar, 183
Avian influenza, 93

B

Backbone, 22, 241, 368, 373
Backpropagation, 316
Behavioral health, 411
Bernoulli circulation, 317
Big data, 9, 85, 95, 116, 134, 163–165, 168–175, 178, 202, 225, 296, 304, 412, 414
Biodata, 69, 101
Biomedical, 19, 78, 166, 173, 177, 382
research, 78, 166, 173
Bitcoin, 2, 5, 11, 12, 15, 42–45, 55, 57, 63, 96, 126, 147, 150, 226, 234–236, 259, 282–284
mining, 45
network, 2
Black-box tests, 352
Blockchain, 1–31, 41–50, 53–67, 69–86, 91, 92, 94–110, 115–138, 145, 147–160, 163, 181, 213–237, 241–276, 279–291, 294–305, 311, 331, 365, 399, 414, 416
applications, 1, 8, 47, 53, 65, 85, 97, 104, 109, 150, 221, 229, 230, 287
architecture, 153
configuration, 305
development, 12, 15
equipment, 43
implementation, 85, 234
infrastructure, 19, 138, 298
innovation, 119, 137
network, 3, 4, 8, 22, 23, 28, 29, 45, 57, 59, 67, 71, 74, 76, 77, 135, 147, 149, 150, 153, 154, 224, 226, 232–234, 242, 272, 282, 284, 287, 299, 302, 304, 305
nodes connectivity, 60
organization, 75
permissioned, 44
permissionless, 44
platforms, 21, 64, 150
protocol, 104
system, 3, 47, 214
technology (BCT/BT), 1–5, 7, 8, 10–12, 14–24, 29, 30, 41–45, 47–49, 53–57, 62–67, 73–78, 80–85, 91, 92, 94, 96–101, 104, 105, 108–110, 115, 116, 121, 123–131, 134, 137, 145, 147–151, 159, 213–224, 227–230, 232–237, 241–254, 256–259, 261, 266–276, 280–291, 294–296, 299, 301–304, 416
tools, 241, 275
transactions, 20
Blockpharma, 8
Blood
glucose level, 165, 175, 289
pressure, 280, 289
Bluetooth component, 292
Bock cloud, 125
Bottom-up summarization (BuS), 338
Braille, 201
Brain storage platforms, 20
Breast cancer, 197
Business
benefits, 252
procedures, 47
process modeling notation (BPMN), 334

C

Cancer genome atlas, 168
Cardiovascular single-photon emission imaging, 195
Caregivers, 10, 200–202, 289, 370, 380
Case diagram, 342
Catastrophe, 78, 217
Centers for
disease control and prevention, 82
Medicare and Medicaid services (CMS), 47, 227
Central authority, 13, 44, 61, 254, 258, 283

Chain logistics, 8
Chinese
skin image database (CSID), 192
vaccine manufacturing, 82
Chronic
ailments, 14
diseases, 190, 199, 201, 336, 380
Ciphertext, 313, 318, 327
policy attribute-based privacy preservation (Cip-PolAttPrivPre), 313, 318, 327
Classification and regression tree (CART), 336
Cleanroom-designed robots, 393
Clinic EMR systems, 292
Clinical
applications, 190, 196
care, 109, 174, 190, 202, 387, 390
decision support system (CDSS), 260
institutes, 3
laboratories, 54, 96, 98
pathway systems, 225
research, 20, 97, 264, 273, 399
studies, 42
trial, 130, 174, 288, 299
activities, 288
Cloud
computing, 85, 95, 170, 298, 300, 305, 355, 358, 414
data protection, 21
signature, 18
storage, 18, 125, 126, 314, 332
Co-App DHS, 105, 106
Collective action theory, 4
Communicable diseases, 91, 94, 332
Communication
overhead (C), 324, 327
systems, 137, 164, 228
Community
fitness management, 80
keys, 45
Company network, 13
Complex
data, 190
networks, 146
Computational
intelligence, 164
medical data (CIMD), 166
models, 164
logic, 117
machine, 163
methods, 196
Computed tomography (CT), 104, 393
Computer, 193, 241, 311, 331, 413
vision techniques, 193
Computerized transaction protocols, 104
Consensus
algorithms, 3, 19, 103, 218
nodes, 43, 218
procedures, 15, 84
processes, 57
rules, 67, 284
Consortium, 44, 76, 150, 235
Contact
tracer, 67, 69–71, 101
tracing, 64, 66–68, 70, 81, 97, 98, 100–105, 107, 109, 110, 332, 333
model, 102
program, 66
records, 68
tracking, 65
Convolutional neural network (CNN), 379
Corona warn app, 106
Coronary artery disease (CAD), 194
Coronavirus, 10, 11, 46, 53, 54, 64, 75–78, 82, 83, 93, 103, 106, 289, 304, 332, 391, 399–401, 418
disease of 2019, 10
epidemic, 77, 78, 82
Counterfeit, 7, 8, 128–131, 136, 145–147, 151, 152, 155, 159, 219, 232, 281, 302, 313
drugs, 7, 145–147, 151, 152, 155, 281
Counterfeiters, 21
COVID-19, 10, 11, 53–56, 62–67, 72–86, 92, 93, 95, 97, 100, 101, 103–108, 110, 146, 177, 279, 289–291, 304, 305, 331–333, 359, 361, 369, 387–389, 394, 399–401, 404, 410, 413, 416
epidemic, 53–55, 62, 65, 66, 78, 85, 290, 359
instances, 80
outbreak, 53, 64, 79, 85, 107
pandemic, 10, 53–55, 63, 75, 76, 78, 84, 85, 92, 93, 95, 97, 107, 108, 146, 279, 304, 333, 359, 387, 389, 394, 416
patients, 63, 291
testing kits, 80

Cryptocurrencies, 44, 45, 48, 62, 233, 236, 272, 282, 303
platforms, 47
Cryptographic
hash, 24, 25, 62, 100, 126, 148, 149, 214, 218, 230
keys, 10, 22
protocols, 22
technique, 57, 62, 67, 71
Cryptography, 24, 44, 217, 270, 281, 284

D

Data
accuracy, 9
alterations, 24
analysis, 11
analytics, 7, 80, 165, 168, 172, 199, 202, 366, 368
breaches, 78, 84, 215, 230, 275
collection, 13, 28, 67, 225, 227, 268
compression techniques, 64
exchange, 42, 45, 73, 85, 92, 129, 176, 260–262, 298, 299
experts, 80
fraud, 73
immutability, 16, 41
integrity, 22, 24, 75, 234, 243, 251, 252, 263, 272
interchange, 299
joining, 171
management, 127, 173
matrix tracking systems, 152
mining, 164–166, 170, 172, 335, 337
misuse, 16
ownership, 302
privacy, 15, 28, 30, 85, 129, 224, 229, 252, 304, 320, 321, 400, 418
processing, 16, 64, 164, 169, 170, 175, 177, 230, 256, 257
issue, 64
production, 20
recovery, 20
repositories, 12, 379
security, 5, 22, 42, 73, 124, 138, 215, 225, 227, 243, 292, 295, 304, 312, 414
sets, 20, 116, 123, 166, 172, 195, 226, 248, 297
sharing system, 73
source, 9, 14, 21, 47, 120, 246, 346
blockchain platforms, 21
storage, 1, 2, 45, 106, 232, 257
transfer, 133, 305
transmission, 200, 289, 312, 317, 327
validation, 303
verifiability, 22
visualization, 82
Database, 9, 5, 15, 19, 25, 26, 29, 42, 45, 56, 75, 78, 84, 99, 116, 117, 124, 126, 148, 149, 152, 163, 166, 169, 177, 189, 192, 224, 230, 246, 250, 256, 274, 281, 282, 287, 288, 296, 298, 303, 338, 339, 341, 343, 345–348, 354, 359, 409, 413
access, 347
Dataset, 17, 115, 163–166, 169, 172, 175, 177, 190, 314, 318, 317, 331, 332, 338, 340, 359, 360
Deadline, 175
Debug, 158
Decentralization, 5, 19, 21, 22, 42, 54, 56, 61, 65, 73, 94, 109, 217, 231, 258, 283
Decentralized
AI systems, 133
application (DApp), 23, 48, 67, 69, 71, 72, 103–105, 145, 153, 154, 157, 232
autonomous organization, 68
database, 153
network, 7, 56, 78, 248, 282, 304
storage, 45, 49, 125, 153, 154
Decision makers, 102, 103
Decontamination, 382, 385, 387, 390
Decryption, 326, 327
keys, 18
time (D), 326, 327
Deep
genomics, 378
learning (DL), 164, 166, 184, 186, 203, 311, 327
algorithms, 311
neural networks (DNNs), 313
Q-learning architecture, 311
DeepMind, 46
Delegated laboratories, 27
Dementia, 199
Demographic groups, 62
Denial of service (DoS), 135
Dental replanting, 370
Dentistry education, 370

Department of telecommunication, 403
Dermatology, 192
Devoid, 68
Diabetes, 54, 190, 293, 337, 338, 387, 407
Diagnosis, 11, 14, 25, 44, 45, 98, 163, 165, 167, 173, 181, 183, 191, 192, 194–197, 202, 260, 265, 267, 287, 289, 299, 302, 312, 336, 360, 369, 371, 388, 389, 399, 412
Diagnostic tools, 14, 178, 367
Digest chains, 56
Digital
 assets, 15
 contact tracing, 63, 64, 81, 85
 data, 44, 54, 97, 127
 health, 1, 2, 6, 9, 10, 31, 42, 194, 202, 359, 377, 399, 400–402, 410–412, 416–418
  passports, 105
  trend, 2, 31
 healthcare, 1, 194, 359, 377, 399, 401, 402, 411, 412, 416–418
 industry, 404, 418
 maturity, 14
 revolution, 30, 399, 400, 406, 410–415, 417, 418
 signature, 58, 59, 271
 technology, 92, 109, 333, 359, 361, 414, 416, 417
 transformation, 399, 413, 415
Digitalization, 168, 192, 401, 402, 404–410, 413, 414, 416–418
Dimension reduction, 172
Directed acyclic graphs (DAGs), 233
Disease
 control, 82
 outbreak, 91
 surveillance, 76, 91–95, 97–100, 109, 110
Dispensation mobile, 79
Disruptive technology, 365
Dissemination, 13, 66, 95, 216, 259, 265, 333
Dissolved oxygen, 390
Distributed
 consensus algorithms, 19
 denial of service (DDoS), 10
 file system (DFS), 23
 ledger, 30, 82, 214, 250, 282
  technology (DLT), 5, 30, 147, 214, 244, 250, 284
 system, 150
Domain, 24, 124, 145, 159, 267, 283, 313, 335, 355, 357, 388, 399
Drug
 industry, 8
 log, 157
 manufacturers, 4
 scientists, 146
 supply chain, 7, 130, 131, 145, 146, 160
  security act, 12
 traceability, 145, 151, 153, 154, 157, 159
 tracing, 160
 use, 183

E

Earthquake, 7
Ebola
 outbreak, 333, 390
 virus, 76, 93, 94, 108
  disease (EVD), 94
Economic outlook, 83
Educational credentials, 75
E-government, 67, 75, 76
E-health, 42, 44, 45, 50, 164, 173, 175, 202, 230, 237, 361, 410
 data, 173
 solution, 361
 system, 45, 237
Electrocardiogram (ECG), 3, 165, 201
Electroencephalogram (EEG), 165, 294
Electromyogram (EMG), 165
Electronic
 components, 54
 devices, 76, 96, 289
 government, 65
 health record (EHR), 19, 20, 26, 45, 47, 120, 122, 123, 126, 127, 171, 172, 175, 190, 221, 227, 229, 250, 260–264, 266, 295, 296, 298, 332, 339, 340, 361, 412
 medical record (EMR), 21, 28, 47, 97, 124, 250, 295, 335
 product codes (EPC), 152
 records, 191, 226, 243, 327
 vaccination license, 73
Electrooculography (EOG), 165
Elimination, 7, 13, 225
E-mail, 356, 403
Embedded sensors, 190
Emergency information, 70

Employ genomic analysis, 172
Encoding, 249
Encrypted
data, 10, 45, 295
medical data, 18
Encryption, 18, 19, 30, 42, 58, 69, 71, 73, 77, 124, 126, 158, 252, 258, 261, 264, 270, 298, 303, 312, 318, 320, 321, 325–327, 341, 355, 356, 358
time (E), 325, 327
Energetic relationship, 125
Energy
consumption, 45, 249, 312
costs, 18
sector, 48
Engineering microrobots, 373
Enterprise Ethereum alliance (EEA), 234
Epidemic, 91, 92, 100, 103, 108, 109, 178, 274, 333, 387
outbreaks, 65
Epochs, 322, 324–326
Equivalent rights, 67
E-Rezept, 81, 108
Estonia, 99, 230, 243, 250
Estonian healthcare system, 231
Ethereum, 2, 17, 23–27, 44, 79, 104–106, 108, 130, 149, 150, 154, 155, 157, 158, 230, 233–235, 253, 257–259, 282, 285, 291, 295
address, 24, 154, 157, 158
blockchain, 23, 25–27, 233, 234, 253, 258, 291
platform, 253, 291
foundation, 108
network, 27, 130, 157, 257
node, 157, 158
wallet, 23
European
antimicrobial resistance surveillance network, 99
Commission, 401
Parliamentary Research Service (EPRS), 97
Union (EU), 8, 220, 297, 401
Event logs, 334
Evidence-based medicine (EBM), 260
Externally owned account (EOA), 265

F

Fast
healthcare interoperability resources (FHIR), 292
transmission, 125
Fatal
coronavirus, 82
diseases, 81
Federated blockchain, 44
Federations, 44
Final model testing, 172
Financial
activity, 47
aid, 116
applications, 50
sectors, 47
transactions, 6, 13, 47, 214, 219, 253
Fitbit, 290
Flebo, 405
Food and Drug Administration (FDA), 146, 220
Frontline health, 78
Fuelband, 290
Fuzzy
decision-making trial and evaluation laboratory, 56
miner, 334

G

Galvanic skin reaction (GSR), 165
Ganache, 257
Gartner hype cycle, 216
Genetics, 20, 164, 288, 366
data, 8, 165, 178, 288, 378
Genomes project, 168
Genomic data, 9
Geographic information, 63, 67
Geriatric mental health research, 190
GitHub repository, 155
Global
blockchain survey, 11
collaboration, 178
compatibility, 42
compliance, 42
disability innovation hub, 201
economy, 83, 224
health crisis, 54

humanitarian operation, 7
standards organization, 234
Globalization, 91
Google
Apple, 104
Scholar, 53, 86
Government accountability office (GAO), 221
Governmental institution sector, 75
Grant lot sale, 156
Graphical user interface, 67

H

Hadoop distributed file system, 169
Hardware resources, 83
Hash
data, 69
function, 10, 59, 96, 159, 263, 291
Heal point, 110
Health
associations, 80
checkup, 292
contract caller, 280, 305
data, 5, 6, 22, 42, 49, 124–126, 137, 168, 198, 216–218, 224, 254, 261, 262, 267, 273, 286, 289, 300, 338
ownership, 5
examination records, 340
information, 41, 173, 295
exchange, 30, 41, 47
management, 21, 265
technology for economic and clinical health (HITECH), 173
innovations, 202
insurance, 6, 13, 26, 127, 131, 229, 242, 245, 246
portability and accountability act (HIPAA), 23, 73, 226, 230, 233, 260–262, 295, 354
level 7 (HL7's), 295
monitoring, 286, 289
officials, 80, 100, 107
organizations, 4, 72, 73, 82, 97, 106, 273, 303
promotion, 56
records, 15, 18, 43, 47, 105, 123, 126, 175, 215, 218, 230, 244, 249, 257, 263, 281, 355
sector, 365
service providers, 257
standards, 275
technology, 82, 106, 378
Healthcare
apps, 21
blockchain, 17, 23, 25, 147, 229, 261, 262, 304
business, 10, 14, 43, 131, 213, 215, 230
companies, 2
division, 133
industry, 2, 4, 10, 13–17, 21, 22, 30, 42, 47, 48, 56, 77, 81, 85, 121, 123, 125, 126, 128, 131, 164, 165, 182, 186, 215, 216, 218, 220–222, 258, 285, 289, 302, 303, 312, 313, 366, 367, 381, 388, 399–402, 409, 410, 412–414, 416–418
information systems, 43
institutions, 3, 95, 96, 256, 264, 274
ledgers, 78
management, 78, 86
organizations, 18, 98, 108, 124, 134, 147, 217, 260, 275, 298, 301, 304
partners, 65, 72, 76
payment process, 13
practitioners, 298
problems, 276
provider, 218, 233, 298
sector, 2, 5, 10, 16, 17, 29, 41, 42, 44, 49, 56, 85, 92, 97, 109, 133, 163, 214, 223, 227, 231, 232, 234, 235, 248, 258, 262, 272, 285, 287, 312, 314, 408, 409, 416, 417
services, 174
solutions, 21
supply chain, 145–147, 160
system, 4, 15, 17, 18, 21, 26, 28, 41–43, 47, 49, 73, 81, 92, 93, 98, 107, 123–125, 127, 133, 151, 191, 215, 217–219, 222, 229–231, 236, 237, 250, 257, 262, 280, 285, 289, 301–303, 311–313, 365–367, 373, 376, 399, 400, 410
technology, 261
wearables, 191
workers, 22, 133, 198, 287, 374, 384
Hematology, 371
Heparin-induced thrombocytopenia (HIT), 337

Hesitance, 12
Heterogeneous, 42, 134, 242, 340
HeteroHER
graph, 339, 340
network, 343
Heuristic miner, 334
Hidden Markov model (HMV), 378
Hierarchical
location, 124
upward reporting, 95
High-quality output, 11
Hindering adoption, 12
Hindrance, 46, 408
History transaction, 151
Holter systems, 293
Human
brain, 185, 186
computer interaction (HCI), 197
robot interaction (HRI), 199
Hybrid approaches, 217
Hyperchain, 82, 106
Hyperledger, 3, 44, 79, 80, 110, 150, 222, 231, 295
based medical chain, 110
fabric, 3, 150
Hypertension, 190

I

Illness progression, 166, 194
Immune protection, 73
Immunity, 76
certification, 105
passport, 62, 74
testing, 73
Immunization, 65, 274
Immutability, 9, 16, 19, 41, 54, 56, 62, 75, 94–96, 103, 109, 148, 149, 157, 158, 217, 218, 220, 224, 231, 234, 262, 282
Incubation phase, 65
Independent
agencies, 92, 94
entities, 69, 146
Indian
Contract Act, 1872, 270
Evidence Act, 1872, 271
Information Technology Act, 2000, 271
Individual
data, 67
genome, 9
Infection verification subsystem, 79
Information
and communication technology (ICT), 134, 183
exchange, 76, 260
security (IS), 15, 78, 122, 135, 245, 262, 264, 295, 313, 348, 351
systems, 334
technology (IT), 14, 41, 125, 147, 214, 221, 222, 226–230, 236, 245, 271, 272, 331, 415
infrastructure, 125, 228, 229
legacy systems, 214, 221
solutions, 147
Innovation sector, 12
Insurance, 2, 13, 14, 22, 25–28, 48, 78, 83, 97, 116, 123, 131, 134, 136, 216, 222, 230, 236, 241–245, 254, 255, 259, 275, 288, 290, 295, 296, 299, 300, 354, 356, 409
claims, 22, 78, 97, 254, 288
companies, 13, 25–28, 131, 236, 244, 254, 255, 259
policy, 13, 27, 242
Integration, 350, 351, 353
testing, 351, 353
Intel, 235, 366, 367, 369, 370
Intelligent
applications, 6
healthcare, 311
Intensive care unit (ICU), 168, 292
International
agencies, 73
business machines, 77
health regulations, 92, 333
quality certification, 402
Internet, 4, 31, 61, 67, 132, 133, 166, 184, 226, 311, 366, 401–403, 411
information services (IIS), 61
of medical things (IoMT), 120, 132, 133, 137
of things (IoT), 4, 9, 10, 14, 31, 62, 66, 67, 94, 97, 120, 124, 132–136, 148, 157, 175, 184, 189, 280, 282, 286, 289–292, 294, 295, 311–315, 327, 366, 367, 411, 414
device, 4, 10, 133, 290, 313
environment, 136
gadgets, 134–136
system, 292

Interoperability, 29, 30, 42, 46, 47, 62, 64, 77, 84, 92, 95, 126, 159, 213, 215, 220, 221, 227–230, 234, 237, 285, 287, 288, 296, 297, 302, 410
Interplanetary file system (IPFS), 69–71, 108, 153–156

J

Java
applets, 349
application, 349
byte codes, 349
compiler, 349
database connectivity, 347
development
kit (JDK) 1.8, 341
tool, 349
interpreter, 349
operating system, 348
program, 349
user interface, 348
virtual machine, 349
Jeopardy, 28
Jurisdiction, 265, 272, 276

K

Keen agreements, 63
Knowledge, 2, 15, 42, 43, 45, 54, 71, 79, 126, 127, 163, 173, 217, 236, 258, 260, 268, 285, 286, 305, 335, 341, 347, 350, 352, 360, 367, 416, 417

L

Lal Pathlabs, 405
Large data analysis methodologies, 190
Ledger, 1, 6, 7, 9, 13, 23, 25, 30, 42–44, 54–56, 82, 83, 96, 115, 125, 128–130, 133, 145, 148, 149, 151, 155–159, 218, 224, 225, 230, 236, 241, 245, 246, 254, 258, 259, 270, 272, 273, 275, 281–284, 286, 288, 299, 320
Legal, 44, 287, 401
contracts, 44
systems, 302
Leverage, 63, 153, 157, 225, 269, 373
Licensed blockchain system, 3
Life-threatening diseases, 394
Light detection and ranging, 369
Limited memory machines, 188
Linux, 3, 158
foundation, 3
Local
area network, 346
health agencies & departments, 92, 99
Lockdowns, 75, 93, 359
Logitech serial mouse, 341
Long assessments, 119
Low
cost, 104, 106, 294
quality traceability, 119
risk, 168

M

Machine
analysis, 178
learning (ML) 14, 94, 95, 98, 164, 165, 168, 173, 176–178, 184–186, 189, 191, 193–197, 199, 202, 203, 242, 275, 287, 313, 314, 332, 333, 337, 366, 367, 379
level byte code, 23
Macintosh, 349
Magnetic resonance imaging (MRI), 373
Magnetoencephalogram (MEG), 165
Malicious assaults, 73
MARIO project, 200
Market inquiries, 79
Mass surveillance system, 67, 79
Master patient identifier (MPI), 220, 237
Mathematics, 19, 383
Maxillofacial operations, 370
Mean absolute error, 320
Mechanomyogram (MMG), 165
Med chain, 104
Media application, 82
Mediator, 116
Medicaid, 47, 220–222, 227–229
fraud, 221
information technology architecture (MITA), 228
program, 221
Medical
applications, 3, 225, 370
block framework, 124
blockchain, 18, 23, 261, 270
care organizations, 45

data, 1, 2, 18, 21, 25, 42, 43, 45, 46, 50, 56, 71, 78, 97, 124–126, 249, 250, 259, 260, 263, 265, 286–288, 291, 304, 305, 312, 314, 338, 358, 366, 400
management, 50
release (MDR), 1, 18
sharing (MDS), 18
transmission, 305
device, 290
tracking, 237
equipment, 2, 83, 98, 133, 191, 219, 231, 232, 294, 311
exam, 56, 260, 339
facility, 18, 292
history, 18, 26, 27, 47, 96, 123, 124, 255, 287, 343, 355–357, 369
industry, 15, 287, 380, 399
insurance, 26, 27, 241–243, 245, 248, 260, 265, 275, 276
contract, 275
notes, 191
professionals, 293, 301
records, 5, 6, 15, 22–25, 30, 42, 45, 69, 73, 95, 101, 104, 123, 125, 126, 165, 172, 230, 232, 256, 259, 260, 274, 287–289, 297, 299, 300, 336, 409
robots, 380
sector, 49, 54, 168, 256–259, 327, 409
sensors, 280, 305
services, 122
source chain, 77
supply chain, 55, 77, 86, 97, 115, 287, 304
treatment, 25, 183, 248, 273, 358
workflows, 24
Medicare, 47, 172, 227, 229, 273
Medications, 7, 77, 81, 92, 108, 115, 117, 118, 128–131, 137, 165, 190, 219, 232, 281, 287–289, 336, 356, 372, 379, 381, 389
Medlife, 402
Megabyte, 2
Menial duties, 370
Mental
health, 181, 183, 190, 191, 198, 335, 389, 411, 412
issues, 190
Mentoring insurance, 42
Merkle tree root hash, 58
Metadata, 24, 44, 58, 255, 290
Metrics, 56
Microfluidic valves, 385
Microrobots, 372, 373
Microsoft, 106, 107, 183, 201, 234, 235, 341, 343, 346
Windows, 341
Middle East respiratory syndrome (MERS), 76, 93
Miners, 2, 23, 29, 45, 54, 96, 214, 235, 282
Minimum-level priority queue, 170
Mining, 18, 45, 54, 59, 65, 84, 85, 137, 164–166, 170, 172, 173, 214, 335, 337, 378
Ministry of Health and Prevention, 231
Misinterpretation, 26
Misuse location, 135
Mobile
app, 106
contact tracing, 66
telepresence functionality, 382
ModelChain system, 136
Modern
digital products (MDP), 409
robotics, 368
technology, 286
Modular robots, 369, 374
Modules, 67, 127, 311, 347, 360, 374
MOODLE platform, 75
Multidisciplinary idea, 17

N

Naive Bayes, 166
Nakamoto consensus protocol, 57
Nanobots, 371
Nanorobots, 371, 372, 375
National
boundaries, 302
Council on Aging (NCOA), 199
government, 80, 95
health service (NHS), 105, 220
Institute of Standards and Technology (NIST), 262, 411
Science Foundations and the White House Office of Science and Technology, 390
Netmeds, 401
Neurodegeneration, 190
Next-generation smart contract, 48

Nipah, 76, 93
Node, 20, 24, 43, 57–59, 84, 96, 99, 102, 125, 147, 157, 196, 233, 258, 263, 264, 275, 284, 292, 296, 302, 304, 320, 324
  connection, 59
Non-profit sectors, 2
Non-reproduction, 158
Non-repudiation, 60
Notary services, 42
Nutrients, 77

O

Off-chain, 25, 62, 69, 100, 108, 154, 288, 294
Oncology, 196
Online
  analytical processing, 170
  databases, 359
  education, 65, 98
  interface, 23
  resources, 160
Open
  access control model, 19
  database connectivity (ODBC), 345
  surgery, 368
Operational management, 104
Optimistic overtones, 16
Optimization technique, 56
Oracle, 106, 107, 346
Oral radiographs, 370
Organization for economic cooperation and development (OECD), 83
Original data, 158, 171, 290
Orthodontics, 370
Outbreak, 11, 54, 55, 91–95, 97–99, 108, 109, 168, 169, 332, 333, 359
  management, 64
Oversight, 12, 131, 376
Oyente tool, 158

P

Pace, 64, 95, 109, 297, 333, 392
Pandemic, 11, 46, 53, 54, 75–78, 80, 81, 91–95, 97–100, 103–105, 108–110, 274, 289, 290, 292, 304, 331, 332, 359, 387, 399, 401, 410
  fighting infrastructure, 53
  level, 95
  management, 54, 332, 359
  research, 292
Paper-based
  contracts, 61, 99, 104
  systems, 92
Paradigm, 23, 43, 126, 132, 134, 138, 195, 216, 297, 299, 332, 411
Parameters, 327
Parent block hash, 58
Pathological aging, 190
Pathology, 196
  AI system, 196
Patient, 22, 28, 69, 71, 101, 129, 163, 173, 174, 191, 228, 241, 279, 286, 296, 300
  approval, 296
  confidentiality, 54, 263, 332
  data, 10, 21, 28, 44, 46, 78, 83, 84, 108, 124, 175, 199, 217, 226, 231, 235, 257, 258, 265, 274, 282, 290, 298, 301, 313, 314, 332, 341
  enrollment, 129
  monitoring (PM), 3, 18, 48, 182, 279, 290, 305
  privacy, 73, 215, 304
  profile analysis, 173
  protection and ACA, 228
  record, 26, 45, 69, 70, 78, 115, 218, 232, 258, 260, 263, 407
  selection, 163
  symptoms, 69
  tracer, 69
Peer-to-peer (P2P), 14, 19, 25, 44, 50, 56, 59, 67, 79, 95, 96, 102, 105–107, 115, 120, 148, 214, 221, 258, 279, 282, 284
  insurance, 50
  network, 19, 25, 56, 96, 102, 214, 279, 282, 284
Percutaneous coronary intervention (PCI), 195
Performance analysis, 327
Permit, 11, 16, 73, 183
Personal
  domains (PSD), 355
  health
    information (PHI), 43, 226, 354, 361
    record (PHR), 126, 332, 356, 361
    signs, 175
  information, 10, 22, 221, 287, 291, 355–357
Personalized medicine, 167, 178, 215, 285, 412

Personnel protective equipment, 62
Pew research center, 202
Pharmaceutical, 7, 21, 81, 128, 219, 232, 281, 286, 291, 298, 300, 371, 378–380, 401
  companies, 7, 130
  innovation, 11
  sector, 8, 138
  supply monitoring, 115
Pharmacies, 27, 131, 146, 148, 152–155, 231, 244, 298
Pharmacogenomics, 167
Pharmacological sector, 131
Pharmacy, 5–7, 26, 30, 41, 53, 91, 163, 213, 273, 279, 286, 296, 365, 399, 401, 402
  line, 5
PharmEasy, 402
Physical
  examination, 191, 355
  illness, 183, 190
Physiological parameters, 133
Picture archive and computer systems (PACS), 193
Plague, 42, 115, 333
Pointless costs, 119
Policyholders, 6
Policymakers, 120
Polymerase chain reaction, 74
Polypyrrole (Ppy), 371
Population, 175
  health, 171, 178, 285
Portable, 3, 191, 192, 203, 374, 383
  electronics, 3
Portal, 353, 354
Post-performance, 269
Potential
  assaults, 63
  drawbacks, 22
  health issues, 9
Powerful computers, 292
Practical byzantine fault tolerance (PBFT), 23, 103
Pragmatic clinical trials (PCTs), 173
Pre-authorization process, 13
Precision, 185, 321
  medicine, 185
Preliminary data, 175
Preventive measures, 92, 94, 388
Primary care, 15
Privacy policies, 66
Private
  blockchains, 233, 302
  system, 57
Professional university, 145, 159, 160
Prognosis, 167, 173, 196
Proliferation, 14, 236, 394
Proof-of-authority (PoA), 4, 291
Proof-of-burn (PoB), 151
Proof-of-deposit (PoD), 151
Proof-of-elapsed time (PoET), 284
Proof-of-importance (PoI), 151
Proof-of-stake (PoS), 151, 284
Proof-of-work (PoW), 3, 149, 234, 284
Protocol registration, 27
Providers, 14, 26, 259, 295
Proxy re-encryption (PRE), 358
Pseudo-anonymous, 42
Public
  blockchain, 3, 44, 60, 62, 150, 219, 232
    systems, 62
  DApp library, 23
  domains (PUD), 355
  health, 168, 169, 172, 174, 359
    agencies, 95
    management, 16
    messages, 359
    officials, 80, 100, 107
  key, 18, 45
    pair, 58
  permission, 44
  private key, 1
  updates, 292
  utilities, 75
Puzzle game, 45

Q

Q-learning, 311–313, 316, 327
QR code, 157, 252
Quality, 98, 119, 181, 266, 287
  control, 138, 195
  management, 287
  of life (QoL), 178, 181–183, 200–203
Quarantine, 66, 68, 74, 75, 77, 83, 85, 100, 101, 105, 388, 390, 399
Quick
  alerts, 99
  data, 55

detection, 91
development, 169, 190, 195
Quicker resolution, 61

R

Radio-frequency, 4, 135
identification (RFID), 312
Radiological assessments, 193
Radiology, 193
Random split, 172
Raw
data, 54, 96, 121, 296
material suppliers, 146
Real-time, 84, 109, 298
data, 67, 77, 96, 97, 99, 109, 132, 176, 296, 298
surveillance system, 99
tracking, 110, 152, 155, 293
uploads, 292
Recipient-oriented transactions, 84
Record
keeping system, 71
managers, 48
Redundancy, 95, 229
Reflex syncope, 293
Reliable
data, 73, 94, 259
management method, 73
sources, 80, 267
Remix
online editor, 158
web IDE, 155
Remote
health monitoring (RHM), 201, 289
monitoring, 9, 10, 97, 169, 202, 215, 293–295, 297, 312, 370
devices, 10
technology, 9
patient monitoring, 279
Research
and development (R&D), 172, 174, 382
environment, 190
gaps, 11
literature, 160
Reserve Bank of India (RBI), 271
Resource, 154, 295
consumption, 18
Restorative dentistry, 370
Retrieve data feature, 70
Roadblocks, 85, 229, 332, 378
Robotics, 188, 197, 374, 392, 394
Robots, 197, 201, 365–369, 372–375, 390–393, 395
Roomie bot, 369, 370

S

Safe issuance, 75
Safeguard, 5, 44, 72, 77, 119, 123, 230, 250, 259, 275
Sanitary facilities, 75
Scopus, 53, 86, 413
Screening, 390
Secrecy, 14, 75, 260–262, 299
Secure
certification, 65, 76, 98
data transmission, 311
system, 80, 137
Security
issues, 69, 84
policy, 41
Self-awareness, 189
Self-monitor, 101, 293
Self-quarantine, 68, 101
Self-report, 68, 101
Self-sovereign identification (SSI), 81, 108
Self-test, 106
Semi-supervised heterogeneous graph, 339, 340
Sensitive data, 2, 13, 84, 282, 291, 356
Sensitivity, 135, 312, 320–323, 327, 336
Sensors, 9, 44, 155, 175, 177, 184, 189, 190, 198–200, 274, 280, 287, 290, 294, 296, 299, 311, 312, 374, 375, 382–384, 386–388, 392
Sequence diagram, 343
Sequential organ failure assessment scores (SOFA), 168
Servers, 317
Service, 47, 49, 174, 215, 227, 403
robots, 200, 370, 374
Severe acute respiratory syndrome (SARS), 93
Shared transmission, 117
Shareholders, 13
Signal-to-noise ratio (SNR), 294
Single nucleotide polymorphisms, 168

Smart
agreements, 17, 62, 130
check, 158
contract, 3, 4, 6, 8, 9, 11, 13, 22–28, 45, 48, 49, 60–65, 68, 76, 98, 99, 101, 103, 104, 106, 124, 130, 133, 148–151, 153–159, 213, 214, 219–221, 229, 230, 234, 235, 241–245, 247–249, 254–261, 265, 267–276, 280, 288, 291, 294, 296, 297
guard, 391
healthcare, 1, 41, 53, 91, 115, 145, 163, 181, 213, 241, 279, 311, 331, 365, 399
home assisted living for the elderly (SHALE), 201
Smartphone, 66, 190, 292, 333, 405, 411
applications, 177, 252
contact tracing, 105
Social
customs, 68
interaction, 66, 183, 201, 202, 380, 389
isolation, 63, 198, 199
robots, 198, 370, 374, 381, 389
security number, 24
Software, 105, 235, 353
applications, 105
integration, 353
Solaris, 349
Solidity, 23, 155, 257, 265
language, 155
programming language, 23, 265
Solitary
consumer needs, 119
point, 73
portion, 115, 117
Sovrin, 81, 108
Spot fraudulent activity, 20
Stakeholders, 27, 43, 55, 74, 104, 121, 126, 148, 152–154, 214, 229, 242–246, 248, 252, 271, 303
participation, 21
Standardization, 137
State-by-state policy changes, 228
Stochastic simulation, 4
Storage
capacity, 42, 62
space, 29
Strategic applications, 17
Strong
AI, 188, 190
discretion measures, 73
Substitute medications, 7
Sun microsystems, 347
Super AI, 187, 188
Superior medical management resources, 285
Supply chain, 4, 7, 8, 21, 22, 47, 64, 65, 74, 76, 77, 83, 93, 94, 103, 115, 116, 118, 119, 128, 129, 131, 138, 145–148, 151–153, 155, 158–160, 214, 216, 219, 221, 222, 224, 232, 234, 237, 276, 286, 288, 289, 291, 300, 302, 366, 375–377
data, 77
management (SCM), 7, 22, 47, 65, 76, 115, 118, 119, 128, 138, 219, 237, 276, 302, 376
Surgical robots, 368
Surveillance, 67, 76, 79, 85, 91–95, 97–100, 109, 110, 131, 274, 288, 332, 387, 390
Sustainability, 42, 231, 291, 303, 359, 417
Swabbing, 389
Swiss hospitals, 231, 232
Symmetric key, 18, 69
Syndromic surveillance systems, 99
System
features, 72
implementation, 69
malfunctions, 44
model, 317
testing, 351, 352
Systemic chemotherapy, 373
Szabo, 61, 265

T

Tackle, 53, 81, 155, 177, 185, 267, 339
Tailored predictors, 191
Tampering, 19, 59, 60, 148, 152, 154, 220, 234
Tamper-proof, 67, 96, 130, 231, 232, 247, 291
Tax collection, 75
Technological
challenges, 57, 287
hazards, 56
platforms, 42
Telehealth, 295, 336
Telemedicine, 54, 79, 98, 107, 183, 194, 200–202, 297, 387, 389, 390

Teleradiology, 1
Therapeutic
  decisions, 14
  development, 11, 105
  information, 25
  robots, 369
Third
  iteration, 15
  party, 101
    administrators (TPAs), 244
    agencies, 18
Three-dimensional (3D), 54, 94, 368, 371, 374, 385, 394
  printing, 94
Traceability, 119, 145, 159
Traceable resource unit, 151
Tracing, 70, 101, 104, 106
Tracking, 53, 91, 94, 146, 220
  systems, 4, 91, 92, 98, 103, 152
Traditional system, 92, 94, 103, 110
Traits, 177, 189, 194, 201
Transaction, 14, 23, 76, 157, 302
  cost theory, 4
  counter, 58
  fees, 75
  per second (TPS), 64
  pool, 45
  section, 58
  transmission techniques, 14
Transcripts, 75
Transmission, 117
Transparency, 4, 19, 22, 42, 46, 48, 54, 56, 61, 73, 74, 77, 94, 96, 108, 109, 116, 137, 152, 153, 214, 217, 221, 231, 232, 235, 243, 244, 254, 256, 257, 281, 286, 288, 299, 300, 303
  feature, 73, 109
Treatment
  adherence, 370
  rank, 83
  strategy, 27, 163, 177
True
  negative rate (TNR), 322
  positive rate (TPR), 321
Trusted
  administrative organization, 69
  authority (TA), 317
Turing-complete scripting language, 48

U

Ultraviolet (UV), 382, 388, 391
  -C Disinfection Robot, 391
  lights, 382
Unauthorized users, 61, 124
Unchangeable
  data, 1
  logs, 105
Undisputable autograph business, 61
Uniformity, 42, 231
Unique
  address, 67
  hash function, 10
  identifier, 69, 108
United Nations Educational, Scientific, and Cultural Organization, 415
Unmanned aerial vehicles (UAVs), 381
Unreliable traceability, 95
User
  authentication, 229
  information privacy, 81

V

Vaccination, 62, 65, 172, 291, 300
  certificates, 63, 65
  development, 82
  information, 82
  policies, 92
  records, 62
Vaccine, 64, 82, 100, 106, 174, 290, 375
  certification, 73
  manufacturing, 82, 290
  specifics, 82
Validation, 13, 57, 69–72, 83, 102, 150, 158, 159, 172, 246, 248, 251, 252, 266, 303, 305, 350
Vendor-neutral archives (VNA), 297
Vietnam Blockchain Corporation (VBCs), 225
Viral
  hot spots, 80
  outbreak, 79
Vision processing unit (VPUs), 370
Visualization, 171

W

Wage payment, 75
Warranty, 271, 405

Wayfinding aids, 370
Wearable, 3, 6, 62, 133, 134, 164, 175, 183, 190, 199–201, 203, 273, 285, 289, 290, 293, 295–298, 311
 medical gadgets, 290
Web-based interfaces, 80
Whereabouts, 78, 232
White
 box testers, 352
 House Office of Science and Technology, 390
Wireless
 body-area network (WBAN), 133
 sensor networks (WSN), 152
Workflow, 42, 121, 170, 177, 182, 193, 195, 231
 tools, 42
World
 economy, 83
 face, 14
 Health Organization (WHO), 53, 78, 80, 82, 86, 92, 96, 106, 107, 128, 146, 147, 165, 182, 245, 332, 336
 wide web (WWW), 267, 403
Worldwide, 16, 74, 75, 118–120, 165, 243, 250, 291, 333, 367, 391, 403
 record, 119

X

X-rays, 29, 193, 230

Y

Y-axis, 322, 324–326
Y-hub, 322

Z

Zika virus, 93
ZKSnarks, 108